"Finally, a book about occupational therapy in the Philippines! This historical book gives a snapshot of our beloved profession. The work does not sugarcoat the challenges this profession faces in a country with limited resources yet shows how Filipino occupational therapists adapt very well amid all odds in changing times. A must read for students, new graduates and seasoned professionals!"

Cristina Ines de Leon Hinlo, OTRP, FOTAP, Owner, Therapy Works, Inc. (Philippines)

"It is a tremendous honour to endorse this groundbreaking book, the first written by and for the Filipino occupational therapy community... The authors sensitively mix local language and culture with professional concepts... encouraging occupational therapists that it is a must to understand and embrace our own backgrounds and values before successfully working with others. By discussing the Filipino context, each chapter calls on us as a profession to be conscious of and committed to transformational change. I would like to thank those involved for their dedication to making this book a reality and congratulate everyone on a remarkable job!"

Samantha Shann, President, World Federation of Occupational Therapists

"Michael, Roi Charles and Caroline, and their intrepid Filipino colleagues have produced such an important work. By taking initiative and leadership to inspire and advance powerful occupational therapy for the Philippines, they have produced an exemplar for how their colleagues from around the World, too, can transform their respective professions into powerfully relevant processes. By producing this magnificent volume of ground-breaking texts, Filipino OTs have contributed to the advancement of occupational therapy worldwide, making this great profession better, for more people."

Michael K. Iwama, PhD, MSc, BScHP, BScOT, Professor, School of Medicine, Duke University School

Occupational Therapy in the Philippines

The first book of its kind, *Occupational Therapy in the Philippines* provides a context to the existing occupational therapy knowledge base from a Filipino perspective. This book acts as a guide for occupational therapists to develop and continually evaluate trusting working relationships with clients and other health and social care professionals, leading to more effective occupational therapy services. It discusses occupational therapy concepts, principles, and practices and illustrates examples of occupational therapy practices based on Filipino case studies, narratives, and evidence, and offers recommendations on how to enrich occupational therapy understanding globally. The chapters delve into theory, education and training, clinical practice, research, case studies, and topical issues. This book is an ideal read for occupational therapy students and practitioners from all areas of practice as well as to those who are interested to know more about occupational therapy.

Michael Sy is an international academic who has significantly contributed to contemporary occupational therapy and science research in the Philippines.

Roi Charles Pineda is a rehabilitation scientist who has done extensive work on occupational therapy, disability sports, and interprofessional education and collaborative practice.

Caroline Fischl is a prominent occupational therapy educator in Sweden and serves as an educational leader in Europe through the European Network of Occupational Therapy in Higher Education.

Occupational Therapy in the Philippines

Theory, Practice, and Stories

Edited by
Michael Sy, Roi Charles Pineda and
Caroline Fischl

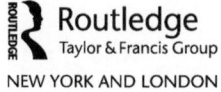
Routledge
Taylor & Francis Group

NEW YORK AND LONDON

Designed cover image: Malayang Abilidad [Unfettered Ability] by Noel
Sadicon. Print on archival paper, 30.48 x 44.45 cm. ©2024

First published 2025
by Routledge
605 Third Avenue, New York, NY 10158

and by Routledge
4 Park Square, Milton Park, Abingdon, Oxon OX14 4RN

Routledge is an imprint of the Taylor & Francis Group, an informa business

Library of Congress Cataloging-in-Publication Data
A catalog record for this title has been requested

ISBN: 978-1-032-34257-3 (hbk)
ISBN: 978-1-032-34256-6 (pbk)
ISBN: 978-1-003-32121-7 (ebk)

DOI: 10.4324/9781003321217

Typeset in Times New Roman
by Taylor & Francis Books

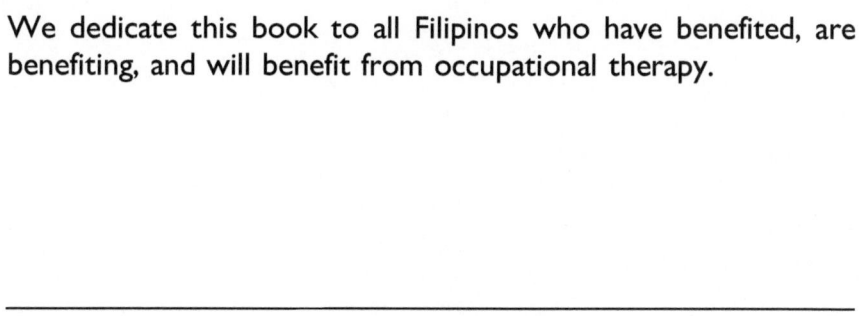

We dedicate this book to all Filipinos who have benefited, are benefiting, and will benefit from occupational therapy.

Contents

SECTION I
Theory Owning and Reclaiming

SECTION 4
Weaving Research, Ethics and Policies for the Future

Figures

Tables

Boxes

Acknowledgments

We would like to thank all the people who have contributed directly or indirectly towards the completion of this book.

We thank our family, friends, and colleagues who have supported us throughout the process of writing the book. We are also grateful to Noel Sadicon who has beautifully created the book's front cover, to occupational therapy students and professionals who supported the completion of select chapters (Kit Sinclair, Micah Therese Del Rosario), colleagues who gave their time and whom we consider as pillars of the occupational therapy profession in the Philippines—Evanina Curran, Corazon Tablan, Ruth Beltran, and Zielfa Maslin—who shared with us their invaluable occupational therapy memories and stories from the past.

Foreword

Ana Malfitano

> Looking at the past must only be a means of understanding more clearly what and who they are so that they can more wisely build the future.
>
> Paulo Freire, 1970, *Pedagogy of the oppressed*

Paulo Freire, an important Brazilian philosopher, understands history as a movement composed of dialectical elements shaped by humans. This means that contradictions are part of it. To interpret history, gain insight into the present, and foresee the future, Freire's ideas are imbued with ontological hope, foundational understandings of our society, and teleological transformation (Rossatto, 2008).

Based on the relevance of understanding history to "wisely build the future," discussions about history, fundamentals, theory, and practices—leading to critical reflections—are important (Freire, 1970). These elements are essential for approaching a profession and its knowledge field, creating opportunities to understand who we are, what we are doing, who benefits from our work, and what we would like to be and do (Farias & Lopes, 2020).

The field of occupational therapy worldwide requires deep reflection on its fundamentals and concepts, developing theories to inform practice in a responsive way (Lopes & Malfitano, 2021). Critical reflections on the locus and purpose of occupational therapy actions are essential to guide us through a conscious process regarding our professional role in our contexts during this challenging historical time. I believe occupational therapists work with occupation, everyday life, activities, and/or ways of life to promote social participation, social inclusion, and/or social emancipation. The social function of professionals is to address local demands, applying their knowledge to ensure a dignified life for all (Malfitano, 2022).

This kind of reflection is referred to as *epistemological curiosity* by Paulo Freire. This means being curious about where knowledge was produced historically, who was involved, why it was reproduced in other contexts, and what interests were involved. For Freire, this epistemological curiosity can lead to *critical curiosity*, promoting solidarity (Rossatto, 2008).

Informed by the relevance of history and envisioning the construction of the future based on epistemological curiosity, this book organized by Michael Sy, Roi Charles Pineda, and Caroline Fischl presents an important path, adding essential elements about the field of occupational therapy worldwide. With the collaboration of 30 Filipino occupational therapists and other professionals, the 15 chapters guide us through an important trajectory: the historical development of occupational therapy in the Philippines and the influence of the colonial process; connections between macro elements related to the country's history and their impacts on the micro sphere, such as in the occupational therapy profession; different fields of practice, from traditional settings to contemporary new places; professional responsibilities in addressing challenges related to our historical time, such as disaster management and poverty; professional education processes; research development, building knowledge to inform practice; and future projections. The book offers the possibility of discussing the profession based on local material, written by local academics and practitioners. It is an important achievement, contributing to the local *epistemological curiosity*, building reflections, opening and diversifying dialogues.

However, it is important to highlight that the relevance of this book extends beyond the local context. While the book primarily impacts Filipino occupational therapists by offering a discussion based on local material written by local academics and practitioners, it also addresses historical processes relevant to the implementation of the profession in what are referred to as Third World countries.

It is crucial to highlight how those discussions about global centers and economic peripheries, including "underdeveloped" countries, reflect historical relationships. No former African, Asian, or Latin American colony can explain its present without acknowledging a history marked by invasions, exterminations, exploitation, trafficking of enslaved people, racism, et cetera. Meanwhile, industrialization and economic prosperity in "developed" countries are partly due to the overexploitation of human and physical resources in Africa, Asia, and Latin America (Monzeli, Morrison, & Lopes, 2019).

This common economic historical aspect also influenced other projects, such as the implementation of occupational therapy. In Latin America, since the 1950s, international cooperation led by the United Nations has started rehabilitation centers and professional training in different countries, including the implementation of our profession. The history of occupational therapy in the Philippines and Latin America reflects the same historical moment—the second half of the twentieth century—during the Cold War, after World War II, in a specific political context aimed at the "Western World." All projects for occupational therapy education were based on models developed in the United States, shaping the profession's beginnings (Monzeli, Morrison, & Lopes, 2019).

These facts help us understand a global project that shows the connection between politics and the implementation of rehabilitation professionals, and our role influenced by the macro context, in the past, present, and future. It underscores the necessity of critical reflections, starting with questions, to critically imagine other possible futures. Therefore, epistemological curiosity related to a local context can contribute to a critical view of occupational therapy worldwide, including its differences, power relationships, epistemological colonization (including vocabulary discussions), and possibilities for the future.

It is my pleasure to invite people from the Philippines and other countries to read this insightful book on the field of occupational therapy. Considering the connection between the local and global, the inseparability of macro and micro elements, and the possibilities for occupational therapists to work beyond what has already been done, we should return to Freire's ideas and develop an ontological hope based on foundational understandings of our society and a vision of teleological transformation.

Let's "wisely build the future" of occupational therapy worldwide, respecting local histories, vocabularies, and developing knowledge that effectively contribute to a world with less inequality and more solidarity.

Good reading!

Ana Malfitano
September 2024

References

Farias, M. N., & Lopes, R. E. (2020). Social occupational therapy: Formulations by Freirian references. *Brazilian Journal of Occupational Therapy*, 28(4), 1346–1356. doi:10.4322/2526-8910.ctoEN1970.

Freire, P. (1970). *Pedagogy of the oppressed*. New York, London: Continuum Books.

Lopes, R. E., & Malfitano, A. P. S. (2021). *Social occupational therapy: Theoretical and practical designs*. Philadelphia: Elsevier.

Malfitano, A. P. S. (2022). An anthropophagic proposition in occupational therapy knowledge: Driving our actions towards social life. *World Federation of Occupational Therapists Bulletin*, 78(2), 70–82. doi:10.1080/14473828.2022.2135065.

Monzeli, G. A., Morrison, R., & Lopes, R. E. (2019). Histories of occupational therapy in Latin America: The first decade of creation of the education programs. *Brazilian Journal of Occupational Therapy*, 27(2), 235–250. doi:10.4322/2526-8910.ctoAO1631.

Rossatto, C. A. (2008). Freire's understanding of history, current reality, and future aspirations: His dream, take on ethics, and pedagogy of solidarity. *Journal of Thought*, 43(1–2), Special Issue on Paulo Freire, 149–161. https://www.jstor.org/stable/10.2307/jthought.43.1-2.149.

Preface

If we have to be honest, none of us editors knew precisely what our 15- or 16-year-old selves were signing up for when we enrolled in an entry-level program in occupational therapy in the Philippines. Prior to the age of broad access to the Internet, our only options were to learn from someone or from a book. There were no local occupational therapy textbooks available back then, which made USA-sourced textbooks the standard reference material. One such book (Willard and Spackman's *Occupational Therapy*) is often referred to as the occupational therapy student's *bible*.

These books were informative and provided the foundational knowledge one needed to learn about occupational therapy then. Generations of Filipino occupational therapy students and practitioners have been informed by these imported books, and this trend will likely continue for decades to come. What quickly becomes apparent when reading these books is how Filipino occupations—the very same occupations we students would encounter in actual Philippine practice settings with real Filipino occupational beings—are unrepresented. This should not, however, come as a surprise because books from the USA naturally prioritize the coverage of USA settings and American occupations. More recent editions of the most popular occupational therapy textbooks have been more conscious of incorporating international examples of occupations and practice settings. Nevertheless, it is unreasonable to expect these books to broadly cover the quirks and nuances of occupational therapy in the Philippines.

The existing vacuum in the literature for a book that comprehensively synthesizes occupational therapy in the Philippines can be, at least partially, attributed to weak and underfunded occupational therapy scholarship that can inform the writing of such a book. Some would-be authors may ask if it is possible to write book chapters on a topic if there is little to no published work about it. This is where we foreground the value of *stories*. While findings from empirical research are undeniably informative for the advancement of a profession, stories can help people make sense of the world and connect individual experiences to the collective. Stories are useful vehicles in communicating messages that invoke not only the intellect but also emotions. It is for these reasons that well-packaged narratives have a place in grant writing and advocacies for policy changes. Furthermore, stories from practice spark questions that research can help answer. This feedback from practice helps guide researchers and scholars on what knowledge is valuable to practitioners, supporting a bi-directional influence between research and practice.

The idea for *Occupational Therapy in the Philippines: Theory, Practice, and Stories* was first conceived in 2019 and it took two years to develop and submit a full book proposal to Routledge. Back then, we were all at various stages of our PhD studies outside the Philippines but were determined to get a book about occupational therapy written by Filipinos for Filipinos and beyond. Even at the start, it was clear to us that this book's intention is neither to reinvent occupational therapy in the Philippines nor replace imported books as standard textbooks in universities. Rather, it is to provide a descriptive, local, and current account of occupational therapy, which can enlighten individuals curious about the profession in general, or about occupational therapy in the Philippines in particular. We believe that this intention is best realized by gathering Filipino researchers, practitioners, educators, and leaders who understand the local context that shapes the profession. We also want to see this book project as a historical landmark in the development and advancement of the occupational therapy profession in the Philippines.

This book is intended for students, practitioners, researchers, and leaders of occupational therapy. While the book is situated in the Philippine context, we believe that our book will be relevant to students and professionals belonging to professions other than occupational therapy. For Filipino occupational therapy students, starting their first year of studies with a reference book authored by Filipinos that is published internationally will be very encouraging. The contents of the book can provide an overview of occupational therapy knowledge drawn largely from a Filipino perspective, preparing them for what lies ahead before they enter the workforce. Practitioners can optimize the book by reflecting on the issues unearthed and critical perspectives offered within the chapters and see how these can influence, shape, and improve their practice, teaching, the policies they create, and the services they provide across all settings. Graduate students (master's and doctoral students) and researchers in occupational therapy can utilize the book as a starting point to develop local studies that will consequently yield empirical evidence. For practitioners, scholars, and students outside occupational therapy, the book can serve as a supplementary reference that provides localized stories and practices that can inform their respective professions.

Guided by Kolb's Experiential Learning Cycle, consisting of a four-stage process, each chapter intends to improve effective learning to all readers. In every chapter, there is an introduction to core concepts and theories in occupational therapy and peripheral disciplines (*abstract conceptualization*), explanation of the concepts through local examples and stories (*concrete experience*), space for thinking and questioning via the critical questions posed by the authors (*reflective observation*), and opportunities to actuate and adapt what they have learned into actual and situated practice and learning level (*active experimentation*). Open educational resources, websites, repositories, as well as suggested individual and group activities are available in select chapters in order to expand the learning experience beyond reading the book.

We organized this book into four sections. Section 1 deals with establishing foundational knowledge on occupational therapy practice in the Philippines, including a multidisciplinary conceptualization of occupations from a Filipino perspective (Chapter 1), a historical account of the profession's development in the country (Chapter 2), and a curation of studies on Filipino occupations through the lens of occupational science (Chapter 3). Section 2 focuses on the education aspect of occupational therapy from undergraduate or entry-level education (Chapter 4) to postgraduate and lifelong learning (Chapter 5), as well as the education of occupational therapy students as healthcare professionals (Chapter 6). The focus shifts to practice aspects of occupational therapy in Section 3. It covers the various practice settings in the Philippines, namely the four traditional practice areas of geriatrics, mental health, pediatrics, and physical rehabilitation (Chapter 7), community-centered (Chapter 8), and emerging practice areas such as technology/telehealth-based (Chapter 9), disaster risk reduction (Chapter 10), and justice work (Chapter 11). Lastly, Section 4 wraps up the book with a discussion of research generation and utilization (Chapter 12), legislation and policy (Chapter 13), and ethics (Chapter 14) in relation to contemporary occupational therapy practice, with a concluding chapter about a vision of the future of occupational therapy in the Philippines (Chapter 15).

All contributing authors have been invited specifically because of their credibility, authority in their respective fields, richness of practice experiences, and connectedness to the Filipino heritage. The editors (Michael, Roi, and Caroline), who were educated and trained in the Philippines and now live and work abroad, hope that this allows them to cocreate a nexus between local and global understanding of occupational therapy.

While the chapters are grouped into thematic sections, readers should also be aware that each chapter has been written separately by different authors, with the understanding that the chapter they wrote could be related to one or more chapters within the edited book. We also anticipate that some readers may find the book lacking in respect of tips and techniques for actual practice, which is totally understandable. At the beginning of the book-writing process, the editorial team attempted to create authoring teams composed of academics and practitioners with the intention of bridging the gap between theory and practice. What this book offers students, practitioners, leaders, and scholars in occupational therapy is a starting point for numerous things: ideas, discussions, conversations, practice translations, and perhaps another story.

Michael, Roi, and Caroline

Editors

Michael Palapal Sy, PhD, OTRP, Senior Researcher, Institute of Occupational Therapy, Zurich University of Applied Sciences, Zurich, Switzerland. Michael is a licensed occupational therapist (Philippines) and a health professions educator with a PhD in occupational therapy from the Tokyo Metropolitan University, Japan. His PhD focused on translating occupational justice concepts into occupational therapy practice in the drug addiction rehabilitation setting in the Philippines. He worked as a private clinician both in the pediatric and community settings in the Philippines and has held various academic positions in teaching in the Philippines. As a senior researcher at the Institute of Occupational Therapy, Zurich University of Applied Sciences, Michael focuses his research on the return-to-work process of people with long COVID, occupational justice, and occupational science. He also teaches for the European Master of Science in Occupational Therapy program. Currently, Michael has external appointments as an academic at Dalhousie University (occupational science), Tokyo Metropolitan University (occupational therapy), University of Southern Queensland (occupational therapy) and University of the Philippines Open University (international health).

Roi Charles Pineda, PhD, OTR, OTRP, Associate Researcher, Department of Rehabilitation Sciences, KU Leuven, Leuven, Belgium. Roi has a professional background in occupational therapy with nearly 15 years of experience in various roles. Early in his career, he was a practitioner in hospital- and home-based physical rehabilitation settings and a clinical instructor for occupational therapy students. He later worked as a university instructor and contributed to the development of the only occupational therapy program in Central Luzon, Philippines. Roi received full scholarships to complete his postgraduate degrees in adapted physical activity (MSc) and biomedical sciences (PhD) from KU Leuven. His postgraduate education allowed him to flourish as a researcher with international collaborations. Currently, his research is focused on physical activity, across the spectrum of top-performance sport to leisure-time physical activity, with relevance to policies and practices for facilitating physical activity participation among persons with disabilities and their inclusion in the Paralympics.

Caroline Fischl, PhD, Reg.OT, OTRP, Assistant Professor, School of Health and Welfare, Jönköping University, Jönköping, Sweden. Caroline earned her bachelor's degree in occupational therapy from the University of the Philippines Manila and her master's degrees in ergonomics and occupational therapy in Sweden. She completed her PhD at Umeå University, focusing on older adults' social participation through digital technologies. Caroline has worked in community and home settings, as well as private clinics and a school in the Philippines. She currently serves as an assistant professor of occupational therapy at Jönköping University, managing the Swedish and international master's programs in occupational therapy. She teaches scientific theory, research methods, and ethics. Caroline also serves as President of the European Network of Occupational Therapy in Higher Education (ENOTHE) and is a member of the executive board of Occupational Therapy Europe. She has co-developed the 2024 European Qualifications and Assessment Reference Frameworks in Occupational Therapy.

Contributors

Deborrah Sadile Anastacio, PhD, Associate Professor, De La Salle University, Manila, Philippines. Deborrah has a master's degree in International Relations and a PhD in Philippine Studies, with a major in Language, Culture, and Media. Her research interests include Philippine studies, cultural heritage, religious studies, the education system in the Philippines, and sustainable development.

Alexa Blas, OTRP, Graduate Student, Asian Institute of Management, Makati City, Philippines. Alexa is an occupational therapist, an operations manager, and a graduate student in Development Management. Her advocacies and research interests include the role of occupational therapists in enabling work and sustainable livelihood as a development intervention.

Paolo Miguel P. Bulan, OTD, OTRP, Professor, Velez College, Cebu City, Philippines. Paolo is a professor of occupational therapy at Velez College, Cebu. He is an occupational therapist and educator with a passion for teaching and research. His published works focus on exploring academic occupations, mental health, and the concept of occupation within the local context.

Kristine Ann M. Carandang, MSc, OTRP, Adjunct Faculty and Data Scientist, Asian Institute of Management, Makati City, Philippines. Kristine is an occupational therapist (Philippines) with postgraduate degrees in international health (diploma) and data science (MSc). She is currently pursuing a doctorate in data science and also serves as a PAOT board director. Her research interests include occupational science, health policy and systems research, and the applications of data science and artificial intelligence in healthcare.

Ricardo Carrasco, PhD, FAOTA, Professor, Nova Southeastern University, Fort Lauderdale, Florida, United States of America. Ric is a professor and founding chair of the Occupational Therapy program at Nova Southeastern University. Originally from the Philippines, he has been an occupational therapist for over 40 years and has qualifications in elementary and special education, commerce, and psychology. He is also a proponent of the SIBOL group.

Christianne Marie Coronel-Andigan, MHlthSc(OT), OTRP, Assistant Professor, Occupational Therapy Program Chair, College of Rehabilitation Science, St. Paul University Iloilo, Iloilo City, Philippines. Chrissy has been an occupational therapist for more than 20 years, with a substantial part of her career spent in academia. She spearheads and teaches in the first BSOT academic program in the Western Visayas region of the Philippines. She also provides direct therapy services for children and families of children with developmental disabilities and serves as an OT resource person for schools, and government and non-government agencies.

Abelardo Apollo I. David, Jr., MOccThy, LPT, OTRP, Assistant Professor, College of Rehabilitation Sciences, University of Santo Tomas, Manila, Philippines. Archie is the founder of several organizations (e.g., REACH Foundation, Inc.) that foster pioneering health and education equity programs in the Philippines. His work in inclusive education and CBR have gained national and international recognition, including the UN Public Service Awards, and are recognized as best practice models.

Charmaine Kristabel De Vera-Fevidal, MSc, Doctoral Student, National Teacher Training Center for the Health Professions, University of the Philippines Manila, Manila, Philippines. Charmaine is a licensed occupational therapist in the Philippines and is currently pursuing a doctorate in Health Professions Education. Her clinical experience includes working in both government and private institutional settings. She has also been the program head of two undergraduate occupational therapy programs in the Philippines.

Icy Fresno Anabo, PhD, Postdoctoral Researcher, Technical Project Manager, Universidad de Deusto, Bilbao, Spain. Icy is an international education consultant specializing in international higher education, educational policy research, student mobility, and graduate employability. With a background in occupational therapy, she practiced in Manila and has conducted research on vocational training, mobility, and employability across Europe. Icy holds a PhD in Education and a Joint Master's in Lifelong Learning.

Ivan Neil B. Gomez, PhD, Associate Professor, College of Rehabilitation Sciences, University of Santo Tomas, Manila, Philippines. Ivan is an academic occupational therapist whose research interests include evidence-based healthcare, neuroscience, and the translation and development of pediatric outcome measures.

Maria Elizabeth Grageda, PhD, PTRP, Associate Professor, Dean, National Teacher Training Center for the Health Professions, University of the Philippines Manila, Manila, Philippines. Maria Elizabeth is a licensed physical therapist specializing in health professions education. She holds a PhD in Education, with a focus on educational research and evaluation. Her scholarly work revolves around clinical education and the evaluation of student performance.

Joel R. Guerrero, OTD, OTR/L, Assistant Professor, Cedar Crest College, Allentown, Pennsylvania, USA. Joel is an internationally educated occupational therapist with over 25 years of experience in academia and clinical settings. He specializes in aging-in-place, dementia care, and care for the homeless, marginalized, and underserved populations. His scholarship focuses on addressing issues related to discharge planning for unhoused patients.

Camille Anne L. Guevara, OTRP, Occupational Therapist III, Mariveles Mental Wellness and General Hospital, Mariveles, Bataan, Philippines. Cami is an occupational therapist specializing in mental health. She works in a psychiatric hospital, leads staff growth initiatives, and is a co-founder of a mental health advocacy group. Her research focuses on occupational justice, substance use rehabilitation, and mental health. She is pursuing postgraduate education in international health.

Jomarx Jocson, OTRP, Program Director, Nurturing Early Skills Therapy Center (NEST), Inc., Cainta, Rizal, Philippines. Jomarx is an occupational therapist specializing in managing children with developmental disabilities. He also manages transitional and vocational programs for the adolescent population. He is currently a clinic manager in a private pediatric clinic.

Maria Menierva Lagria, OTRP, Program Chair, Department of Occupational Therapy, Silliman University. Minnie is an occupational therapist with extensive community development experience in Africa and Asia. She spent several years in Namibia providing community-centered rehabilitation for people with communicable diseases. In 2015, she returned to the Philippines to teach as an instructor at Velez College Cebu and help develop a community relocation program for families displaced by Typhoon Yolanda in Bantayan, Cebu.

Mark Oliver S. Llangco, PhD, FHEA, Associate Professor, University of the Philippines Los Baños, Los Baños, Laguna, Philippines. Mark Oliver is a Filipino sociologist and educator. He teaches quantitative and qualitative social research courses in the Department of Social Sciences at the University of the Philippines Los Baños and chairs the university's Research Ethics Board.

Diana Jane A. Luib, JD, OTRP, Former Chair for Political Advocacy Committee on Legislations, Philippine Academy of Occupational Therapists, Inc., Makati City, Philippines. Diana is an occupational therapist in the Philippines. She completed her occupational therapy degree at the University of the Philippines and her Juris Doctor degree at San Beda College. She is an advocate of the Occupational Therapy Law and other laws for persons with disabilities in the Philippines.

Pauline Gail V. Martinez, MIH, OTRP, Occupational Therapist, Blue Wing Care Professionals, Brisbane, Australia. Pauline is a Filipino occupational therapist who works with clients across various age groups. She is also an educator and researcher with published works on occupational science, occupational therapy education, and interprofessional collaboration.

Kim Gerald G. Medallon, PhD, OTRP, Associate Professor, Internship Supervisor, College of Rehabilitation Sciences, University of Santo Tomas, Manila, Philippines. Kim is an occupational therapy educator and a part-time pediatric clinician. He holds a Master of Health Professions Education degree and a PhD in Educational Administration (2023). Kim serves as the Pedagogical Lead and Internship Supervisor for occupational therapy at the university. His research interests include the cross-cultural adaptation of OT tools and inclusive education.

Teresita C. Mendoza, MEd, OTRP, FPAOT, Retired Professor, College of Allied Medical Professions, University of the Philippines Manila, Manila, Philippines. Teresita is a licensed occupational therapist in the Philippines with a master's degree in education specializing in guidance and counseling. Her interest areas include psychosocial occupational therapy, mental health, and community-based education. She is also a Fellow of the Philippine Academy of Occupational Therapists.

Paulin Grace Morato-Espino, PhD, MA, OTRP, Assistant Professor, College of Rehabilitation Sciences, University of Santo Tomas, Manila, Philippines. Pau is an occupational therapist who works with children with developmental disabilities and their families, an educator at the University of Santo Tomas preparing future occupational therapists, and a researcher. Her research interests include play, screen time, and the well-being of young Filipino children.

Arden A. Panotes, OTRP, Occupational Therapist, Everyday Independence, Australia. Arden is an occupational therapist and a graduate student of health professions education. She now works as an occupational therapist in Australia. Arden remains active in doing research and advocacy work regarding family involvement in therapy, use of telehealth in service delivery, and student development.

Terry Peralta-Catipon, PhD, Department Chair, California State University, Dominguez Hills, Carson, California, United States of America. Terry has a PhD in Occupational Science with an interest in ethnographic research, particularly in the areas of Filipino migrant adaptation, community wellness programs for older adults, and defining cultural occupations.

Karen S. Sagun, MRS, MSOT, OTR, OTRP, Faculty College of Rehabilitation Sciences, University of Santo Tomas, Manila, Philippines. Karen leads the Quezon City KABAHAGI Center, a government program empowering underserved children with disabilities and their families. Through participatory research and consultancy, she develops evidence-based strategies that transform lives, championing disability-inclusive policies and enhancing the quality of life for marginalized communities.

Oliver Santos Trinidad, MBE, OTR/L, Program Director, Ability Builders for Children Early Intervention Program, Bronx, New York, United States of America. Oliver is a licensed occupational therapist in New York with a master's degree in education in Mind, Brain, and Education (MBE). He has participated in research and written on health, Filipino personality, and corruption using Filipino indigenous psychology methods and concepts.

Sally Jane Uy, MEd, MBAH, OTR, OTRP, Senior Lecturer, College of Allied Medical Professions, University of the Philippines Manila, Manila, Philippines. Sally is a licensed and registered occupational therapist in the Philippines and in the United States, with over 30 years of experience in various practice settings. Sally currently specializes in older adult health and wellness in community-based settings and continues to be an OT educator, advocating for lifelong learning and service.

Daryl Patrick Yao, PhD(cand.), MS(OT), Doctoral Researcher, Department of Disability and Human Development, University of Illinois Chicago, Chicago, Illinois, United States of America. Daryl is a licensed occupational therapist in the Philippines and a PhD candidate in Disability Studies. He holds a master's degree in occupational therapy from Tokyo Metropolitan University. His master's thesis explored the integration experience of Filipinos with spinal cord injuries through an occupational justice perspective. He advocates for an accessible and inclusive society through an organization of persons with disabilities.

Anna-Liza Yap Tan Pascual, MRS, OTRP, Director, Restart Hope in Children in Conflict with the Law, Manila, Philippines. Anna has worked with pediatric clients for the past 31 years across multiple settings, populations, and countries. After working with orphans in China, she transitioned to working with "spiritual orphans" when she returned to the Philippines.

Constantine L. Yu Chua, MD, OTRP, Associate Professor, College of Medicine, University of the Philippines Manila, Manila, Philippines. Cons is a licensed occupational therapist who also pursued a career in medicine and psychiatry. He is currently a child and adolescent psychiatry consultant involved in private clinics and teaching. His work bridges and integrates occupational therapy, human development, medical neuroscience, and mental health.

List of abbreviations

ABM	Accountancy, Business, and Management
ADHD	Attention Deficit and Hyperactivity Disorder
ADL	activities of daily living
AHA	American Heart Association
AOTA	American Occupational Therapy Association
BP	Batas Pambansa
BSOT	Bachelor of Science in Occupational Therapy
CBR	community-based rehabilitation
CCHP	Comprehensive Community Health Program
CEDEFOP	European Centre for the Development of Vocational Training
CHED	Commission on Higher Education
CICL	children in conflict with the law
CK	Content Knowledge
CMO	CHED Memorandum Order
CoP	Communities of Practice
CPD	Continuing Professional Development
CPG	Clinical Practice Guideline
CPSP-CATS	Career Progression and Specialization Program and Credit Accumulation and Transfer System
CRPD	Convention on the Rights of Persons with Disabilities
DDOP	disaster and development occupational perspective
DepEd	Department of Education
DESA	Department of Economic and Social Affairs
DOH	Department of Health
DOLE	Department of Labor and Employment
DOST	Department of Science and Technology
DRR	disaster risk reduction and response
DSWD	Department of Social Welfare and Development
EBP	evidence-based practice
EO	Executive Order
ESeC	European Socio-economic Classification

FGD	focus group discussion
GA	General Assembly
GAS	General Academic Strand
GCP	Good Clinical Practice
GSIS	Government Service Insurance System
HEI	higher educational institution
HERDIN	Health Research and Development Information Network
HUMSS	Humanities and Social Sciences
ILO	International Labour Organization
IRB	Institutional Review Board
ISCO	International Standard Classification of Occupations
ISSP	International Social Survey Program
JJWC	Juvenile Justice Welfare Council
LGU	local government unit
MARCH	Medical Action for Relief, Counseling and Health
NBCOT	National Board for Certification in Occupational Therapy
NCCDP	National Commission Concerning Disabled Persons
NCMH	National Center for Mental Health
NDRRMC	National Disaster Risk Reduction and Management Council
NHIP	National Health Insurance Program
NOH	National Orthopedic Hospital
OJHQ	Occupational Justice Health Questionnaire
OT	occupational therapy
OTAP	Occupational Therapy Association of the Philippines
OTION	Occupational Therapy International Online Network
OTPF	Occupational Therapy Practice Framework
OTSA	Occupational Therapy Students Assembly
PAASCU	Philippine Accrediting Association of Schools, Colleges, and Universities
PAOT	Philippine Academy of Occupational Therapists
PARM	Philippine Academy of Rehabilitation Medicine
PCAU	Philippine Civil Affairs Unit
PCK	Pedagogical Content Knowledge
PD	Presidential Decree
PDAO	Persons with Disabilities Affairs Office
PEARLS	Practice, Education, Advocacy, Research, and Leadership in Synergism
PhilHealth	Philippine Health Insurance Corporation
PHREB	Philippine Health Research Ethics Board
PHRR	Philippine Health Research Registry
PJOT	Philippine Journal of Occupational Therapy
PK	Pedagogical Knowledge
POC	Philippine Orthopedic Center

POJF	Participatory Occupational Justice Framework
PQF	Philippine Qualifications Framework
PRB	Professional Regulatory Board
PRC	Professional Regulation Commission
PT	physical therapy
PWD	persons with disabilities
RA	Republic Act
RCOT	Royal College of Occupational Therapists
SAGE	South African Guideline Evaluation Clinical Practice Guideline Development
SAMP	School of Allied Medical Professions
SDG	Sustainable Development Goal
SIBOL	Sowing, Informing and Building Occupational Science for Living
SLP	Speech and Language Pathology
SSS	Social Security System
STEM	Science, Technology, Engineering, and Mathematics
SWOT	Strengths-Weaknesses-Opportunities-Threats
TCK	Technological Content Knowledge
TEACH	Therapy, Education and Assimilation of Children with Handicap
TESDA	Technical Education and Skills Development Authority
TK	Technological Knowledge
TPaCK	Technological Pedagogical and Content Knowledge
TPK	Technological Pedagogical Knowledge
UHC	Universal Health Care
UN	United Nations
UNDRR	United Nations Office for Disaster Risk Reduction
UNESCO	United Nations Educational, Scientific and Cultural Organization
UNFPA	United Nations Population Fund
UNFPA	United Nations Population Fund
UNICEF	United Nations International Children's Emergency Fund
UNISDR	United Nations International Strategy for Disaster Reduction
UP	University of the Philippines
UP-CAMP	University of the Philippines—College of Allied Medical Professions
USA	United States of America
USC	University of Southern California
WFOT	World Federation of Occupational Therapists
WHO	World Health Organization

Chapter 1

Occupation and occupational therapy

The evolution of these concepts from a Filipino perspective

Michael Sy, Roi Charles Pineda, Deborrah Sadile Anastacio, Mark Oliver Llangco, Kristine Ann M. Carandang and Michael Wilson Rosero

Chapter objectives

1 Explore the multidisciplinary conceptualization of occupation from historical, sociological and linguistic perspectives
2 Propose a reimagined definition of the terms "occupation" and "occupational therapy" to be applied and used in contemporary occupational therapy practice in the Philippines

In a typical occupational therapy session in the local practice arena, you would hear and observe the following dialogues:

Scenario 1: Practitioner talking with the mother of a pediatric client

THERAPIST: *Hello po. Ako po si Maria, ang 'yong occupational therapist.* [Hello. I am Maria, your occupational therapist.]
CLIENT: Hello, Teacher Maria.
THERAPIST: *May ideya po ba kayo sa occupational therapy?* [Do you have an idea about occupational therapy?]
CLIENT: *Wala po. Ngayon ko lang po 'yan narinig.* [No, it is my first time hearing about it.]
THERAPIST: *Ang occupational therapy po ay isang propesyong pangkalusugan na sumusuporta sa mga taong mayroong kapansanan dahil sa sakit, aksidente, o karamdamang pisikal at mental.* [Occupational therapy is a health profession that supports people who has a disability due to sickness, accidents, or physical and mental conditions.]

Scenario 2: Client who had a stroke asking what occupational therapy is

CLIENT: *Doc, ano po ba ang occupational therapy?* [Doctor, what is occupational therapy?]

DOI: 10.4324/9781003321217-1

THERAPIST: *'Nay, 'di ho ako doktor. Ako po ang occupational therapist n'yo. Layunin po ng occupational therapy na matulungan kayong muling magawa ang mga gawaing kailangan at gusto n'yong gawin. Tulad na lamang po ng mga gawaing may kinalaman sa pag-aalaga ng inyong katawan—pagkain, pagbihis—o 'di kaya mga gawaing bahay.* [Ma'am, I'm not a doctor. I'm your occupational therapist. The goal of occupational therapy is to help restore your ability to do the activities you need and want to do, such as self-care activities—eating, dressing—or household chores.]

CLIENT: *Iba pa ba 'yan sa physical therapy?* [Is that different from physical therapy?]

THERAPIST: *Opo, 'Nay. Bagamat pareho po kaming tumutulong sa rehabilitasyon n'yo, iba ho ang occupational therapy sa physical therapy.* [Yes, ma'am. Although we both help with your rehabilitation, occupational therapy is different from physical therapy.]

The nuances of the responses will also be largely influenced by the occupational therapist's education, training, workplace environment, paradigm preference, culture, language spoken, and age associated with the generation he or she belongs to. While we know that it is impossible to have a uniform definition of occupational therapy, it is crucial to communicate the profession to clients with a shared perspective drawn from the therapeutic use of occupations (meaningful activities), as well as provide context-focused examples. However, the concept of occupation needs some degree of ambiguity to encompass the multidisciplinary perspectives inherent to the concept, based on what Breines (1995) believes is a deliberate choice by the professions' founders. Confounded by the recent developments in contemporary and critical occupational therapy, this creates a conundrum towards the development and advancement of the occupational therapy profession today.

The word "occupation" has been a debatable terminology when used and applied in the occupational therapy profession and theorized in the occupational science discipline. Deconstructing the concept "occupation" in the Philippine context is important in understanding how Filipino society understands the role of occupational therapy in contemporary times. Doing so can potentially sustain the efforts of Filipino occupational therapists to advance and promote the profession towards the twenty-first century. Concretely, understanding where the concept "occupation" came from and how it had been interpreted through the years can help occupational therapists and other professionals better communicate occupations as a therapeutic and transformative action to service users and the general public. In this chapter, it is our aim to deconstruct the concept "occupation" from historical, linguistic, and sociological perspectives. To do this, the chapter was written by authors with backgrounds in occupational science, sociology, Philippine studies, data science, and occupational therapy. We conclude by discussing how we can reimagine the definitions of "occupation" and "occupational therapy" and make them a proposition for use in the current and future praxis of the profession in the Philippines.

Historical perspective

The Spanish language heavily influenced the Filipino language due to the colonization of Spain for over three centuries. The word "occupation" is translated into Spanish as *occupacion* in *Vocabulario de la Lengua de Tagala* (1860) by Juan de Noceda and Pedro Sanlucar. Referred to as one of the oldest for the Tagalog language, this dictionary defines the words *abala* [busy], *ligalig* [restless], *gaua* [action connoting productivity], and *libang* [leisure] as equivalents to the term *ocupacion*. Notably, each word redirects to one another and conveys any activity that is given time and attention without the concept of obtaining financial income. The reason can be explained by the Philippines' pre-colonial social structure known as the *barangay*.

Barangay is the unit of society consisting of less than one hundred families, headed by a *datu* [barangay leader] (Pearson, 1969). In the Luzon area (northern part of the Philippine archipelago) they were divided into four social classes: *maginoo* [noble], *maharlika* [warrior], *timawa* [freeman], and *alipin* [slave] (Scott, 1980). The four classes had a client-patron relationship as service is rendered to pay feudal dues. In addition, individuals from each class had differing rights that influence their client-patron relationship (Scott, 1980). A *datu* is part of the *maginoo* and is responsible for organizing the barangay's labor force (Pearson, 1969). A title of a *lakan* or *rajah* is given to the *datu* if he (at that time, this title was only given to men) gained power and controlled more territories other than his original barangay. Peace and order are maintained through kinship and treaties between the *datus*. *Maharlika* rendered military service, while the *timawas* are described as common farming people with the ability to pay feudal dues through agricultural labor (Scott, 1980). The *alipin* is categorized into two subclasses: *aliping namamahay* (someone who had property rights but worked on a land and offered tribute and labor to a master) and *aliping saguiguilid* (depended totally on a master).

Leadership in the barangay was organized based on functions such as *datu* [chieftain], *babaylan* [priestess], *panday* [blacksmith], and *bayani* [warrior] (Salazar, 1996). The *datu* had a broad responsibility spanning from the political and military to economic aspects of the community. The *babaylans* were the knowledge bearers, ritual performers, and spiritual intermediaries between the people and the spiritual realm. The *bayanis* facilitated peace, order, and protection of the whole barangay against any external threats, while the *pandays* were skillful artisans who crafted weapons for wars as well as tools for farming and household keeping.

With this historical point of view, the concept of "occupation," that is, engagement in meaningful activities, largely depended on ancient Filipinos' sociopolitical function within the barangay system. These functions have shared values of productivity and contribution to the community, with underlying restrictions due to the pronounced existence of social classes. At that time, meaningful activities did not necessarily mean promoting health and well-being as what we perceive today. For instance, being a warrior entailed killing other human beings to gain territorial lands to achieve respect from one's community, and spiritual intercourses led by the babaylans entailed using plant-based psychedelics that would induce a trance to connect to the spiritual realm. Both examples were regarded as valuable and socially acceptable to ancient Filipinos, which if done today would be criminalized, or done in clandestine situations.

During the Spanish colonization, the scattered and independent barangays were merged to create larger communities through the establishment of the *encomienda* system. This system was introduced by the Spanish colonizers to control the labor system between the Spanish colonizers and the colonized people characterized by the indigenous, native, and non-Christian people from the barangays. In this new system, the barangays were pushed centrally to settle in *pueblos*, a community that is within hearing distance of the church bells. The progressive entry of Spanish missionaries and migrants brought Christianity into the archipelago, which in turn created economic, religious, and social changes. Although Anderson (1976) considered the encomienda system as the "the earliest and, for half a century, the most important system in order in Filipino society and labor," this new system devolved the barangay system, and instituted a communal slavery to occupy the native Filipinos, who were later called *indios*, a derogatory term that showed inferiority.

While the colonized communities became more centralized, this allowed the Spanish to gain more power and control over the conquered native Filipinos (Demeterio, 2010). This century-long process of invasion is called "Spanish occupation," which has a negative connotation and induces historical trauma. One way to sustain and progress the colonial occupation was establishing partnerships between the Spanish colonizers and the *datu*s to co-share the leading of the conquered lands. Meanwhile, the *bayani*s were stripped of their military prowess, and the *babaylan*s and *panday*s were marginalized and eventually lost their function as spiritual and cultural forebearers of the community. Another process of Spanish occupation was through the Catholic Church, which replaced the spiritual function of the *babaylan*s and led in establishing priest-governed hospitals, asylums, almshouses, orphanages, and schools (Almanzor, 1966). Through these institutions, basic education and occupational training based on Spanish ideals and values were employed to galvanize the colonial order. The Filipinos who were mainly educated and trained to integrate into the new colonial system originally come from the *Maginoo, Maharlika*, and *Timawa* social classes. To a certain extent, their day-to-day actions and activities started to be shaped and hybridized from their indigenous past and colonized present, which perpetuated throughout the American and Japanese colonization during the nineteenth and twentieth centuries, and until today.

Linguistic perspective

The Philippines is a linguistically diverse country of over 100 mutually unintelligible languages, with eight languages, Tagalog, Cebuano, Ilokano, Hiligaynon, Bikol, Samar-Leyte, Kapampangan, and Pangasinan, comprising the mother tongue of 85% of the population (McFarland, 2008). This diversity, however, has hindered communication among language groups, necessitating a *lingua franca*. The language of its colonizers, first Spanish and later English, served this purpose. As declared by the Philippine Constitution of 1987, the current national language is Filipino, which is based on the variant of Tagalog spoken in Metro Manila (Sibayan, 1991).

However, English continues to hold a position of prestige in most of the *controlling domains* in the Philippines. These domains such as law, mathematics, science and technology, and education dictate what language to learn to effectively participate in these domains (Sibayan, 1991). Aside from resistance from the non-Tagalog language groups in adopting Filipino rather than English, Filipino is still an insufficiently intellectualized language; that is, Filipino lacks the terminology for use in those aforementioned controlling domains (Sibayan, 1991). For these reasons (and likely also the cause), English remains the dominant language of education, including health professions education.

Because the language of occupational therapy education in the Philippines is English, there has been no impetus to use the Filipino language despite the potential detriment to client-therapist communication (Fischl, 2005; Grecia et al., 2011; Pineda, 2022). In the more than 50 years of existence of occupational therapy in the Philippines, few studies have taken the task of intellectualizing the Filipino language for occupational therapy. This is consequently reflected in the persistent absence of a definition and/or translation of occupational therapy in Filipino or any other Philippine languages (WFOT, 2018). One of these few studies was by Fischl (2005), which proposed a register of translated occupational therapy terms in Filipino for use during client-therapist interaction. Moving beyond translation, Grecia et al. (2011) employed a lexical approach to arrive at a Filipino structural definition of occupation (translated as *mahalagang gawain* [important activity] in their study). They found that Filipino speakers view occupations as positively and negatively experienced physical activities that satisfy needs for happiness, fulfillment, and calmness and reflect Filipino food culture. Both studies used *gawain* [task, activity] as the Filipino translation for occupation, but the implication of such a choice was never examined.

In usual practice, Filipino occupational therapists often simply use the terms "occupation" and "occupational therapy" while communicating with clients in Filipino. For example, the official Filipino translation of the 2024 World Occupational Therapy Day theme was *occupational therapy para sa lahat* [occupational therapy for all], which contrasts with other languages (WFOT, 2024). This unassimilated lexical borrowing is accepted as standard orthography for newly borrowed English words (Komisyon sa Wikang Filipino [Commission on the Filipino Language], 2013) and is facilitated by the common language practice of *Taglish* or code-switching between English and Filipino (Baklanova, 2017). It is unclear, however, how using these loanwords influences clients' understanding of these terms, considering that "occupation" may mean something different to clients.

One attempt to examine potential meanings of "occupation" in Filipino is through the use of dictionary analysis. Using contemporary English-Filipino and Filipino-English dictionaries, we identified four categories of definitions of "occupation" (Table 1.1). The *first category*

Table 1.1 Categories of English to Filipino translations for occupation

1: Being busy with something	2: Means of livelihood	3: General purpose–oriented activities	4: Occupying a place
dibersyon [diversion]	*empleyo* [employment]	*bokasyon* [vocation]	*okupasyon* [occupation]
inaatupag [taken cared of]	*hanapbuhay* [livelihood]	*gawain* [task, activity]	*pag-okupa* [occupy]
libangan [recreation]	*ikinabubuhay* [livelihood]	*tungkulin* [responsibility]	*pagsaklaw* [taken control of]
kaabalahan [busy doing]	*okupasyon* [occupation]		*pagtira* [residence in a place]
pagpapalipas-oras [killing time]	*opisyo* [work]		*pamamalagi* [stay at a place]
	pinagkakakitaan [livelihood]		*pamumusesyon* [take possession of]
	propesyon [profession]		*pananahanan* [residence in a place]
	trabaho [work]		*pananakop* [invasion]
			pananalakay [attack; invasion]

refers to the act of being busy with something within a dedicated period. These words can be interpreted as a hobby without the direct involvement of gaining an income and can serve as a distraction that brings entertainment and/or relaxation to a person or group. The *second category* encompasses words related to activities meant to gain a living income. The *third category* refers to a broad category of general purpose–oriented activities that fulfill a personal commitment, a sense of duty, or even a calling to fulfill one's life purpose, but do not necessarily generate resources. Finally, the *fourth category* pertains to the act of occupying a place, which can have a negative connotation when the act involves force. Notable across the categories is that all words refer to the act of doing something in line with one's intention.

To further the results of a dictionary analysis, an ongoing corpus linguistics study by Pineda (2022) has been examining the Filipino conceptualization of "occupation" based on the occurrence of keywords in authentic (i.e., naturally occurring rather than intentionally constructed for the study's purpose) layperson discourse from print media. The study's corpus of print media consists of texts from news articles and web pages from 2011, 2014, 2016, 2020, and 2021. Initial analysis was performed on the four keywords—*trabaho, hanapbuhay, gawain*, and *tungkulin*—that represent the aforementioned second and third categories of definitions of occupation. Findings revealed that Filipinos generally relate "occupation" to work productivity or denote social responsibility that can vary from religious activities, livelihood pursuits, hobbies, and even illicit doings or work. The dictionary and corpus linguistics analysis support key elements of Grecia and colleagues' (2011) Filipino structural definition of occupation, except the food-related aspect.

The study findings from Pineda's (2022) on-going work reinforce the point that "occupation" cannot be captured by a single Filipino word, although *gawain* appears to be the most encompassing out of four words used in the initial analysis. Moreover, the variety of Filipino translations alone suggests that occupational therapists should be cautious in the choice of Filipino words to use when communicating about occupations with their clients. How these are used in print media provides further support as to why it has been a challenge for occupational therapists to explain what occupational therapy is in Filipino. Accordingly, at least for now, it seems that Filipino occupational therapists should be more intentional in their choice of Filipino words to better communicate the idea of engaging in activities to earn a living, to obtain personal fulfillment, to enjoy, or simply to live. This intentionality must be done to cover the essence of occupations as "meaningful everyday activities," and to ensure that clients understand what occupational therapists do.

Sociological perspective

The definition of occupation is consequential in how research and practice in different fields (e.g., occupational science, occupational therapy, sociology of occupations) are mapped and developed. The concept of occupation has different meanings in various contexts. From a sociological perspective, the word "occupation" is largely attributed to the second category of definition in Table 1.1, pertaining to the means of livelihood.

In the field of sociology, an example of a cross-national survey that directly asks about occupation and occupation-related topics is the International Social Survey Programme. The question items in Table 1.2 were used in a cross-national survey of more than 40 countries, including the Philippines. These questions allow us to encounter and reflect on at least two ways of conceptualizing occupation. The basic questionnaire written in English is translated into different languages, including four major Philippine languages: Tagalog, Ilokano, Bisaya, and Hiligaynon. The Filipino translation in the right column provides an insight into how the concept of occupation is understood and operationalized by social science researchers and how it is communicated to survey participants.

When understood narrowly, especially in economics or sociology, "occupation" may be defined as a specific work role within a system of labor market classification undertaken by a person consistently as a source of income and identity. Occupation is what people consider to be their main economic activity, usually outside the household, and is consistent with a formal job classification, and in which they receive income. We discuss below six key points that need to be highlighted regarding the narrow working definition of "occupation."

Firstly, an occupation describes a person based on their economic activity, i.e., the production of goods and services. When researchers ask people about their occupation, they are asking about the work that they are doing (*trabaho*). In Survey Question 2, the survey respondent is expected to mention a specific job title, such as laundry worker, farmer, occupational therapist, professor, or Chief Justice of the Supreme Court.

Secondly, people engage in their "specialized work role" (White, 2006, p. 420) to earn money (Johnson, 2000). Those who reported that they are in "paid work"—whether as an employee, self-employed, or working in a family business—in Survey Question 1 will be able to identify a specific job title in Question 2. Here, occupation refers to a source of livelihood. To the question, "What is your source of income or livelihood?", some people may be involuntarily excluded from this category because, in reality, there are people who are working but are not in paid employment. These people could include family members who are doing unpaid housework, as well as the unemployed, students, unpaid trainees, and retirees. From a sociological standpoint, they do not have an occupation.

Table 1.2 Sample survey question items asking about a respondent's "occupation"

English	Filipino translation
Question 1	
Which of the following best describes your current situation? (SHOW CARD)	*Alin po sa mga sumusunod ang pinaka-naglalarawan ng inyong kasalukuyang kalagayan?* (SHOW CARD)
If you temporarily are not working for pay because of temporary illness/parental leave/vacation/strike, etc., please refer to your normal work situation.	*Kung kayo ay pansamantalang hindi nagta-trabaho para sa bayad dahil kayo ay pansamantalang maysakit/naka-maternity o paternity leave/bakasyon/o naka-strike, at iba pa, mangyari po na tukuyin ninyo ang inyong normal na sitwasyon sa pagta-trabaho.*
1. In paid work, as an employee, self-employed, or working for your own family's business	*1. Nagtatrabaho bilang empleyado, self-employed, or working for your own family's business*
2. Unemployed and looking for a job	*2. Walang trabaho at naghahanap ng trabaho*
3. In education (not paid for by employer), in school/student/pupil, even if on vacation	*3. Nag-aaral*
4. Apprentice or trainee	*4. Apprentice or trainee*
5. Permanently sick or disabled	*5. Permanenteng may sakit o baldado*
6. Retired	*6. Retirado*
7. Doing housework, looking after the home, children, or other persons	*7. Gumagawa ng mga gawaing bahay, nag-aalaga ng bahay, nag-aalaga ng anak o ibang tao*
8. Other	*8. Iba pa*
Question 2	
What is/was your occupation, i.e., what is/was the name or title of your main job?	*Ano po ang inyong kasalukuyang trabaho/ dating trabaho – o ano po ang posisyon o designasyon ninyo sa inyong pangunahing trabaho/ sa inyong pangunahing trabaho dati?*
If you work for more than one employer, or if you are both employed and self-employed, please refer to your main job.	*Kung kayo ay nagta-trabaho sa higit sa isang employer o amo, o kung kayo ay parehong nagta-trabaho sa employer o amo at self-employed, pakitukoy ang inyong pangunahing trabaho.*
If you are retired or not currently working, please refer to your **last main job**.	*Kung kayo ay retirado o retired na, o hindi na kasalukuyang nagta-trabaho, pakitukoy ang inyong pinakahuling pangunahing trabaho.*
• Verbatim: _____	• *Verbatim*
• Don't know, inadequately described	• *Hindi alam, hindi nailarawan ng maigi*
• No answer	• *Walang sagot*

Source: International Social Survey Program 2019—Social Inequality V Questionnaire (Filipino) (ISSP Research Group, 2022).

Thirdly, there is also the implicit assumption that occupations are economic activities done outside the household. But during and even after the COVID-19 pandemic, work-from-home (Galanti et al., 2021), hybrid work (remote work combined with work in an office; Lund et al., 2020), and online work arrangements have become increasingly popular and prevalent in the contemporary working world. Hence, we argue that the performance of one's occupation (i.e., activities that produce economic gain) need not be done exclusively outside the household or remotely.

Fourth, occupational titles situate individuals within a systematic classification or division of labor wherein occupations are grouped and ranked according to some criteria. One official classification is the International Standard Classification of Occupations, which is approved by the International Labour Organization Governing Body. Under this classification, occupations are organized in a hierarchy based on skill level (i.e., range and complexity of the tasks involved) and skill specialization (i.e., knowledge applied, tools and equipment used, materials worked on or with, and the nature of the goods and services produced). The latest version published in 2008 identifies ten major groups of occupations:

1   Managers
2   Professional
3   Technicians and associate professionals
4   Clerical support workers
5   Service and sales workers
6   Skilled agricultural, forestry, and fishery workers
7   Craft-related trades workers
8   Plant and machine operators and assemblers
9   Elementary occupations
10   Armed forces occupations

In the International Standard Classification of Occupations, an occupational therapist is classified under the "Professional" group. Alternatively, the European Socio-economic Classification is an occupation-based measure of social class (Rose & Harrison, 2007). Depending on whether people are involved in short- or long-term labor contracts, and whether they are in service relationships or intermediate forms of employment regulation, individuals may be classified under a salariat (e.g., large employers, scientists, administrative managers), intermediate (e.g., administrative assistants, self-employed in agriculture, precision instrument makers), or working class (e.g., shop workers, plumbers, messengers) category.

Fifth, a person's occupation is socially consequential in terms of income, prestige, and identity. As already mentioned, people engage in short- or long-term occupations to earn money. Different occupations are economically rewarded differently. Table 1.3 shows a sample of specific job titles of

Table 1.3 Sample job titles and salary

Specific Job Title[a]	Salary Grade[a]	Basic Salary in 2024[b] (in Philippine pesos)
Laundry Worker I	1	13,000
Occupational Therapist I	11	27,000
Assistant Professor I	15	36,619
Chief Justice of the Supreme Court	32	331,954

Note: [a]Based on Index of Occupation Services, Occupational Groups, Classes, and Salary Grades, CY 2022 Edition, Volume II. [b]Based on Step-I Salary grade specified in RA 1146 "Salary Standardization Law of 2019" An Act Modifying the Salary Schedule for Civilian Government Personnel and Authorizing the Grants of Additional Benefits, and for other Purposes.

civilian government personnel in the Philippines with their associated salary grade and basic salary received in the year 2024.

Finally, the income associated with each occupation is not only based on the skills and preparation involved in performing the job. Judging by the salary grade described in Table 1.3, certain occupations receive higher prestige (e.g., esteem and honor) than other occupations. Carpentry and law are essential fields of practice, but lawyers are accorded more prestige than carpenters. Adopting formal and official occupational classifications previously discussed meant that some people in paid work may also be involuntarily excluded. Occupational classifications only include "legitimate" occupations and exclude morally stigmatized jobs such as sex work, professional gambling, or psychic reading (Ashforth & Kreiner, 2014). Occupations are important because they translate into monetary rewards and social (dis)incentives (e.g., prestige or stigma).

A broad definition of occupation is also possible, as seen in Survey Question 1. In general, the term occupation refers to how a person engages in broad forms of activity or inactivity, whether paid or unpaid. The employed and self-employed are engaged in economic activities and are paid. Students and retirees are not in the labor force and are unpaid. Although a student may receive a daily monetary allowance from parents and retirees may also receive a pension, these people groups are still considered to be economically inactive and are not receiving money in exchange for producing goods and services. Moreover, apprentices and trainees may or may not be paid. In contrast to the narrow definition, this broader definition of occupation includes economic and household activities. Care work (i.e., looking after children or sick household members) and housework (e.g., washing and ironing clothes, gardening, house cleaning) are activities to which different people devote time. Family members (e.g., mother, father, grandparents) who are doing care work and housework are generally unpaid, whereas a non-family member working as a domestic worker is and should be paid. The *Kasambahay* Law (RA 10361) defines *kasambahay* as "any person engaged in domestic work within an employment relationship." Under this law, a *kasambahay* receives the existing regional minimum wage and is entitled to a 13th month pay.

Within this broad definition of occupation, its temporal dimension is progressive or lifelong. In the Philippines, a person undergoes basic education between the ages 5 and 18. Those who decide to pursue higher education are expected to complete a university degree typically in four years. An educational qualification may be completed in under four years or may extend to six years or more. After gaining a qualification, a student becomes a "graduate" and now actively looks for remunerative economic activity. After doing one job after another, they may develop a career that spans decades and, eventually, retire. Nevertheless, this broad operational definition of occupation still describes a person in relation to work—before (e.g., student, never worked), during (e.g., employee, employer), and after (e.g., retirees, permanently disabled after an accident at work) employment in specific job positions. It describes a person's relative position in a hierarchical division of labor.

An even broader definition may be advanced to support charting research and practice in occupational science and occupational therapy. Occupations (in plural form) refer to "the everyday activities that people do as individuals, in families, and with communities to occupy time and bring meaning and purpose to life" (American Occupational Therapy Association, 2020, p. 7). This broader definition frees the term from the economic labor criterion captured in the narrow and broad definitions. The broader definition identifies ADL (e.g., bathing, feeding, and sexual activity), instrumental ADL (e.g., care for others, financial management, shopping, meal preparation), health management, rest, and sleep, education, play, leisure, and social participation alongside work as occupations of a person. The broader definition is fundamental for researchers and practitioners of occupational science and occupational therapy. But, in a country where such fields are only gaining popularity, clients and stakeholders have yet to become more familiar with occupations as "meaningful everyday activities." In everyday usage, the general public are still more accustomed to conceptualizing occupation as "paid work" (*trabaho, hanapbuhay*) or general situation in relation to work (*pinagkakaabalahan*).

Reimagining the concept of occupation in contemporary occupational therapy theory and practice in the Philippines

We have used a multidisciplinary approach to be more intentional in addressing questions from occupational therapy through occupational science scholarship (Sy et al., 2024). In our attempt to deconstruct the concept of occupation from different disciplinary perspectives, it remains challenging to make a conclusion of how occupation should be defined for use in occupational therapy theorization and practice in the Filipino context. However, we are certain about one thing, the concept of occupation will keep on evolving as we continue to shape the history of our profession.

As you read through the next chapters of this book, you will see the broad range of "occupation" that is viewed through a Filipino lens. This variety is influenced by practice setting, epistemological standpoint, and authors' experiences and expertise. It is not our intention to prescribe a specific definition or way of how occupation should be understood or communicated. Rather, we would like our readers to be critical and reflect on how we can convey the meaning of occupation to our clients, service users, and stakeholders for them to recognize the role of occupational therapists. Here are some questions that we can ask ourselves, or with colleagues:

- Should we continue to use the unassimilated terms to refer to the profession (occupational therapy), ourselves (occupational therapists), and our domain (occupation) in conversing in Filipino, or do we use another term in its place (*gawain*)?
- Do we need to reconsider using our own Filipino language in practice, rather than English, or should we optimize our capacity to be fluent in mixing both languages? Consider how this influences (or how it is influenced by) the socioeconomic class of service users our profession caters to.
- Do we need to reconsider perceiving occupation as only positive, health-promoting, and socially acceptable? What if you encounter a client who uses illicit drugs or engages in sex work; how can these non-sanctioned occupations be considered and integrated in your occupational therapy practice?

Instead of answers, perhaps you may have more questions after pondering these questions. However, it is our hope that, after reading this chapter, you will have a more nuanced and critical understanding of the profession, which will in turn help you develop your clinical and professional reasoning and decisions.

Conclusion

This chapter established the long-standing conundrum of defining the concept "occupation" in the Philippine context. Hence, the need to examine occupation from multiple perspectives—history, linguistics, sociology, and occupational science—was necessary to locate where the challenges lie. In this chapter, we highlight how indigenous Filipino occupations were highly based on social, cultural, political, and spiritual functions—all sharing the values of productivity and community contribution. From a linguistic standpoint, we acknowledge that Filipino is a complex language but does not have a direct translation of the word "occupation." We propose four categories to define occupation from a Filipino language perspective: being busy with something, means of livelihood, general purpose–oriented activities, and occupying a place. Lastly, from a sociological perspective, we have agreed that the term occupation is largely attributed to work and employment. This strong attribution reinforces the challenge of making the role of occupational therapy profession vague, misunderstood, and highly stereotyped. We end the chapter with some reflective questions in order to guide practitioners from all fields in being more intentional in our use of words and terms, to promote the value of meaningful occupations to the lives of the people we support and serve.

References

Almanzor, A. C. (1966). The profession of social work in the Philippines: Historical background. *International Social Work*, 9(4), 27–34. doi:10.1177/002087286600900407.

American Occupational Therapy Association. (2020). Occupational Therapy Practice Framework: Domain and process—fourth edition. *American Journal of Occupational Therapy*, 74(2), 7412410010p1–7412410010p87. doi:10.5014/ajot.2020.74S2001.

Anderson, E. A. (1976). The encomienda in early Philippine colonial history. *Asian History*, 14(2), 25–36.

Ashforth, B. E., & Kreiner, G. E. (2014). Dirty work and dirtier work: Differences in countering physical, social, and moral stigma. *Management and Organization Review*, 10(1), 81–108. doi:10.1111/more.12044.

Baklanova, E. (2017). Types of borrowings in Tagalog/Filipino (with special remarks on the Ortograpiyang Pambansa, 2013). *Kritika Kultura*, 28, 35–54.

Breines, E. B. (1995). Understanding "occupation" as the founders did. *British Journal of Occupational Therapy*, 58(11), 458–460. doi:10.1177/030802269505801102.

Demeterio, F. P. A. (2010). Ang demokratikong sistema at ang mga modelo ng pamumuno sa Pilipinas [The democratic system and models of governance in the Philippines]. *Kritike*, 4(1), 28–49.

Fischl, C. (2005). Pag-unlad ng wikang Filipino sa sakop ng occupational therapy [Development of the Filipino language in the domain of occupational therapy]. *Philippine Journal of Linguistics*, 36(1–2), 28–32.

Galanti, T., Guidetti, G., Mazzei, E., Zappalà, S., & Toscano, F. (2021). Work from home during the COVID-19 outbreak. *Journal of Occupational and Environmental Medicine*, 63(7), e426–e432. doi:10.1097/JOM.0000000000002236.

Grecia, A., Miciano, E. A., Reyes, R. S., & Tiu, A. L. (2011, November 21–24). *Towards defining the structural meaning of occupation from the Filipino perspective using lexical adjectives* [Conference presentation]. 5th Asia Pacific Occupational Therapy Congress, Chiang Mai, Thailand.

ISSP Research Group. (2022). International Social Survey Programme: Social Inequality V—ISSP 2019. GESIS, Cologne. ZA7600 Data file Version 3.0.0, doi:10.4232/1.14009.

Johnson, A. G. (2000). *The Blackwell dictionary of sociology: A user's guide to sociological language* (2nd ed.). Blackwell.

Komisyon sa Wikang Filipino [Commission on the Filipino Language]. (2013). Ortograpiyang Pambansa [National Orthography], *Kautusang Pangkagawaran Blg.* 34, s. 2013. https://www.deped.gov.ph/2013/08/14/do-34-s-2013-ortograpiya ng-pambansa/.

Lund, S., Madgavkar, A., Manyika, J., & Smit, S. (2020). *What's next for remote work: An analysis of 2,000 tasks, 800 jobs, and nine countries.* McKinsey Global Institute.

McFarland, C. D. (2008). Linguistic diversity and English in the Philippines. In M. L. Bautista & K. Bolton (Eds.), *Philippine English: Linguistic and literary perspectives* (pp. 131–156). Hong Kong University Press.

Pearson, M. N. (1969). The Spanish "impact" on the Philippines, 1565–1770. *Journal of the Economic and Social History of the Orient*, 12(2), 165–186. doi:10.2307/3596057.

Pineda, R. C. (2022, August 28–31). *Filipino conceptualization of occupations: A corpus-based and critical discourse analysis* [Conference presentation]. 18th World Federation of Occupational Therapy Congress, Paris, France.

Rose, D., & Harrison, E. (2007). The European Socio-economic Classification: A new social class schema for comparative European research. *European Societies*, 9(3), 459–490. doi:10.1080/14616690701336518.

Salazar, Z. (1996). The babaylan in Philippine history (P. Domingo-Tapales, trans.). In *Women's role in Philippine history: Selected essays* (2nd ed., pp. 209–222). University of the Philippines University Center for Women's Studies.

Scott, W. H. (1980). Filipino class structure in the sixteenth century. *Philippine Studies*, 28(2), 142–175. https://www.jstor.org/stable/42632521.

Sibayan, B. P. (1991). The intellectualization of Filipino. *International Journal of the Sociology of Language*, 1991(88), 69–82. doi:10.1515/ijsl.1991.88.69.

Sy, M., Ganholm Valmari, E., & Baldissera, A. (2024). Crossdisciplinary approaches as applied in occupational science. *Journal of Occupational Science*, 1–9. doi:10.1080/14427591.2024.2367574.

WFOT. (2018, May). *Definitions of occupational therapy from member organisations.* https://wfot.org/checkout/1213/32569.

WFOT. (2024, May). *World Occupational Therapy Day 2024—translated logos.* https://wfot.org/resources/world-occupational-therapy-day-2024-translated-logos.

White, K. (2006). Occupation. In B. S. Turner (Ed.), *The Cambridge dictionary of sociology.* Cambridge University Press.

Chapter 2

History of occupational therapy in the Philippines

Oliver Santos Trinidad, Teresita C. Mendoza and Michael Sy

Chapter objectives

1   Review events that constitute the history of occupational therapy in the Philippines since its inception until the present
2   Recognize the pivotal events, people, and places in the past that shaped present-day occupational therapy in the Philippines
3   Appreciate the stories from those who built the foundations of occupational therapy in the Philippines (re)told by Filipino occupational therapists

History and its meaning: Connecting the past and present of occupational therapy in the Philippines

In the Filipino language, the word "history" translates to *kasaysayan*, which is derived from the word *saysay*, connoting value and meaning. In this sense, the history of occupational therapy in the Philippines should be approached as a retelling of past events, people, and places valuable and meaningful to Filipino occupational therapists.

A profession's past informs its identity and maps the pathway towards progress. Reviewing historical archives, accounts, and artifacts within the health professions points to possible medical advancements that can improve patient care, education, and policy-making (Kushner, 2008). In occupational therapy, historical research uncovers often-neglected issues, opens dialogues, and identifies potential partnerships for the advancement of the profession (Sy et al., 2021).

In the book *The Philippines: A Past Revisited*, the nationalist historian Renato Constantino explains that history's value arises from its ability to reveal in the present the forces that impede real progress (Constantino & Constantino, 1975). The narratives constituting this chapter encourage readers to connect critical historical events, people, and places to what the profession is now. More importantly, readers are urged to reflect on how

DOI: 10.4324/9781003321217-2

the profession's past and present can pave the way to making occupational therapy more effective and relevant today for Filipinos.

From custody to care: The use of activities in mental health

Initially established in 1782 as a shelter for abandoned children, the elderly, and the poor, the *Hospicio de San Jose* began caring for non-violent individuals with mental illnesses in 1810 (see Figure 2.1; Paular, 1991). As a community shelter, it was not equipped to provide medical treatment. Paular (1991) reports that little to no therapy beyond rudimentary psychoanalysis, such as the method of catharsis, was provided. Instead, the shelter mainly focused on custodial support for self-care and daily living activities.

In the past, a person's institutionalization was due to concerns about potential self-harm or harm to others and worries about the individual causing public disturbances (Camagay, 1988). In some instances, confinement had political undertones. For example, a female member of the *Pulahanes*, an indigenous religious group engaged in active rebellion against the Spanish and later the Americans, was labeled "insane" and admitted to the *Hospicio*.

By 1910, the *Hospicio* also served orphaned or abandoned young people, who were being prepared for adulthood by teaching them vocational skills

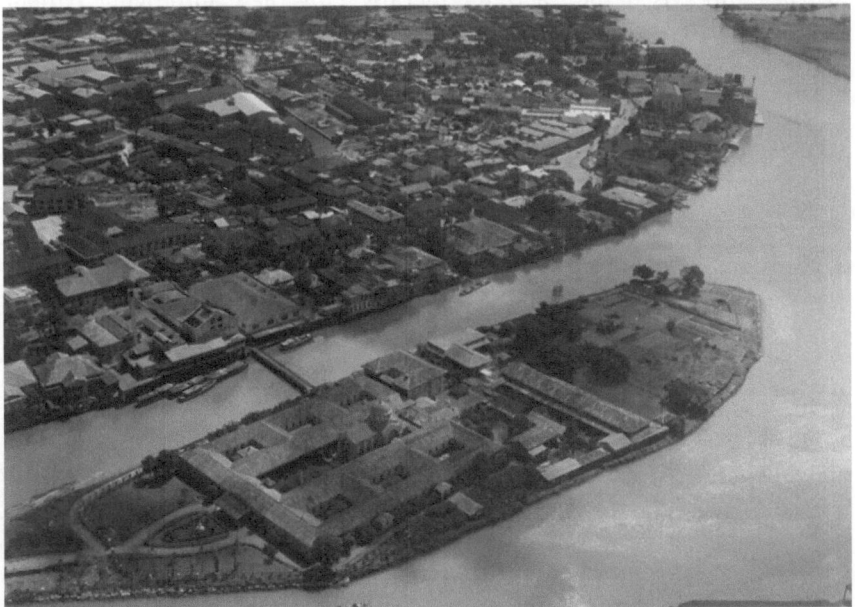

Figure 2.1 The Hospicio de San Jose in 1944. War Department U.S. Army Air Forces (1941–1947) Philippine Island—Manila [still photograph]
Source: National Archives at College Park, College Park, Maryland. https://catalog. archives.gov/id/68156579. Reproduced with permission of the U.S. Library of Congress and the Theodore Roosevelt Center.

like carpentry, tin-smithing, rope-making, farming, and gardening (Camagay, 1988). However, there was no mention that this training was also provided to those with mental illness. As late as 1922, people with mental illness were treated more as prisoners than patients. For instance, posting a guard armed with a club to "discipline" patients was a common practice.

With the arrival of the Americans in 1898 came a new perspective in providing treatments. Patients with mental illness were transferred to hospitals, including the *San Lazaro Hospital* in Manila. Founded in 1577, the San Lazaro Hospital is the oldest continually existing hospital in the Philippines (see Figure 2.2). It was taken over by the Americans after the sham Battle of Manila which led Spain to cede the Philippines to the United States. At that time, it was the primary institution for infectious diseases such as leprosy but was also charged with the care of patients with mental illness.

In 1923, six years after occupational therapy was founded in the United States, a department that promoted the principles of occupational therapy was already established in the San Lazaro Hospital's "Insane Department" (Philippines Bureau of Health, 1923, 1924). The United States Veterans' Bureau set up a small industrial shop for former soldiers and civilians who showed signs of improvement. A *teacher* supervised the "activity therapy" for these improving patients that included gardening, cleaning the premises, and repairing rattan parts of beds and chairs.

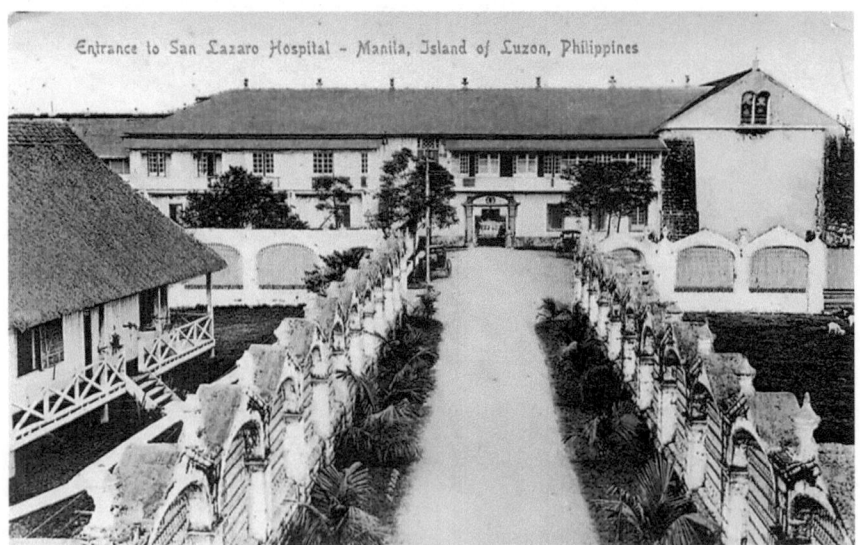

Figure 2.2 Postcard of the San Lazaro Hospital entrance circa 1909–1910

Even though providing these activities was encouraged, a report in 1923 by Dr. Jose Fernandez revealed that very little treatment was being done. Dr. Jose Fernandez, a Filipino beneficiary of the *Pensionado Act*, which allowed him to train at the Boston Psychopathic Hospital, recounted that hospitals treated patients primarily with medical remedies such as sedation and water therapy consisting of showers, douches, and cold baths that could last six hours. The following year, the activities promoted at San Lazaro Hospital were discontinued due to lack of funding, and 50 patients were transferred to the *Bilibid Prison Hospital* to continue this activity therapy.

As San Lazaro Hospital closed its short-lived activity therapy unit, the use and promotion of "occupations" to treat patients with mental illness continued in the *Insular Psychopathic Hospital*. Founded in 1925 in Mandaluyong City, the Insular Psychopathic Hospital was later renamed the National Mental Hospital in 1928 before taking its current name, the *National Center for Mental Health (NCMH)*, in 1986. The hospital advocated for "push therapy" based on the "total push" approach. Total push encompassed a blend of psychosocial and pharmacological treatments, employing a collaborative strategy involving doctors, nurses, and therapeutic technicians to counteract a "prison stupor," a pronounced withdrawal from social interactions (Myerson, 1939). The use of arts and crafts activities like loom weaving, painting, and pottery as treatment modalities was introduced during this time. These arts and crafts activities were seen to alleviate mental illness and facilitate the patients' eventual return to societal roles by teaching them work skills.

Crafting wellness: Occupational therapy in the fight against tuberculosis

In the American colonial period, tuberculosis, or the "greatest scourge of all diseases in the Philippines," posed a significant health threat in the Philippines (Moralina, 2009). Concerned Filipinos and Americans established the *Philippine Islands Anti-Tuberculosis Society* in 1910 to respond to this threat.

The Society inaugurated its health facility, the *Santol Sanatorium*, eight years later in 1918 (see Figures 2.3 and 2.4). The sanatorium opened an *Occupational Therapy Department* in 1926 to cater to charity patients. A resident physician was assigned the task of managing the department. This newly established section was dedicated to offering a variety of activities such as basketry, making lampshades, embroidery, cross-stitching, and crochet, all of which, as the society's history claims, have widely recognized therapeutic benefits. The crafts produced by these charity patients were then sold to defray the costs of their confinement.

According to the Philippine Islands Anti-Tuberculosis Society (1926), incorporating the Occupational Therapy Department signified the sanatorium's commitment to adopting new treatment approaches to boost patients' mental and physical health. Additionally, the activities were seen as a way of

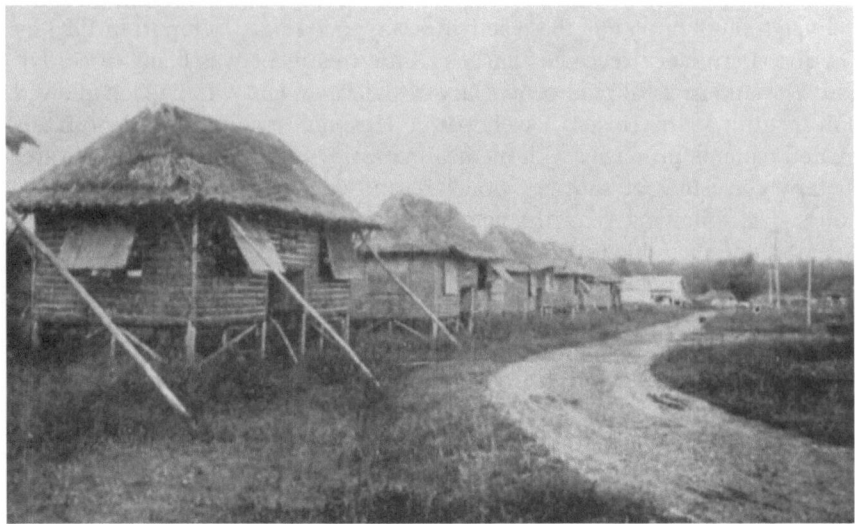

Figure 2.3 The old nipa houses that became the Santol Sanatorium

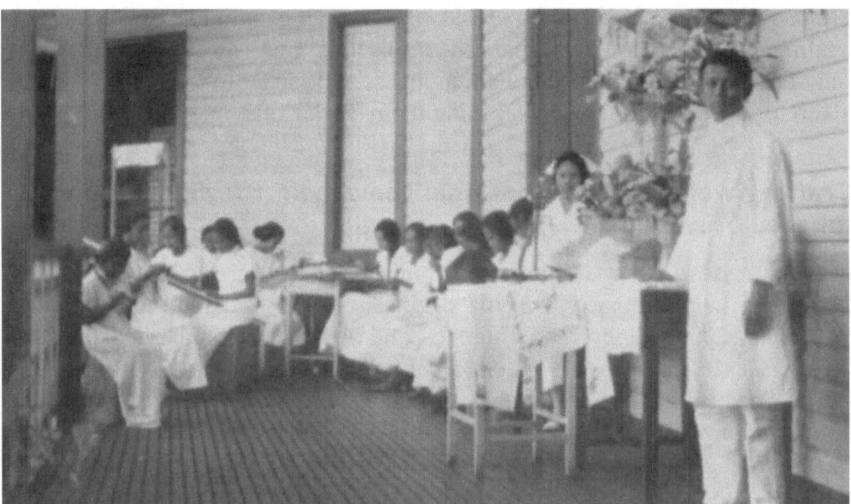

Figure 2.4 Female patients at the Santolan Sanatorium Occupational Therapy Department

imparting vocational instruction and recreation. During this period, occupational therapy continued to be mentioned and discussed as a treatment for other diseases such as leprosy, alcoholism, psychosis, manic depression, and other mental illnesses in several issues of the *Philippine Journal of Science*. However, it can be said that occupational therapy did not exist as a profession at that time and was largely misunderstood and unappreciated.

The roots of professional occupational therapy after the war

In the closing months of World War II, the continual shelling and bombing leveled Manila, destroying almost all of its civil and health infrastructures. The war decimated the population and maimed hundreds of thousands of civilians across the islands. The lack of a skilled workforce and the almost non-existent civil and health infrastructure threatened to plunge the country into chaos. Hoping to avert the crisis, General Douglas McArthur directed the formation of 30 Philippine Civil Affairs Units (PCAUs) tasked with rebuilding the war-torn nation as early as 1944.

In 1945, when the total liberation of the Philippines was announced, the PCAUs sprang into action. Filipino citizens and foreign advisors educated in medicine, nursing, law enforcement, agriculture, labor relations, and administration took the lead in organizing, staffing, and administering the PCAUs (Smollar, 2015).

Box 2.1 *Inutil: The Linguistic Legacy of Philippine Colonization* **by Oliver S. Trinidad**

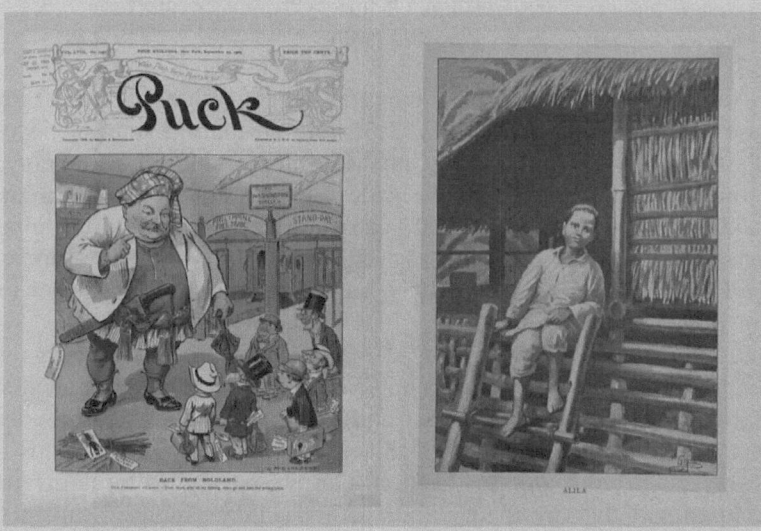

Figure 2.5 On the left, US President "Taft Back from Bololand." A bolo is a native Filipino weapon used in the Filipino-American War. On the right is an illustration from the book *Our Little Philippine Cousin* with the caption "alila," which translates to "servant"
Source: Library of Congress.

The study of language provides lessons relevant to occupational therapy practice in the Philippines. Traces of the historical experience of colonization can be found in the words related to disability. Disability is translated in Filipino as *walang silbi* and *inutil*. *Silbi* comes from the Spanish root word *servir*, which means "to serve," and the word *wala* denotes "the lack of." Thus, being *walang silbi* denotes a person who is unable to serve. *Inutil*, a direct borrowing from Spanish, literally means "useless." In contemporary Filipino usage, these words refer to the disabled, weak, and aged.

Historian Marco Lagman, while researching *vecindarios* (civil registers) during the 1800s, found that the Spanish civil government listed disabled people as any of the following: *inutil fisicamente* (physically useless), *inutil y pobre* (useless and poor), and *sexagenario y inutil* (in their 60s and useless). A more neutral Spanish word, *discapacitado* (incapacitated), could have been used instead of *inutil* and *walang silbi* to refer to those with disabilities. It is telling that both terms ascribe a person's worth to their usefulness to the colonizer.

In contrast, the native Filipino word *may-kapansanan*, also used to refer to a person with a disability, carries a more neutral connotation. *Kapansanan* is a weakness, impediment, or an injury. *Kapansanan*, together with the prefix *may-*, translates to *a person who* has a weakness, impediment or injury. Unlike an *inutil*, *may-kapansanan* can be helped to adapt to or regain the lost ability; he or she is not useless, and his or her worth as a human being remains intact.

PCAU No. 1 deserves a special mention in occupational therapy history because it operated the *PCAU No. 1 General Hospital*. Established within the Psychopathic Hospital (now NCMH) compound in Mandaluyong City, the hospital rehabilitated the war's Filipino and American military and civilian casualties. In 1946, it was renamed the National Orthopedic Hospital (NOH), changing names several more times until it became the *Philippine Orthopedic Center* in 1989, as it transferred to its current location in Banaue, Quezon City.

Among the Filipinos who played leading roles in rehabilitating war casualties was a team of nurses, namely: Conchita Abad, Fe Isaac-Saño, and Gliceria Andaya. Abad, Isaac- Saño, and Andaya took up the enormous task of helping countless civilians and soldiers whose minds and bodies were marred by military action. Despite having no formal training in occupational therapy theory and methods, they practiced prosthetics, orthotics (splinting), and arts and crafts under the supervision of two American occupational therapists, Elizabeth Nachod and Mary Berteling (Nachod, 1947). The three also founded and staffed the occupational therapy department at the NOH in 1946.

While occupational therapy departments existed in San Lazaro Hospital and the Santol Sanatorium in the 1920s, in those earlier days, occupational therapy was equated with arts, crafts, and vocational skills training.

The department founded by Abad, Isaac-Sano, and Andaya signaled a shift to a more contemporary and professionalized occupational therapy practice that incorporated arts and crafts with the developing scientific understanding of medicine, human anatomy, and kinesiology.

Up to this point, occupational therapy has yet to emerge as a recognized profession in the Philippines. This changed with the efforts of Abad and Isaac-Saño of the NOH and was reinforced. This shift was reinforced by the return of Charlotte Aspuria, a Maui-born Filipino who returned to the Philippines in 1954 after getting a degree in occupational therapy in the United States. The efforts of these women pioneers led to the founding of the first school of occupational therapy in the Philippines as well as the first professional association of the profession. Both institutions marked the birth of the occupational therapy profession in the country.

Floro, Abad, and the genesis of the School of Allied Medical Professions (SAMP)

In 1956, the Philippine Government, through Dr. Benjamin Tamesis of the NOH, invited Dr. Henry Kessler, a United Nations Technical Assistance appointee, to survey rehabilitation services in the country. Kessler (1957) recommended creating a school dedicated to training occupational therapists and physical therapists.

Seizing on the recommendation, Dr. Tamesis proposed the formation of the school to then Health Secretary Elpidio Valencia. The University of the Philippines (UP) was designated to develop the program. Nevertheless, several obstacles remained. The greatest among them was the availability of trained occupational therapists to develop the curriculum and provide instruction and training to prospective students. Two parallel journeys by two exceptional women, one in the United States and the other in the Philippines, solved this challenge.

Several years back, Charlotte Aspuria, who was studying for a bachelor's in education at the University of Hawaii, became aware of a scholarship to study occupational therapy at the Wisconsin Milwaukee Downer College (see Figure 2.7). Seeing the potential of the new profession, she applied and was accepted for the scholarship, consequently obtaining a degree in occupational therapy in 1949. She passed the certification examination and became the first formally educated Filipino occupational therapist.

In the Philippines, Abad, still working at the NOH, became one of the first recipients of a Fullbright scholarship in 1948. Abad studied occupational therapy at the *Philadelphia School of Occupational Therapy* at the University of Pennsylvania. She completed her degree in 1950, returned to the Philippines, and reorganized the occupational therapy section at the NOH (Soriano, 2018; Alto, 2018).

D-4 Honolulu Star-Bulletin Thursday, Nov. 10, 1966

Maui girl boosts therapy in P.I.

By LIGAYA FRUTO

The occupational therapy training program is well underway at the University of the Philippines, thanks to a Maui-born Filipina.

M r s. Charlotte Aspuria Floro, chairman of the university's Department of Occupational Therapy in the S c h o o l of Allied Medical Professions, College of Medicine, is in Honolulu on the next to the last lap of her 4½ month fellowship in Europe and America.

T h e fellowship is sponsored by the United Nations And World Health Organization. Her last stop is Japan.

Occupational therapists no longer work in the confines of a four-by-four-foot clinic, Mrs. Floro said.

O.T.'s (as she put it) now bring their programs for rehabilitation t o the people and work closely with the community.

"For instance, on mental health, we don't have to work with patients in a mental hospital," she said.

"We work in community clinics or, in the case of children, particularly, we go to the homes in the company of trained nurses."

Occupational therapists play great roles in the work adjustment aspects of rehabilitation, she added, developing systematic ways of improving the work potentials of the handicapped.

Mrs. Floro, who went to school on Maui and the University of Hawaii and received her bachelor of science degree from the Milwaukee-Downer College in Wisconsin, started the Philippine occupational therapy program shortly after she obtained her master's degree at the University of the Philippines.

She has been living in the country of her parents since she married Francisco Floro, a Filipino businessman, over 10 years ago in San Francisco.

She was there as a first

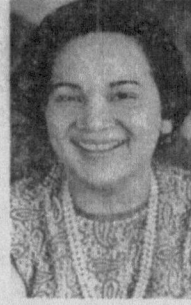

Mrs. Charlotte Floro

lieutenant in the Women's Medical Specialist Corps at Letterman. Before going to the Mainland, she worked at the Hawaii State Hospital.

"When we started the U.P. occupational therapy training school," she said, "we had only two students. That was four years ago. Now we have more than 50 students, and our program is very internationally involved.

"We get either technical assistance or material aid from such agencies as the United Nations International Children's Emergency Fund, Colombo Plan and the World Health Organization.

"We h a v e two Peace C o r p s therapists and an American W.H.O. consultant to help us. The Peace Corpsmen were specially recruited for our program and serve as instructors in clinical training."

Since the Philippines is a developing nation and occupational therapy is an emerging profession there, the U.P. is not only concerned with providing training for prospective O.T.'s but must also help develop community programs t h a t can absorb the new graduates.

As president of the O.T.

Association, she has helped p r o v i d e the initiative in m a k i n g the community aware of its responsibility in organizing and administering rehabilitation centers.

"We're proposing a comprehensive, w o r k-oriented rehabilitation complex that will offer services and lead in developing work potentials among the handicapped," she said. "We feel we're losing a huge amount of human resources and talent among the handicapped, and this is wasteful."

Mrs. Floro and Mrs. Violet Kam, director of Lanakila Crafts, are working out what they call a "helping hands a c r o s s the Pacific program."

Under this arrangement, rehabilitation centers in the Philippines can furnish handicrafts that can be finished in Hawaii.

Mrs. Kam and Mrs. Floro, who went to the same school and have visited each other's workshops, believe that the abundance of products and talent in the Philippines can provide Hawaii's handicapped with enough incentive and activity to help in their rehabilitation.

"T h i s close cooperation among people with similar backgrounds a n d similar problems can be of mutual benefit in more ways than one," Mrs. Floro said.

Figure 2.6 A newspaper feature of the interview with Charlotte Aspuria-Floro in 1966
Source: Uploaded by shortechinacea at Newspapers.com, dated 28 May 2018.

In 1954, Charlotte Aspuria also returned to the Philippines. Now married, she took her husband's name and became Charlotte Floro. Abad and Floro used to correspond via mail when they were in the United States but never met each other in person. However, to their mutual surprise, both

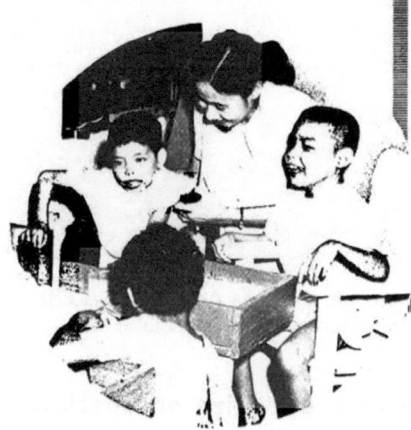

Wellesley College, conducts a private gym class for children at the Rizal Memorial Stadium at Manila. Here the children demonstrate confidently on the balancing beams.

Filipino Educators Put U.S. Training To Work

The pictures on these pages tell the story of how Filipino scholars who studied in the United States under educational exchange grants from this Government are using the skills they acquired to help the children of their country. Whatever their special field of instruction may be, these teachers are all demonstrating through their work the message of democratic education—the importance of each individual student and his role in co-operative community action.

Cerebral-palsy victims pretend to blow out the candles on an imaginary birthday cake. Conchita Magdaluyo-Abad, chief nurse of the Occupational Therapy Department of the Philippine National Orthopedic Hospital, studied at the Philadelphia School of Occupational Therapy.

Figure 2.7 A newspaper feature of Conchita Abad providing occupational therapy services for children with cerebral palsy in 1952

discovered they lived in the same village in Quezon City, which was then the Philippines' capital city. Hearing of the plans to start an occupational therapy school in the Philippines, the two approached Dr. Tamesis and volunteered to lay the groundwork for the development of the school.

From 1959 to 1961, Floro and Abad worked together to draft the occupational therapy curriculum based on their coursework experiences in the United States and the integration of liberal arts courses mandated by UP. In 1962, the developed curriculum was approved by the UP College of Medicine Curriculum Committee and UP Board of Regents. Dr. Tamesis obtained PhP 50,000 worth of funding for the school from the *Philippine Charity Sweepstakes* and the President of the Philippines' Contingent Fund. He also arranged to house the fledgling school at a newly constructed wing of the NOH. At the start of the academic year, the occupational therapy program at SAMP, under the leadership of Dr. Guillermo Damian, admitted its first cohort. The program claims to be the first school in the Asian region to offer a baccalaureate degree in occupational therapy (Sy et al., 2021; Alto, 2018).

Among the first cohort of occupational therapy students were Evanina Estrada and Corazon Tablan, both sponsored by the *Elk's Cerebral Palsy Project* (see Figure 2.8). Both were then obliged to work at Elk's after graduation. Attesting to its international caliber, the *World Federation of Occupational Therapists* recognized SAMP's occupational therapy program in 1963 and approved it in 1968.

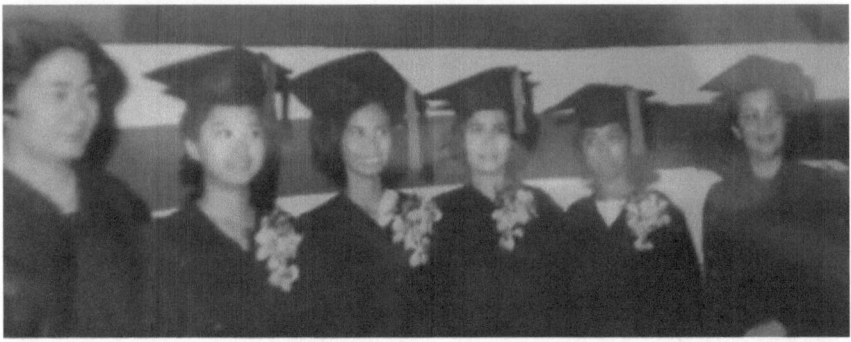

Figure 2.8 The first SAMP OT graduates from the left, Conchita Abad with Eva Estrada next to her, and from the right, Charlotte Floro and Corazon Tablan next to her

The start of the legislative journey to recognize occupational therapy

The Occupational Therapy Association of the Philippines (OTAP) was established in 1963. OTAP's mission was to promote and advance ethical and professional occupational therapy practice, education, research, dissemination of knowledge in rehabilitation, and collaboration with other professionals (OTAP, 1965). The founding officers and members of OTAP were Charlotte Floro (President), Conchita Abad (Vice President), Corazon Tablan (Secretary), Fe Isaac-Saño (Treasurer), and Evanina Estrada (Public Relations Officer). OTAP's first headquarters was in a small building along Maria Clara Street, Quezon City.

OTAP was indispensable in lobbying legislation to recognize occupational therapy as a profession in the Philippines. Republic Act (RA) 5680, also known as "An Act Creating the Board of Examiners for Physical Therapists and Occupational Therapists" or *The Philippine Physical Therapy and Occupational Therapy Law* passed in 1969, can be considered one of OTAP's landmark victories. Isaac-Saño chaired this legislative process and closely coordinated with Representative Jose Aldeguer to mandate the creation of the first *Board of Examiners* for the occupational therapy and physical therapy professions. With the passing of this law, the Professional Regulatory Commission named the examiners in June 1973, with Dr. Jose Mendoza as the board chairperson and Henry Pit-og, Fe Isaac-Saño, Josefina Rabino, and Conchita Abad as board members. The first board examination happened a month later, yielding the first cohort of licensed occupational therapists: Corazon Tablan, Agnes Uyengco, Aida Quodala, Curie Rubio, Cynthia Isaac, Marylynn Querouz, Monica Clemente, Lilia Marcelo, Nerissa Pesigan, Corazon Miranda, and Delia Ramos. The PRC website remains the online portal to find all registered occupational therapists in the Philippines.

The 1960s and 1970s: A period of exchange and expansion

The founding of SAMP and OTAP cemented the professionalization of Filipino occupational therapists. This pivotal event leveraged both institutions to facilitate exchanges between Filipino occupational therapists who were sent overseas for training and foreign consultants who conducted capacity building opportunities in the Philippines.

One of the first recorded encounters was in 1965 when Fredericka Foulks from the *World Health Organization* arrived to reify recommendations to improve SAMP's occupational therapy curriculum. From 1968 to 1969, Wanda Mayberry and Charlotte Erikson from the *United States Peace Corps* and Berendean Ruth Anstice from the *United Kingdom Colombo Plan* went to the Philippines to teach and train in SAMP.

Anstice also assisted Filipino occupational therapists in obtaining scholarships through the Colombo Plan. The first scholars, Susan Baladad-Villegas and Corazon Tablan-Santos, were sent for a short-term scholarship at *Dorset House of Occupational Therapy* (now *Oxford Brookes University*) in Oxford, England. Founded in 1930, the Dorset House is known as the first school for occupational therapy in the United Kingdom. The fellowship grant to Villegas at the Dorset House was focused on the observation of teaching and training occupational therapy students in classrooms, hospitals, and rehabilitation centers. At the same time, Santos honed her skills and knowledge in providing occupational therapy for children with cerebral palsy.

In 1972, Zielfa Bayoneta-Maslin finished her *Teaching Diploma in Occupational Therapy* with the UK College of Occupational Therapists and the Polytechnic of North London. When she returned to the Philippines in 1974, she researched the status of occupational therapy in the country. Marylynn Querouz assisted her in the first part of the study. The study revealed that the number of agencies and hospitals offering occupational therapy services has ballooned from six to 23. Furthermore, in 1974, SAMP conferred diplomas to 68 occupational therapists, the total graduates since the BSOT program has been offered in UP.

Opportunities to practice in various settings became available to occupational therapists who stayed in the country. At that time, these practice areas included aged-care homes, private clinics for children with special needs, hospitals, mental health institutions, drug rehabilitation centers, and leprosariums. Additionally, more occupational therapists diversified their roles beyond medical and clinical settings to serve as consultants in special education schools, business and industry, higher education, and policy development (Trinidad & Sison, 1995).

Community immersion and empowerment in the turbulent 1970s

The Philippines in the 1970s was engulfed in social, political, and economic upheavals, with the situation worsening as President Ferdinand Marcos declared martial law in 1972. Amid this tumult, Filipino occupational therapists and rehabilitation professionals focused on the urban and rural poor communities impacted by the political chaos.

The UP Manila established the *Comprehensive Community Health Program* (CCHP) in Bay, Laguna, as part of the UP College of Medicine in 1964. It became a full-fledged university program in 1970. CCHP was designed to respond to the primary healthcare needs of the community. The colleges in UP Manila, namely allied medical professions, medicine, nursing, pharmacy, and public health, send their students for community fieldwork.

In 1973, the Department of Physical Therapy of SAMP joined the CCHP. Maria Lucia Magallona started the training for physical therapy interns. After three years, the Department of Occupational Therapy joined CCHP through the leadership of Teresita Camiling. At that time, these students rotated in the community for eight weeks and interacted with other health science students. This laid the groundwork for the community-based rehabilitation (CBR) program that exists today.

Despite the phase-out of the CCHP in 1988, the different units of UP Manila developed partnerships with various communities to sustain their students' field practice. The CAMP moved to Montalban, Rizal, to set up its CBR. The CAMP CBR sharpened occupational therapy students' competencies in community health and their ability to meet the needs of individuals with disabilities despite limited resources (read more about community-centered occupational therapy in Chapter 8).

Championing inclusivity: The legislative and grassroots push for Filipino disability rights

The success of the capacity-building efforts among the local champions of the profession, through collective or individual efforts, was demonstrated through their involvement in policy and legislative work. The advocacy focused on integrating and including Filipinos with disabilities in their communities.

One of the local champions is Fe Isaac-Saño. She returned to the Philippines in 1964 to upscale her current work on orthotic and prosthetic services at the NOH. Most importantly, she applied her overseas education by advocating for the increased participation of Filipinos with disabilities in sports, performing arts, and business. Specifically, Isaac-Saño dedicated her career to establishing groups that foregrounded the inclusion of Filipinos with disabilities into the community. She was highly involved in forming and training the Philippine Paralympic Team for the Tokyo Paralympics in 1964, founded the "Philippine Dancing Wheelchairs" in 1966, and, with Sister Valeriana Baerts, co-established the Philippine Council of Cheshire Homes for the Disabled, now the Philippine Council of Organizations on Disability and Empowerment Inc. (Bondoc, 2005). Sister Valeriana was a Belgian missionary and founded the *Tahanang Walang Hagdanan, Inc.* [House with No Steps] in 1973. This non-profit organization spearheaded the training and employment of people with paraplegia by making crafts, packaging, and manufacturing wheelchairs (Trinidad & Sison, 1995). Charlotte Floro, alongside other Filipino advocates, also led a technical group that drafted Presidential Decree (PD) 1509 in June 1978 to create the *National Commission Concerning Disabled Persons* (NCCDP). The NCCDP protected the rights of Filipinos with disabilities by adopting an integrated long-term National Rehabilitation Plan and institutionalizing the National Council on Disability Affairs. Chapter 13 provides a more comprehensive discussion on legislations related to Filipino persons with disabilities (PWDs).

Opportunities and challenges: The rise of occupational therapy schools in the 1980s and 1990s

The loss of trained occupational therapists to emigration has been a problem in the Philippines since the inception of the profession. Bayoneta-Maslin and Molina-Gonzales (1974) reported that 60% of the first-generation Filipino occupational therapy graduates have already left the country to work abroad, leading to shortages of occupational therapists in the country.

In 1984, Marylynn Querouz, then-president of the OTAP, realized that the country needed another occupational therapy school. Although the plan later proved prescient and heralded the boom in OT schools in the 1990s, according to Querouz in an interview in 1995 with the first author, the proposal met with some opposition from some who feared that the move would dilute the quality of graduates and produce an oversupply of occupational therapists. Querouz countered that OTs would create their demand and allow the fielding of occupational therapists in the provinces. After numerous consultations and negotiations, Querouz co-established an occupational therapy program in Perpetual Help College Laguna (now University of Perpetual Help System, Laguna Campus) in 1985.

By 1986, despite the initial euphoria of the EDSA revolution that toppled Ferdinand Marcos Sr. from power, the economic situation continued to worsen, and the future looked bleak for most Filipinos. Hence, starting a new life overseas became more attractive. At this time, the *Individuals with Disabilities in Education Act* and the *Americans with Disabilities Act* legislations were passed, which spurred a boom in hiring foreign occupational therapists.

Taking advantage of this opportunity, more occupational therapy schools opened their doors. During the 1990s, there was at least one school in the three primary island groups in the country, with the number of schools peaking by some estimates at as many as 33. Coinciding with this increase in the number of schools, legislative changes that would negatively impact migration were brewing in the United States. By the mid-to-late 1990s, the United States healthcare system faced budgetary shortfalls due to the exploding costs of reimbursements and fraudulent activities by health facilities. The *Balanced Budget Act* was passed in 1997, limiting reimbursable OT services. Because of the drop in reimbursement, numerous rehabilitation professionals, including occupational therapists, were laid off. Moreover, immigration requirements in the United States have become more stringent for healthcare professionals. Additionally, a master's degree in occupational therapy became the minimum qualification to work as an occupational therapist in the United States in 1999.

These restrictions almost completely blocked Filipino occupational therapists from working in the United States. The recruitment process came to a standstill, and unemployment and underemployment of occupational therapists in the Philippines ensued. However, in the next few years, more Filipino occupational therapists sought work in other developed countries such as the United Kingdom, Australia, and Canada (Pineda et al., 2023).

21st century: Renewed optimism, participation, and growth

In the early 2000s, many Filipino occupational therapists in the Philippines responded to the drop in demand for occupational therapists abroad by exploring possibilities to develop, sustain, and strengthen the profession's identity and relevance. Their efforts included entrepreneurial ventures to provide jobs for occupational therapists and political actions that redefined occupational therapy's identity, popularity, and reach in the economic, legislative, and academic arenas.

In the field of legislation, the Occupational Therapy Association of the Philippines continued its lobby for the profession's autonomy by having its law separate from the physical therapy profession. Then OTAP President Delia Pabalan, along with her counterparts from the *Philippine Physical Therapy Association* and the *Philippine Association of Speech Pathologists*, advocated for repealing RA 5680 and worked tirelessly towards passing separate legislation governing the OT profession. This move received pushback from the *Philippine Association of Rehabilitation Medicine*, the official organization of physiatrists who succeeded in opposing the ratification of the Occupational Therapy Law in the mid-2000s.

In 2008, a group of occupational therapy students from UP and five other schools led by Michael Sy organized the first *Occupational Therapy*

Student Officers' Assembly, an inter-collegiate meeting attended by 100 occupational therapy students (Sy et al., 2021). This group is now called the *Occupational Therapy Students Assembly*, and has served as the student arm of OTAP since 2012.

OTAP, now reorganized as the Philippine Academy of Occupational Therapists (PAOT), persisted in pursuing the profession's independent status through its success in passing the RA 11241. Known as *The Philippine Occupational Therapy Law of 2018*, RA 11241 recognized occupational therapy as an independent healthcare profession, positioning occupational therapists as primary healthcare providers distinct yet allied with other healthcare professions.

The law strengthened the capacity of occupational therapy schools to develop their own post-graduate programs, providing growth opportunities to local occupational therapists (read Chapters 4, 5, and 6 to learn more about education and continuing development for Filipino occupational therapists).

Floro eschewed imprisoning occupational therapy within the confines of a "four-by-four-foot clinic." Occupational therapists in the 21st century found relevance beyond clinical work. The PAOT led this effort by establishing a Disaster Risk Reduction and Response team that provided therapy, relief operations, and psychosocial first aid to survivors of natural disasters in the country (Bulan & Eturma, 2018; read Chapter 10 for more discussion on the involvement of Filipino occupational therapists in disaster risk reduction and response).

As the second decade of the 21st century drew to a close, occupational therapists succeeded in establishing occupational therapy as an independent profession. With the help of social media, it became increasingly recognized by the Filipino public. However, just a few months into 2020, it became clear that with the emergence of COVID-19, the country faced a catastrophic once-in-a-century event.

Attesting to the resilience of the Filipino OT, the profession quickly pivoted to online means to continue making a difference in the lives of individuals and families. Schools initiated online classes and training opportunities. Individual professionals migrated to telehealth as the primary means of providing continuity of service. Even CBR efforts persisted through a virtual CBR program initiated by the Angeles University Foundation in Pampanga (Musni et al., 2021) and the KABAHAGI Program, a social enterprise spearheaded by occupational therapist Karen Sagun (Quezon City Government, 2024).

Now that we are at the tail-end of a pandemic, it is hard to judge its long-term effects on the profession and the individuals who depend on it. However, it is not difficult to imagine that Filipino OTs will continue to innovate, adapt, and seek relevance to serve the nation and continue to write the history of the profession.

Conclusion

In this chapter, we traced our profession's history to the Spanish colonial era, when occupations were used as custodial care in a hospice for orphans, the elderly, and people with needs. From self-care support and arts and crafts, the profession was medicalized during and after the World Wars to facilitate its recognition towards professionalization. This political maneuver provided scholarships, budget, and governmental support to the tentmakers of the occupational therapy profession.

In the 1970s, the emergence of the community-based approach in occupational therapy was considered a form of resistance to the biomedicalization of the profession. This pivot allowed Filipino occupational therapists to reimagine their professional identity as health professionals and community workers who are always part of a more extensive health and social care team.

Veering away from our historical roots of promoting meaningful occupations as diversional and recreational, our profession developed and became even more recognized publicly. Given that occupational therapy has been in the consciousness of Philippine society in the past century, we hope that Filipino occupational therapists do not merely recall our past milestones and challenges, but instead use these historical moments to critique the knowledge and practices that we have today in order to further the profession for the next generation.

Questions and reflective actions

1   Gather your peers and schedule a meeting with your program's lead or a senior faculty member. In that meeting, discuss the history of the OT program in your school, their local "OT Inspiration," and their thoughts about the past, present, and future of the OT profession in the Philippines.
2   Discuss the historical theme of migration, the reasons for the departure, the impact of "brain drain" on local occupational therapy practice, and solutions that could be employed to balance personal choice and equitable services to Filipinos needing occupational therapy.
3   How can you build on the critical historiographical works as an educator or academic? Create a literature review with a research group to identify gaps, links, and unwritten events that add to, supplement, or contradict the published historiography.

References

Alto, A. M. D. (2018). Cultivating transformative leaders in public health. *Health Ripples: UP Manila Health and Life Magazine*, 4(2), 2–5.

Bayoneta-Maslin, Z., & Molina-Gonzales, A. (1974). The S-A-M-P Story, 12th Foundation Day, 1st Alumni Homecoming, School of Allied Medical Professions, College of Medicine, University of the Philippines System, November 8.

Bondoc, S. (2005). Occupational therapy in the Philippines: From founding years to the present. *Philippine Journal of Occupational Therapy*, 1(1), 9–22.

Bulan, P. M. P., & Eturma, C. M. (2018). Practising occupational therapists' attitudes towards disaster management. *World Federation of Occupational Therapists Bulletin*, 74(2), 99–105. doi:10.1080/14473828.2018.1533154.

Camagay, M. L. T. (1988). The Hospicio de San Jose: Institutional care for mental patients. *Philippine Studies*, 36(3), 365–371. https://www.jstor.org/stable/42633101.

Constantino, R., & Constantino, L.R. (1975). *The Philippines: A past revisited*, Vol. 1. Tala Publishing Services.

Kessler, H. (1957). (rep.). The rehabilitation of the handicapped in the Philippines (pp. 4–45). *United Nations Technical Assistance Administration*.

Kushner H. I. (2008). Medical historians and the history of medicine. *Lancet*, 372 (9640), 710–711. doi:10.1016/s0140-6736(08)61293–61293.

Moralina, A.R.O. (2009). State, society, and sickness: Tuberculosis control in the American Philippines, 1910–1918. *Philippine Studies*, 57(2), 179–218. http://www.jstor.org/stable/42634008.

Musni, M. P. A., Cayanan, K. K. S., Espino, E. A. A., Martinez, P. G. V., & Galang, M. M. R. F. (2021, September). Serving the Capampangan community amid a pandemic crisis through community-based rehabilitation. *OTAPahina*, 6(1).

Myerson, A. (1939). Theory and principles of the "total push" method in treating chronic schizophrenia. *American Journal of Psychiatry*, 95(5), 1197–1204. doi:10.1176/ajp.95.5.1197.

Nachod, E. (1947). Occupational therapy with Filipino amputees. *American Journal of Occupational Therapy*, 1(2), 92–95.

OTAP. (1965). *By-laws of the Occupational Therapy Association of the Philippines (OTAP)*. College of Allied Medical Professions.

Paular, R. P. (1991). Mental illness in the Spanish colonial period: 1865–1898. *Philippine Studies*, 39(4), 525–533. https://www.jstor.org/stable/42633282.

Philippine Islands Anti-Tuberculosis Society. (1926). A brief history of the Santol Tuberculosis Sanatorium since its establishment in 1918 up to 1926. Retrieved October 8, 2023, from https://nla.gov.au:443/tarkine/nla.obj-15949671.

Philippines Bureau of Health. (1923). *Report*. Manila Bureau of Printing.

Philippines Bureau of Health. (1924). *Report*. Manila Bureau of Printing.

Pineda, R. C., Abad-Pinlac, B., Yao, D. P. G., Toribio, F. N. R. B., Josephsson, S., & Sy, M. P. (2023). Unraveling the "greener pastures" concept: The phenomenology of internationally educated occupational therapists. *Occupational Therapy Journal of Research*. Advance online publication. doi:10.1177/15394492231205885.

Quezon City Government. (2024, June 26). Quezon City Kabahagi Center for children with disabilities. Retrieved November 6, 2022, from https://quezoncity.gov.ph/departments/qc-center-for-children-with-disabilities-kabahagi/?fbclid=IwZXh0bgN hZW0CMTAAAR08ttDJEYNclhF6mVzw2-GwcqQ8DJnwt75scPd6bwpQRBfh 8hvbSpUWdMA_aem_xxcZmXltwS13o8K2cBOgXA.

Smollar, D. (2015). "Hard, bitter, unpleasantly necessary duty": A little-known World War II Story of the Philippines. Retrieved November 6, 2022, from https://docslib.

org/doc/269244/hard-bitter-unpleasantly-necessary-duty-a-little-known-world-war-ii-story-of-the-philippines.

Soriano, J. P. (2018, March 24). 1948 Pinay scholar honored at Fulbright 70th Anniversary. *GMA News Online*. Retrieved November 20, 2022, from https://www.gmanetwork.com/news/lifestyle/content/647778/1948-scholar-awarded-at-fulbright-phl-s-70th-anniversary/story/.

Sy, M. P., Yao, D. P., Panotes, A., Kaw, J., & Mendoza, T. (2021). Contemporary history: Progress and resilience of occupational therapy in the Philippines (2004–2020). *World Federation of Occupational Therapists Bulletin*, 79(1), 80–93. doi:10.1080/14473828.2021.1995226.

Trinidad, O. S., & Sison, E. M. M. (1995). The history and development of occupational therapy in the Philippines (1945–1995) [Unpublished undergraduate thesis]. Department of Occupational Therapy, University of the Philippines Manila.

Chapter 3

Occupational science

A basis for understanding Filipino occupations

Ricardo Carrasco, Terry Peralta-Catipon, Caroline Fischl and Michael Sy

Chapter objectives

1 Describe the purpose of occupational science and its relationship to occupational therapy
2 Discuss the historical beginnings of the occupational science in the Philippines
3 Curate studies that investigated occupations from a Filipino perspective
4 Analyze the case of Filipina domestic workers in Hong Kong and their occupations
5 Outline helpful strategies in practicing occupational science

Occupational science is the systematic study of human activities, also largely termed as "occupations," and how they influence health and well-being of individuals and collectives (Clark et al., 1991). While it has been defined as new or emerging, occupational science today is a distinguished social science field that underlines the centrality of occupations studied through pluralistic lenses, perspectives, and contexts (Kinsella, 2012). This chapter begins with describing the purpose of occupational science and how that has changed over time alongside its disciplinary development. The next section provides a critical discussion about the relationship between occupational science and occupational therapy, followed by a short history of occupational science in the Philippines. Aligned with the book's aim of highlighting the Filipino perspective, a curation of selected studies investigating Filipino occupations is provided. The chapter ends with some helpful strategies to start practicing occupational science.

The purpose of occupational science

Since its inception in the 1980s, the purpose of occupational science has been to produce foundational knowledge about occupation that serves to inform the practice of occupational therapy (Clark et al., 1991). As a developing basic science, it has survived transitions in declaring its

DOI: 10.4324/9781003321217-3

disciplinary role, especially in situating itself in occupational therapy practice and other disciplines that study humans as occupational beings. Occupational science formed a basis to study humans who perform occupations and to inspect closely the basic aspects of human engagement such as who, what, when, where, why, and how. Doing so enhances the credibility in adapting occupations so that participation is transformed into meaningful engagement by human beings, consequently creating a synergy between the foundational basic science and the applied science of occupational therapy (Polatajko, 2014). This synergistic entanglement results in a deeper understanding of how each human occupies time in conveying roles, routines, rituals, and habits to achieve their activities of daily living and occupational experiences with goals of productivity, pleasure, restoration, and social connectivity (Atler et al., 2015).

Occupational therapy and occupational science: Beyond a synergistic relationship

Viewing occupational science (basic science) as the theoretical backbone of occupational therapy (applied science) and seeing occupational therapy as the translation of the knowledge produced via occupational science has always been a dominant discourse. While espousing this synergistic relationship between occupational therapy and occupational science has afforded benefits to both fields, this way of thinking can be self-limiting. On one hand, occupational science can be seen to only have a scholarly and practical relationship with occupational therapy. On the other hand, understanding and appreciation of occupational science appears to be more common among occupational therapy educators and researchers, widening the gap between occupational scientists and occupational therapy practitioners. There is a misconception that academics are the only ones capable of doing occupational science, whereas those in clinical practice are only bound to do occupational therapy. This is not the case, however, as clinical reasoning in occupational therapy involves critical appraisal of and reflections related to the underpinnings of the profession, that is, the analysis of human doings.

In the past three decades, there have been trends on the types of studies born out of occupational science. They range from exploring nuanced understandings of occupations, examining the biological/physiological basis of occupations, to illuminating social, historical, political, and cultural aspects of occupations. However, some occupational science scholars have questioned the direction of the academic discipline. Unlike a regulated profession (like occupational therapy) that focuses on monitoring current practice to increase professional autonomy and to serve as gatekeeper of professional boundaries, occupational science as an academic discipline seeks to expand the discourses around occupation as a construct. These discourses are intended to influence the development of practices, scholarship, and policies beyond the borders of health care and occupational therapy, as well as other disciplines that utilize occupational science knowledge. Likewise, as an academic discipline, occupational science can study human occupations without the intention of creating or building on knowledge for interventional goals as applied in occupational therapy. In other words, the relationship between occupational science and occupational therapy can be loose and not necessarily synergistic.

Contemporary occupational science allows for an emancipatory way of (co)producing a knowledge base that can be freely enmeshed with those coming from disciplines fostering multi-, inter-, trans-, and post-disciplinary knowledge generation (Sy et al., 2024). Recently a project by Pineda (2022) examined the contemporary meaning(s) of "occupation" from a Filipino context (see Chapter 1 to learn the details on this trans-disciplinary project). This project highlighted the value of occupational science with the help of applied linguistics, data science, Philippine studies, and occupational therapy in addressing a complex issue of our daily reality. The research gap that motivated the project was to ask the question: why is "occupational therapy" not easily understood, resulting in its invisibility or inaccessibility to many ordinary Filipinos? This project can be considered both trans-disciplinary and post-disciplinary. On one hand, it is trans-disciplinary because the project harnessed knowledge from different disciplines and attempted to provide empirical evidence regarding the incongruence of the meaning of "occupation" using the vernacular language in comparison to how "occupation" means in occupational therapy. On the other hand, it is post-disciplinary because the findings challenge dominant discourses and assumptions about "occupation," hence proposing to reimagine the definition of "occupational therapy" in the Philippine context by, for example, using the word "activity" rather than "occupation" when communicating occupational therapy to service users.

SIBOL: The beginnings of occupational science in the Philippines

It has been written in several books how occupational science started at the University of Southern California (USC) in 1989, carrying with it the conceptualization of "occupation" that embodies a Western ideal (Kantartzis & Molineux, 2011). In the next decades, occupational science expanded to other Westernized regions of the world where key scholars were born not just to promote the academic discipline, but also to scrutinize it to help it further develop (Hammell, 2015). Despite this, occupational science has started to spew its seeds into countries to the east, including the Philippines.

The undergraduate education of occupational therapy in the Philippines has placed scant emphasis in studying occupational science. Concepts in occupational science are often introduced early in the educational programs, but the curriculum's focus shifts towards the preparation for clinical and practical skills used for patient care competencies. At the end of the occupational therapy program, students are typically expected to do a bachelor's thesis related to occupational therapy, with selected theses using occupational science concepts as part of the theoretical framework—but not the focus.

While the awareness about occupational science in the Philippines is in its infancy, some Filipino occupational therapists made attempts to advocate it through occupational science research and advocacy. By using occupational science as a disciplinary framework in their doctoral dissertation, some Filipino occupational therapists were able to initiate the development of occupational science in the Philippines (Sy et al., 2021). These scholars investigated the intersections between occupational concepts (i.e., occupational identity, occupational belonging) and migration of Filipino domestic helpers in Hong Kong (Peralta-Catipon, 2009, 2012) and Filipinos using illicit drugs within a political context of the "war on drugs" (Sy et al., 2020). These research studies have since been communicated in local and international conferences and publications, consequently encouraging more local discourses in occupational science. Although local occupational scientists continue to conduct small-scale research here and there, the growth of the academic discipline in the country can be characterized as more sporadic than developmental.

In 2018, a small group of Filipino occupational therapists and occupational scientists met during the World Federation of Occupational Therapists (WFOT) Congress held in Cape Town, South Africa to form the SIBOL group (see Figure 3.1). SIBOL stands for "Sowing, Informing and Building Occupational Science for Living." Also, *sibol* is a Filipino word that literally translates as *growth* or *sprout*, which characterizes the current status of occupational science in the Philippines. The group, led by Ricardo C. Carrasco and Peñafrancia E. Ching, began as a study group that held a series of online meetings to discuss occupational science topics. After completing the series, the study group conducted a Strengths-Weaknesses-Opportunities-Threats (SWOT) analysis to determine what is needed beyond the creation of an online study group. The SWOT analysis directed the group to do two things: to collaborate in disseminating occupational science information to fellow Filipinos and to establish an occupational science special interest group. The SIBOL group approached the Philippine Academy of Occupational Therapists (PAOT) to request the recognition and sustainability of the group by making it one of PAOT's special interest groups. In 2021, during the PAOT's celebration of World Occupational Therapy Day, SIBOL became known as the *PAOT Special Interest Group in Occupational Science.*

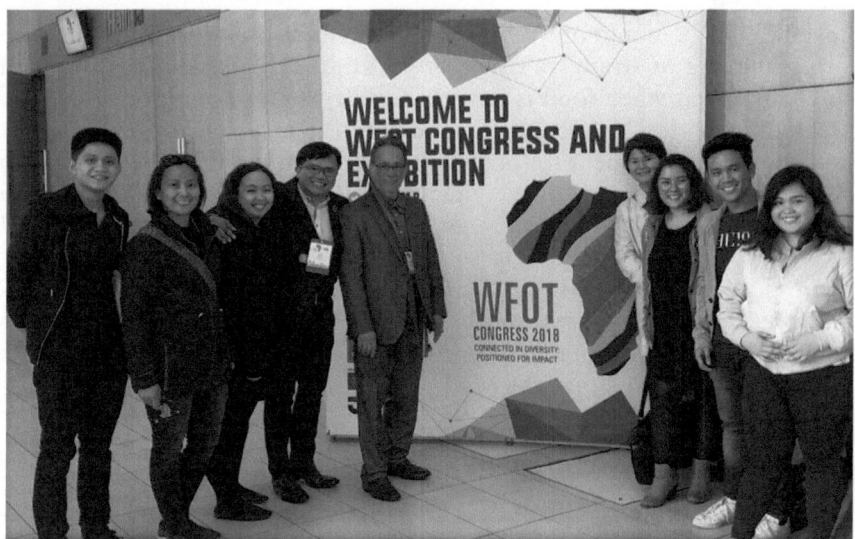

Figure 3.1 Filipino occupational therapists who were at the WFOT Congress in Cape Town South Africa, 2018. They were part of the formation of the SIBOL group. From left to right are: Japet Diaz, Caroline Fischl, Thea Sheila O. Alonto, R. Lyle Duque, Ricardo Carrasco, Peñafrancia Ching, Maria Lucia Nañagas, Rod Charlie Delos Reyes, and Nikki Caballo

The nuances of Filipino occupations: An occupational science perspective

Occupational scientists have long acknowledged that occupations are socially, culturally, historically, and politically constructed. These constructions define the form, function, and meaning of occupations (Zemke & Clark, 1996). *Form* refers to the observable aspects of occupation. *Function* deals with the purpose of the occupation in relation to development, health, and well-being. *Meaning* pertains to an individual's experience of the occupation.

To elaborate, we take eating as an example. The form of eating would differ among various social classes, contexts, and geographical parts of the Philippines. One may observe people eating using the hands, with a spoon, or with a spoon and fork; eating different kinds of foods with different spices; sharing with others or eating alone; eating at home or outside of the home; and so on. The function of eating can be for satisfying hunger, physical growth, or complementing socialization. Meanings attributed to eating include "growing up strong, energetic, beautiful, or intelligent" (often said to Filipino children and adolescents as encouragement to eat, influenced by socially acceptable images of adulthood), being part of a family or group ("A family that eats together, stays together" is a common Filipino belief), and showing hospitality to acquaintances or strangers (*Kain na* [let's eat] or inviting everybody and anybody to eat when food is served). Eating can also manifest from *hiya* [sense of propriety] by accepting food even if one is not hungry so as not to cause embarrassment for or to gain favor from the inviter, or a need to feel connected to one's home country and alleviate *pangungulila sa bayan* [homesickness], which is often experienced by Filipino migrants and overseas Filipino workers.

In the following texts, we provide more examples of occupations (hidden doings, doings towards becoming beautiful, and indigenous doings) from a Filipino context to ascertain how occupations are indeed figured and situated.

Hidden Filipino occupations

Filipino occupations are also characterized by hidden and non-sanctioned doings. A critical work by Sy and colleagues (2023) aimed to illuminate the non-sanctioned Filipino occupations through analyses of secondary data from popular media portrayals and published works. The occupations that were examined include *pagpag* [consumption of food waste], *pangangalakal* [dumpster diving], *panlilimos* [mendicancy], bomb-recycling, small-scale mining, graveyard-digging, *sisid* [free-diving to collect resources—pearls and sea urchins], *nga-nga* [betel chewing], *sabong* [cockfighting], *sugal* [gambling—*jueteng* and tong-its], and sex work. This study revealed the need to iteratively use insider and outsider lenses; the entanglement of power relations, choice, and occupations; and the natural consideration of the concepts of *paghihirap* [suffering] and *hiya* [sense of propriety] in order to choose doings, intentionally participate, sustain belongingness, and possess pride in hard work to fulfill cultural and familial expectations.

The occupations of people who desire to be beautiful

The understanding of beauty as a dimension of occupation has also been a novel contribution to occupational science. Using the dark side of occupation as a conceptual framework, Sy, Martinez, and Twinley (2021) explored essential and hidden occupations within the context of modern-day beauty pageants. In their critical essay, the concept of physical beauty was considered a determinant towards occupational performance, participation, and justice. In a culture where physical beauty is adorned, people and collectives who desire to be and become beautiful will engage in any occupations (whether health-promoting or health-compromising) in order to maintain the agency to choose what occupations they can participate in.

Indigenous Filipino occupations

Although largely influenced by neoliberalism, colonialism, and globalization, Filipino occupations cannot be fully described without understanding indigenous doings. A study by Bulan et al. (2022) aimed to explore the conceptualizations of indigenous occupations of the Ati tribal community within an occupational therapy fieldwork module in the Cebu Province. Framing research on educational experiences using an occupational science perspective revealed how indigenous occupations (e.g., making of herbal remedies or ethnomedicines, crafting talismans and amulets, chanting, dancing, singing, just to name a few) are largely participated from a collectivistic point of view. These indigenous doings are inter-generational, spiritually driven, crucial in preserving traditional customs and rituals, and genderless.

Other examples of preserved traditions are influenced by Catholic religious practices such as *novenas*, expressed through nine evenings of prayers and *simbang gabi* [nine early morning church services before Christmas]. *Batok*, the indigenous Filipino tattooing practice, also unearths the nuanced understanding of how Filipinos engage in occupations from a cultural and historical perspectives (Ramirez et al., 2022). This occupation was suppressed during the Christianization and colonization of the Philippines by the Spaniards for more than 300 years. Understanding *batok* from an occupational science perspective revealed the re-emergence of the *Kapwa* concept (the concept defining the connection between oneself and others among the Filipino community), decolonization, and resistance. Drawn from the conceptualization of transgressive occupations (*ocupaciones transgresivas*) (Tolvett & Dreyer, 2014), engaging in *batok* is perceived to reclaim a Filipino custom and assert one's identity as a Filipino.

In Table 3.1, we provide studies that analyzed occupations from a Filipino perspective and relate them to the proposed framework on occupational science knowledge and research directions by Hocking (2000). It is our intention to partly provide researchers, educators, practitioners, and students alike a synthesis of the occupational focus and research focus of the exemplar studies mentioned to guide occupational science scholarship in the Philippines.

The case of Filipina domestic workers: Seeing the occupation of domestic work from individual to collective perspectives

Drawn from the doctoral dissertation of Peralta-Catipon (2009, 2012), she embarked on an ethnographic enquiry to investigate Filipina domestic workers who spend their Sundays at Statue Square in Hong Kong. Every Sunday, Hong Kong's Central District undergo weekly transformations when thousands of Filipina domestic workers occupy Statue Square and

Table 3.1 The occupational and research focus of select occupation science studies from the Philippines

Authors	Article title and source	Occupational focus	Research focus*
Peralta-Catipon (2012)	Collective occupations among Filipina migrant workers: bridging disrupted identities DOI: 10.3928/15394492-20110805-01	Spending time with fellow countrymen on Sundays	1, 2, 3
Sy, Bontje, Ohshima, & Kiepek (2020)	Articulating the form, function, and meaning of drug using in the Philippines through the lens of morality and work ethics DOI: 10.1080/14427591.2019.1644662	Illicit drug using	1, 3
Sy, Carrasco, Peralta-Catipon, Yao, Dee, & Ching (2023)	Shedding light on hidden Filipino occupations as portrayed by mass media and scholarly resources: A critical interpretive synthesis DOI: 10.1080/14427591.2023.2182348	Consumption of food waste, dumpster diving, mendicancy, bomb-recyling, small-scale mining, graveyard-digging, free-diving to collect resources, betel chewing, cockfighting, gambling, and sex work	1, 3
Sy, Martinez, & Twinley (2021)	The dark side of occupation within the context of modern-day beauty pageants DOI: 10.3233/WOR-205055	Using illicit beauty products, cosmetic surgery routine, weight control regimen, sex work and escorting	1, 3
Bulan, Pestaño, & Sy (2022)	Exploring indigenous occupation: Reflections from a fieldwork experience in an Ati Community in Southern Cebu https://journals.whitingbirch.net/index.php/JPTS/article/view/1738	Making herbal oils, handicrafts, singing, chanting, dancing	1, 2, 3
Ramirez, McCarthy, Cabalquinto, Dizon, & Santiago (2022)	Batok: The exploration of Indigenous Filipino tattooing as a resistive collective occupation DOI: 10.1080/14427591.2022.2110145	Batok or the traditional Filipino tattooing practice	1, 2, 3

Note: Legend: 1—Essential elements of occupation, 2—Occupational processes, and 3—Relationship of occupation to other phenomena several blocks around its vicinity. Sunday was the typical one-day-a-week "holiday" among foreign domestic workers. For Filipinas, they met with their friends at designated areas in and around the Square where they engaged in various leisure activities. In the realm of occupational science, gathering at the Square was an "occupation."

Form. Feeling socially isolated living in their employers' homes during their two year-contracts, the women built social networks during their holidays. "Taga saan ka sa atin?" [From where are you back home?] was a typical means of introduction, which allowed them to build a *barkada* [close set of friends] who also hailed from their hometown. They then agreed to meet at a regular *tambayan* [hangout spot] where they engaged in various leisure activities such as sharing food, reading each other's letters from home, playing cards, or talking about their past week's work experiences throughout the day.

Function. The *tambayan* became a territorial refuge for the workers, which enhanced their sense of agency because it allowed them to engage in activities that they otherwise could not in their employers' homes. They also performed an array of non-work activities that seemed to counterbalance their week of grueling work and limited time for rest and leisure. As such, gathering at the square functioned to alleviate their experiences of occupational deprivation (inability to engage in occupations of choice) and occupational imbalance (see Figure 3.2). Further, regular engagement in collective activities with peers established social structures depicting homelife, such as being an *ate* [older sister] to newcomers; the close

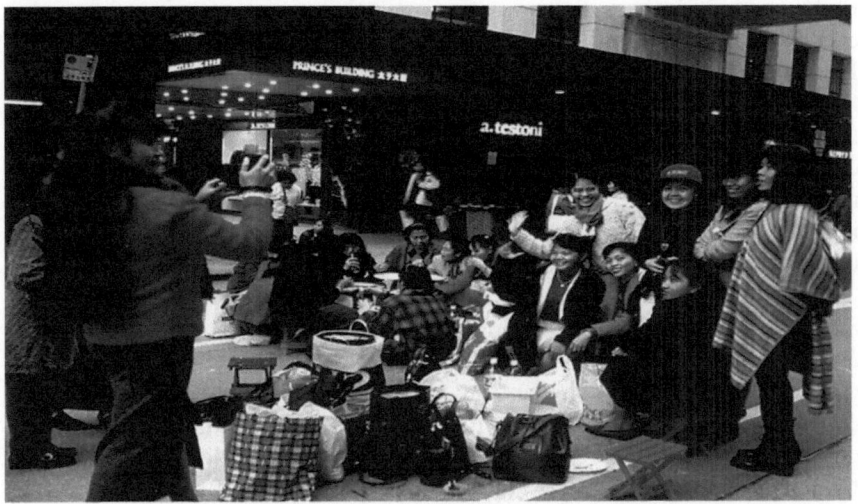

Figure 3.2 A peer group of Filipinas in Hong Kong engaging in various occupations at Central District during their day off from work
Source: Photo taken from Nery (1997) with permission.

barkada became a family and other friends from the same province became a clan. Local merchants and various entrepreneurs offered services and goods that catered to their needs that transformed the downtown metropolis into a provisional society and a "home away from home," which alleviated occupational alienation (sense of isolation and estrangement from society) and marginalization (sense of disempowerment caused by overt discrimination).

Meaning. As a provisional society, landmarks and structures became icons familiar to all that always elicited a grin or smile upon mere mention, such as the statue (they called the black man) in the middle of the square and the two lion statues across the street. Similarities in their plight resulted in the emergence of their own secret lexicon (e.g., "aerobics" meant outside work, "international" meant having a holiday on a different day every week) as well as roles and practices, such as mentoring newcomers and serving as a courier of goods (*padala*) and news to and from families back in their hometown. These icons, lingo, roles, practices, and shared experiences allowed for the emergence of a rich subculture, which provided a socio-cultural context that enabled the women to bridge disruptions in their sense of selves.

Filipina domestic workers have been found to experience multiple stress factors amid their complex living and working conditions (Choy et al., 2022). And in addition to the rigorous week of work and limited personal time and space in their employers' homes, the workers' difficulties came from homesickness and their inability to fulfill maternal duties, demotion in social status since many of them are teachers or office workers in the Philippines, and overt discrimination with the stigma of being a "maid," exemplified by derogatory terms such as "ban mui" (Filipino girl) in Hong Kong and "DH" (domestic helper) in the Philippines. However, when friends came back from the Philippines with news from home, they were told stories of how their family was doing well and their newly built home or purchased *jeepney* or *sari-sari* (variety) store from the hard-earned money they regularly sent. As a result, the square became a venue for identity transformations from the disenfranchised status of being a "maid" to being an *ate*, a mentor, and a breadwinner.

Defining the form, function, and meaning of spending Sundays at the Square among the workers allowed for a deeper understanding of their adaptation process. As an occupation, gathering at the square was not merely diversionary nor simply a time to rest. As occupational beings, the workers' collective engagement led to the emergence of a provisional society and subculture, which provided a socio-cultural context that bridged disruptions in their previous roles, statuses, and identities. The focus on the socio-cultural aspects of occupational engagement can inform occupational therapy practice in how collective occupational engagement can influence adaptation, health, wellness, and/or psychological adjustment.

Additionally, the women's adaptive responses displayed the nuances of the Filipinos' collectivistic nature with an interdependent sense of selves (Markus & Kitayama, 1991). In contrast to more Western and independent identities, Filipinos are sensitive to the opinions of others as well as social and cultural expectations. These are displayed in various other Filipino traits and concepts, such as *hiya* [sense of propriety], *pakikisama* [control of one's own desire for the benefit of others], and *pakikipagkapwa-tao* [treating others as fellow human beings]. As such, this highlights the importance of understanding occupations at a population level. Results from this study can guide policies on international migration, sustainable and decent work provisions for all, and social welfare specific to migrants.

Practicing occupational science

Many could be curious as to how one could become an occupational scientist. Although doing a graduate degree in occupational science is one pathway, this is not always the case. The practice of occupational science is not confined in academic work, but can be done in the process of knowing, learning, exchanging, and acting underpinned by an occupational science perspective. Doing occupational science is also not limited to occupational therapists, but can be done by anyone who is interested in studying and learning about human activities. In other words, the intentional action of foregrounding the centrality of human activities to understand health of people, organizations, and societies characterizes the practice of occupational science. Hence, we provide concrete and practical strategies that one can engage in the practice of occupational science:

1 Listen to podcasts that highlight occupational science topics
2 Watch documentaries and investigative journalism that depict certain occupations that interest you and reflect on their form, function, and meaning
3 Attend free webinars or conferences that talk about occupational science
4 Share your insights about occupational science during your team meetings, seminar sessions, and events in your workplace
5 Reach out to an occupational scientist and schedule a conversation with him or her regarding a certain occupation that interests you or occupational science
6 Enroll in an elective course, or graduate program that focuses on or relates to occupational science
7 Embark on occupational science research as a member of a small research group, or as an independent study or thesis/dissertation

Conclusion

Occupational science research in the Philippines is still emerging, which could only mean that there is a fertile ground for scholarly growth. Themes and topics to be explored in occupational science from a Filipino context can now consider methodological and epistemological framing underpinned by contemporary and critical occupational science perspectives that engender the need to examine occupations from a populational and collective configurations (Farias & Laliberte-Rudman, 2019; Laliberte-Rudman, 2013). Staying true to the multidisciplinary nature of occupational science (Hocking & Whiteford 2012), it is pivotal that occupational science scholarship is grounded in intersecting disciplines that cultivate knowledge of human occupation not limited to occupational therapy. Doing occupational science research and scholarship is also not confined in informing occupational therapy, but also critiquing it and informing the practices in other disciplines.

Reflective actions and questions

1   As a student, identify one or two occupations that you really enjoy doing apart from studying. Make a short outline of its form, function, and meaning. Then, plan within your weekly or monthly schedule when you could participate in this occupation again. After engaging in this identified occupation three or four times, go back to your outline and reflect and note if the form, function, and meaning remained the same or changed.

2   As a practitioner (in the community or clinical practice), you may have reflected on the value of occupational science in actual practice. You then decided to share this with your colleagues, but do not know how and where to begin. Look into your annual work calendar and identify a time when you could propose to have a one-hour discussion on occupational science with your colleagues in the next three months. If possible, you can consult someone with occupational science expertise and co-plan the discussion. The plan should contain the following parts: rationale, discussion goals, benefits to your team and workplace, and program outline.

3   As a researcher/academic, what strategies mentioned above have you used to learn more about or practice occupational science? To the strategies that worked, you can encourage your students or peers to also do the same and discuss other potential ways to learn about occupational science. Moreover, if you are planning to do research on occupational science, you can email or reach out to an occupational scientist whose works you have already read and schedule an online meeting to discuss how to commence your research ideation.

References

Atler, K. (2015). An argument for a dynamic interrelated view of occupational experience. *Journal of Occupational Science*, 22(3), 249–259. doi:10.1080/14427591.2014.887991.

Bulan, P. M., Pestaño, N., & Sy, M. P. (2022). Exploring indigenous occupation: Reflections from a fieldwork experience in an Ati Community in Southern Cebu. *The Journal of Practice Teaching and Learning*, 19(3). https://journals.whitingbirch.net/index.php/JPTS/article/view/1738.

Choy, C. Y, Chang, L., & Man, P. Y. (2022). Social support and coping among female foreign domestic helpers experiencing abuse and exploitation in Hong Kong. *Front. Commun.*, 7, 1015193. doi:10.3389/fcomm.2022.1015193.

Clark, F. A., Parham, D., Carlson, M. E., Frank, G., Jackson, J., Pierce, D., Wolfe, R. J., & Zemke, R. (1991). Occupational science: Academic innovation in the service of occupational therapy's future. *The American Journal of Occupational Therapy: Official Publication of the American Occupational Therapy Association*, 45(4), 300–310. doi:10.5014/ajot.45.4.300.

Farias, L., & Laliberte-Rudman , D. (2019). Challenges in enacting occupation-based social transformative practices: A critical dialogical study. *Canadian Journal of Occupational Therapy. Revue canadienne d'ergotherapie*, 86(3), 243–252. doi:10.1177/0008417419828798.

Hammell, K. W. (2015). Respecting global wisdom: Enhancing the cultural relevance of occupational therapy's theoretical base. *British Journal of Occupational Therapy*, 78(11), 718–721. doi:10.1177/0308022614564170.

Hocking, C. (2000). Occupational science: A stock take of accumulated insights. *Journal of Occupational Science*, 7(2), 58–67. doi:10.1080/14427591.2000.9686466.

Hocking, C., & Whiteford, G. E. (2012). Introduction to critical perspectives in occupational science. In G. Whiteford & C. Hocking (Eds.), *Occupational Science: Society, Inclusion, Participation* (pp. 1–7). Wiley Blackwell. doi:10.1002/9781118281581.ch1.

Kantartzis, S., & Molineux, M. (2011). The influence of western society's construction of a healthy daily life on the conceptualization of occupation. *Journal of Occupational Science*, 18(1), 62–80. doi:10.1080/14427591.2011.566917.

Kiepek, N. C., Beagan, B., Laliberte-Rudman, D., & Phelan, S. (2019). Silences around occupations framed as unhealthy, illegal, and deviant. *Journal of Occupational Science*, 26(3), 341–353. doi:10.1080/14427591.2018.1499123.

Kinsella, E. A. (2012). Knowledge paradigms in occupational science: Pluralistic perspectives. In G. Whiteford & C. Hocking (Eds.), *Occupational Science: Society, Inclusion, Participation*. Wiley Blackwell. doi:10.1002/9781118281581.ch6.

Laliberte-Rudman, D. (2013). Enacting the critical potential of occupational science: Problematizing the "individualizing of occupation. *Journal of Occupational Science*, 20(4), 298–313. doi:10.1080/14427591.2013.803434.

Markus, H. R., & Kitayama, S. (1991). Culture and the self: Implications for cognition, emotion, and motivation. *Psychological Review*, 98(2), 224–253. doi:10.1037/0033-295X.98.2.224.

Nery, M. (1997). *Hanapbuhay Hong Kong*. Global Exponents Publishing House.

Peralta-Catipon, T. (2009). Statue Square as a liminal sphere: Transforming space and place in migrant adaptation. *Journal of Occupational Science*, 16(1), 32–37. doi:10.1080/14427591.2009.968663.

Peralta-Catipon, T. (2012). Collective occupations among Filipina migrant workers: Bridging disrupted identities. *OTJR: Occupation, Participation and Health*, 32(2), 14–21. doi:10.3928/15394492-20110805-01.

Pineda, R. (August 30, 2022). *Filipino conceptualization of occupations: A corpusbased critical discourse analysis* [Oral presentation]. World Federation of Occupational Therapists Congress, Paris, France.

Polatajko, H. J. (2014). A call to occupationology. *Canadian Journal of Occupational Therapy*, 81(1), 4–7. doi:10.1177/0008417414522767.

Ramirez, C., McCarthy, K., Cabalquinto, A., Dizon, C., & Santiago, M. (2022). Batok: The exploration of indigenous Filipino tattooing as a resistive collective occupation. *Journal of Occupational Science*. doi:10.1080/14427591.2022.2110145.

Simangan, D. (2018). Is the Philippine "war on drugs" an act of genocide? *Journal of Genocide Research*, 20(1), 68–89. doi:10.1080/14623528.2017.1379939.

Sy, M. P., Bontje, P., Ohshima, N., Kiepek, N. (2020). Articulating the form, function, and meaning of drug using in the Philippines from the lens of morality and work ethics. *Journal of Occupational Science*, 27(1), 12–21. doi:10.1080/14427591.2019.1644662.

Sy, M. P., Carrasco, R., Peralta-Catipon, T., Yao, D. P., Dee, V., & Ching, P. E. (2023). Shedding light on hidden Filipino occupations as portrayed by media and scholarly resources: A critical interpretive synthesis. *Journal of Occupational Science*. doi:10.1080/14427591.2023.2182348.

Sy, M. P., Granholm Valmari, E., & Baldissera, A. (2024). Crossdisciplinary approaches as applied in occupational science. *Journal of Occupational Science*, 1–9. doi:10.1080/14427591.2024.2367574.

Sy, M. P., Martinez, P., & Twinley, R. (2021). The dark side of occupation within the context of modern-day beauty pageants. *Work (Reading, Mass.)*, 69(2), 367–377. doi:10.3233/WOR-205055.

Sy, M. P., Yao, D. G. P., Panotes, A. A., Kaw, J. X., & Mendoza, T. C. (2021). Contemporary history: Progress and resilience of occupational therapy in the Philippines (2004–2020). *World Federation of Occupational Therapists Bulletin*. doi:10.1080/14473828.2021.1995226.

Tolvett, M. P., & Dreyer, C. S. (2014). Significados de la ocupación en jóvenes infractores de la ley, participantes de programas de inclusión social en Chile. *Ocupación Humana*, 14(2), 5–22. doi:10.25214/25907816.46.

Twinley R. (2013). The dark side of occupation: A concept for consideration. *Australian Occupational Therapy Journal*, 60(4), 301–303. doi:10.1111/1440-1630.12026.

Yerxa, E. J. (2000). Occupational science: A renaissance of service to humankind through knowledge. *Occupational Therapy International*, 7, 87–98. doi:10.1002/oti.109.

Zemke, R., & Clark, F. (Eds.) (1996). *Occupational Science: An Evolving Discipline*. F. A Davis.

Chapter 4

Becoming a Filipino occupational therapist

The undergraduate story

Paolo Miguel P. Bulan, Arden Panotes, Pauline Gail V. Martinez and Michael Sy

Chapter objectives

1 Outline the different requirements to complete an undergraduate degree in occupational therapy (OT) in the Philippine context
2 Describe the profile of undergraduate students studying OT in the Philippines in terms of gender, cultural-linguistic background, and socio-economic status
3 Describe curricular and extra-curricular experiences of occupational therapy students in the Philippines
4 Critique OT education and training against the middle-classist, ableist, and colonial influences

Before entering an occupational therapy program

The occupational therapy education in the Philippines is considered the first bachelor's degree program of its kind in Asia (Sy et al., 2021). Since the 1960s, obtaining a high school graduate diploma or having ten years of primary and secondary education has been the minimum requirement to enter an occupational therapy program. However, in 2016, by virtue of the Enhanced Basic Education Act of 2013, students enrolling for university needed to have two more years of education, which is more popularly called "senior high school." In this envisaged educational reform, high school students were given four tracks: academic, technical vocational and livelihood, sports, and arts and design. Since occupational therapy education in the Philippines can only be offered in higher education institutions, the first track is the typical pathway to apply into an occupational therapy program.

In the recent cohort of senior high school graduates, those who took the academic track were given two years of additional education consisting of clearly defined courses that are focused on a specific knowledge base, called "strands." There are four strands for the academic track: Accountancy, Business and Management (ABM); Science, Technology,

DOI: 10.4324/9781003321217-4

Engineering, and Mathematics (STEM); Humanities and Social Sciences (HUMSS); and General Academic Strand (GAS). While the occupational therapy admission process would prefer students who completed STEM and HUMSS strands, some programs are more lenient in accepting students who completed other strands. Although admissions are typically based on test scores, some programs involve a one-on-one interview with the applicant as part of the admission decision. In these interviews, apart from good study habits as reflected in above-average marks in secondary education, typically applicants with past experiences in volunteering in the community and socio-civic organizations would likely have an edge for admission.

In some cases, there are applicants who are seeking a career shift. They are typically more mature in age and some already have a bachelor's degree or a professional license from a different field. They are called "second coursers." These applicants are welcomed in occupational therapy programs since they add not only diversity but allow occupational therapy to be an inclusive career opportunity to more people.

Overview of occupational therapy education in the Philippines

In the Philippines, to become a registered occupational therapist, you are required to complete a bachelor's degree in occupational therapy offered by a recognized higher educational institution and successfully pass the national licensure examination. To date, there are approximately 20 educational programs offering occupational therapy, of which only one program is publicly funded.

The most recent policies, standards, and guidelines for occupational therapy education in the country was instituted in 2017 to reflect a curriculum following outcomes-based education (Commission on Higher Education [CHED] Memorandum Order [CMO] No. 52 series of 2017). Outcomes-based education is a framework for curriculum, instructional design, and quality assurance that emphasizes the achievement of identified learning outcomes. The shift towards outcomes-based education has entailed designing teaching and learning activities within occupational therapy courses based on and directed towards achieving these learnings outcomes. The ambition was to ensure that these outcomes, when achieved, become a set of competencies that should be possessed by an entry-level occupational therapist.

Most outcomes in OT education in the country relate to the role of an occupational therapist as a general clinical practitioner. This was accentuated by the adjustment to OBE, with several courses focusing on clinical knowledge and skills in evaluation and intervention for different client populations, such as that of mental health, physical dysfunctions, and pediatrics. Despite this, taught content within the curriculum slowly shifted from illness to well-being orientation, medical to biopsychosocial paradigms, mechanistic to occupation-centered models and principles, and individual service to community service (Cabatan & Duque, 2020; Uy, 2019).

The occupational therapy programs in the Philippines are also guided by the World Federation of Occupational Therapists (WFOT) minimum standards for entry-level occupational therapy education. Currently, there are five approved education programs in the Philippines (World Federation of Occupational Therapists, 2024). Other local accrediting agencies such as the Philippine Accrediting Association of Schools, Colleges, and Universities (PAASCU) also help in shaping and maintaining the standards of entry-level occupational therapy education. The accreditation process is entirely voluntary on the part of the higher education institution.

Requirements to complete occupational therapy education and training

For many years, occupational therapy education in the Philippines could be completed in four to five years. With the recent changes in higher education policies, all programs are now completed in four years, encompassing courses from general education, basic sciences, clinical sciences, occupational therapy (professional course work), and a ten-month internship. The prescribed four-year occupational therapy bachelor's degree curriculum in the Philippines can be freely accessed via CHED's official website (2017).

The first three years of the program constitute classroom lectures and laboratory sessions. Teaching-learning activities and assessments are mostly done on-site, while some formative coursework and assessments are now done online. In recent years, more courses are conducted in hybrid arrangements to optimize the use of technology, learning management systems, and simulation applications and equipment. Towards the end of the program, students are expected to complete fieldwork hours in different clinical settings before they embark on the ten-month internship. Alongside these clinical courses, students are expected to complete an undergraduate thesis. The thesis topics are typically faculty-led and are done in pairs or in small groups. An overview of thesis topics from occupational therapy students in the past years are summarized in Chapter 12.

The ten months of internship amounts to a total of 1,200 hours of clocked hours for each occupational therapy student, also called "interns." The WFOT minimum standard of having at least 1,000 clocked hours has been the same for over 60 years and has yet to be supported by formal evidence (Thomas et al., 2019). The occupational therapy internship, usually termed as "placement" or "fieldwork" overseas, involves both clinical and non-clinical training opportunities for interns. On the one hand, the clinical training (Commission on Higher Education, 2017) includes training in major practice settings such as children's care, physical rehabilitation, mental health, and community-based rehabilitation (CBR). On the other hand, the non-clinical internship, normally called "enrichment rotation," includes training opportunities that develop competencies to become an administrator, manager, educator, researcher, community organizer, and an advocate (Sy et al., 2021; see Figure 4.1). The clinical training in each major practice setting would typically entail two months, whereas non-clinical training lasts for at most one month per area.

Throughout the internship, the interns are ideally supervised by a licensed occupational therapist employed either as a clinician or a clinical educator in the accredited institution providing the internship. However, in some cases, within role-emerging or non-clinical internship opportunities, students can be co-supervised by someone who is not necessarily an occupational therapist but is available to conduct the training process to achieve specific internship learning outcomes. The role-emerging internship opportunities have become more relevant recently due to the shortage of practice education placements and occupational therapy supervisors (Overton et al., 2009). The expansion of internship opportunities to areas where occupational therapy services are not typically provided has enriched not only the contemporary occupational therapy curriculum but has allowed for the development of new skills for interns towards early-career advancements (Thew et al., 2018). In one international student exchange program, clinical and role-emerging opportunities were combined through an individualized study plan. These Filipino occupational therapy interns spent four days per week at a hand and plastic surgery clinic while collaborating with knowledge engineers once a week for the development of a

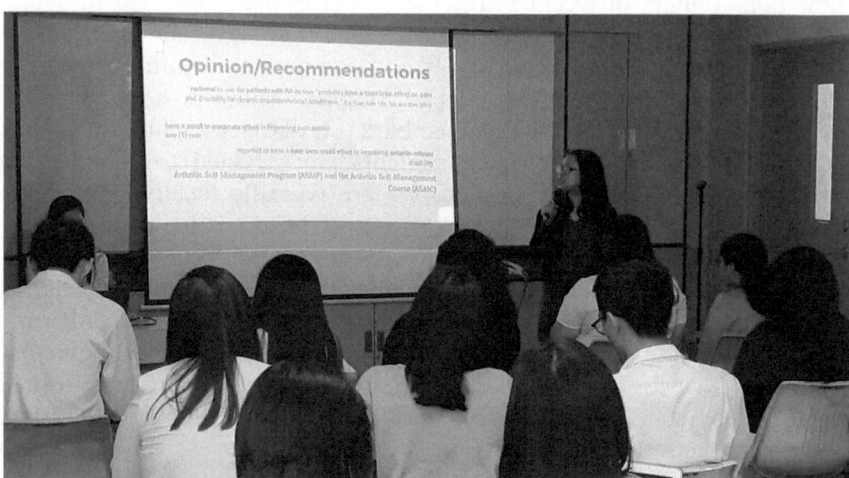

Figure 4.1 An occupational therapy intern delivering a mini lecture to fellow students to practice public speaking as part of the academic rotation

digital technology. Reflections from the students revealed the value of role expectations, understanding professional identity, openness to learning, and developing personal responsibility (Panotes et al., 2015).

On top of the course work, internship program, and the undergraduate thesis, some occupational therapy programs offer additional courses for two purposes: board examination preparation and meeting eligibility requirements to take the American licensure examination, more popularly known as the National Board Certification in Occupational Therapy, Inc. (National Board for Certification in Occupational Therapy, 2023). These additional courses are on top of the minimum prescribed curriculum by the CHED. However, a select number of programs continue to offer these additional courses to ensure that they equip their students both for the local and international qualifications.

Preparation for the national licensure examination

Occupational therapy programs in the Philippines are developed based on the minimum standards set by WFOT and CHED. When these minimum standards are met, programs are allowed to enrich them according to the university's values, mission, vision, and priorities. As subjective as it is, the programs differ in terms of quality, accreditation level, and standards. This situation necessitates a gatekeeping mechanism through a board examination to ensure that only those who passed are qualified to practice the profession. Passing a national licensure examination is not unique to occupational therapy but is mandated by law across all recognized health professions.

To prepare an occupational therapy graduate for the examination, one is given the option to review on his or her own or enroll in a review center. A review center is a private enterprise that is usually external to the higher education institution offering the occupational therapy educational program. While it remains optional for students to enroll in review centers, some occupational therapy programs partner with these review centers to facilitate ease in monitoring the passing rates of their graduates. Although enrolling in review centers is not unique in the Philippines, it has become a popular trend among occupational therapy students who want to have an emotional safety net throughout the process of becoming an occupational therapist.

The national examination to qualify as occupational therapists in the Philippines lasts for one and a half days. The examination is constituted of 600 test items, answerable through a multiple-choice arrangement. The examination has three major parts: 1) anatomy, physiology, and kinesiology; 2) medical and rehabilitation sciences, and 3) occupational therapy practice. With the implementation of the *The Philippine Occupational Therapy Law* of 2018, the scope of the occupational therapy licensure examination (OTLE) will cover basic sciences and health sciences integrated in the domains of occupational therapy applications in three sets.

Filipino occupational therapy students

While it is important to have an overview of the Filipino OT students in terms of demographics and contexts, it is crucial to open a critical discourse on the female orientation of the profession, the classism (middle-class worldview) that is being perpetuated within the profession, and the bias of getting students from largely urban areas across the country. We also would like to open a discussion about the admission policies and the motivation of most students taking occupational therapy as a "passport" to go and work abroad.

Demographics. In a typical occupational therapy program, a class consists of 20 to 40 students. In most programs, only one class is being sustained per year. Recent statistics indicate that there are approximately 1,000 students enrolled in occupational therapy programs across the country (World Federation of Occupational Therapists, 2022). This number, however, is still not enough to meet the needs of the Filipino population. The country still has a 0.5 occupational therapist per 10,000 population ratio, falling behind the average worldwide average ratio of 0.9 occupational therapist per 10,000 population (Carandang & Delos Reyes, 2018).

Sex and gender. Most students are female, which is not surprising since it is known that 89% of occupational therapists are female (World Federation of Occupational Therapists, 2020). The class composition still has more female students than male (Bulan et al., 2024), which is also reflected in the most recent workforce survey where 75% of Filipino occupational therapists are female (Carandang & Delos Reyes, 2018). Although the reason for this gender distribution is not exactly known, the societal perceptions of occupational therapy as a predominantly female profession, coupled with traditional gender norms of caring and nurturing, could potentially influence the fact that more women are convinced to study occupational therapy.

According to the 2023 Global Gender Gap Index reported by the World Economic Forum (2023), the Philippines is number 16 (out of 146 countries) around the world, which indicates gender parity across four dimensions: economic opportunities, education, health, and political leadership. Despite this high gender parity based on a positivist measurement, it is important for Filipino occupational therapists to be cognizant of the impact of covert power differentials and oppressive structures that subordinate female-dominated, feminine, and feministic professions, like occupational therapy (Karaba Bäckström et al., 2023; Lima, 2021). For instance, in the Philippines, occupational therapy as well as other caring and nurturing professions were historically subordinated by the medical profession, which is considered a masculine profession (Lima, 2021; Bondoc, 2005). It is imperative that Filipino occupational therapy students become aware of this reality during their education and training so that they grow into a profession where they learn about gender parity, gender as a social construction, and occupational therapy as intrinsically political. Doing so can concretely allow occupational therapy students to embrace professional autonomy as part of their professional identity where occupational therapists work *with* and not *under* medical doctors. Despite the passing of the new law (i.e., RA 11241), this matter of power differentials remains in the gray zone, that is, whether occupational therapists can receive direct referrals or continue to see a doctor's referral as a requisite to legally assume practice.

Cultural and linguistic backgrounds. In recent years, occupational therapy programs are now available in the three major island groups of the country: Luzon (north), Visayas (central), and Mindanao (south). Most occupational therapy programs are situated in the northern island (i.e., three in the central region and one in the southern region) and are likely to be domiciled in highly urbanized cities. Students who come from more rural areas internally migrate to these cities throughout the whole duration of the program.

The primary mode of teaching in all occupational therapy programs in the country is American English. However, conversations in the classroom and patient care are normally mixed between American English and the vernacular language where appropriate. While there are more than 100 Philippine languages, major language groups relevant to occupational therapy programs are Bisaya, Cebuano, Hiligaynon, Ilocano, Kapampangan, and Tagalog. This interesting cultural diversity among occupational therapy students challenges them to embrace bilingualism and enact flexibility in language use as necessary, especially for patient care.

Although most Filipinos can understand, read, and write basic English, we cannot discount the fact that within occupational therapy education and training—although not consciously recognized—Philippine English is often used. Philippine English is a nativized variety of English close to American English but is also commonly referred to as the "standard" or "educated" English in the Philippine context (Martin, 2020). While not institutionalized or legitimate, Philippine English continues to be closely attributed to Western concepts and discourses resulting in the patronization of Americanized concepts and preferences at the expense of Filipino ideals and values (Dela Cruz, 2022).

The influence of English language use in occupational therapy education and training has an implicit connection to how Western-based conceptualizations and practices are more preferred, or seen as more evidence-based, than the indigenized thinking and doing that are embedded in practice. This preference to use Philippine English, however, undervalues the use of the national languages to connect and communicate better with clients of the profession in practice.

Social class and socio-economic status. Being admitted in an occupational therapy program in the Philippines is considerably competitive and costly. In other words, social and economic considerations are important factors that shape an occupational therapy student's values and goals, which are characterized by middle-class standards.

As mentioned earlier in this chapter, only one program offers free matriculation fees for occupational therapy students, while the rest of the programs require students to pay every semester unless a recipient of a full scholarship. This implies that students in occupational therapy programs would typically come from middle-income families who can afford to send their children to private universities. On top of the tuition and matriculation fees, students will need to pay for dormitories, food, books, transportation, and other school-related expenditures monthly. Students typically study full-time, but we cannot discount the fact that there are some students who also do part-time jobs to support their education.

Several foreign studies have described that occupational therapy students come primarily from lower and middle-class backgrounds (Newfield et al., 2019; van Rensburg, 2011; Beagan, 2007). We do not have statistics to concur that it could be the same in the Philippines, but investing in higher education is a highly regarded value for most middle-class Filipino families (Zialcita, 2020). Knowing that occupational therapy education in the Philippines is largely influenced by Western ideals, underpinned by middle-class, ableist, and imperialist theoretical assumptions (Hammel, 2011), there could be a possibility that more students belonging to middle-class backgrounds would likely resonate or connect to a university program such as occupational therapy. This can be confounded by the fact that students have been exposed to role-modeling at an early age because some of their parents and relatives could belong to the healthcare industry or, in some cases, could have been exposed to a close family member who had been receiving occupational therapy services while growing up.

Another unique characteristic among Filipinos in the middle-class bracket is having a family member who is an Overseas Filipino Worker (OFW), allowing the family to belong to the middle and upper middle-income group (Zialcita, 2020). This brings in another characterization of occupational therapy students in the Philippines, which is the motivation to work abroad for "greener pastures" (Pineda et al., 2023). While this motivation is valid and culturally bound, this could affect the trajectory of their learning goals and study habits of the students especially when they intend to take the licensure examination for overseas employment. Having the mindset of working and migrating abroad could potentially reinforce embracing the Western standards in occupational therapy practice, and thereby hampering the movement of decolonizing occupational therapy education and training in the Philippines.

If some students see the occupational therapy program as a passport to work abroad, some see it as preparation for medical school. In the Philippines, even today, going to medical school requires a student to finish a bachelor's degree from any program in the arts or sciences, or to complete a two-year accelerated pre-medical program at selected universities. A longitudinal study revealed that Filipino medical students would most likely have a pre-medical background in the natural sciences (Catabijan et al., 2016). However, this does not discount the fact that applied and health sciences become popular pre-medical tracks to take, including occupational therapy, because of its pragmatic advantages while in medical school: obtaining a professional license in a field and exposure to clinical training. Although there is no way to control the trajectory of students after completing occupational therapy school, promoting occupational therapy as a good preparation for medical school is adversarial to the goal of the profession to increase its workforce, and could potentially perpetuate the biomedicalization of occupational therapy (Turcotte & Holmes, 2023) in the Philippines.

Learning to be and becoming an occupational therapist

The occupational therapy education constitutes a constellation of courses that involve the intersection of social sciences, biomedical sciences, and rehabilitation sciences. These courses are provided in traditional and hybridized teaching-learning arrangements within and outside of the classroom.

More recently, there are interprofessional education learning outcomes, modules, and programs that are now being integrated within the occupational therapy curriculum (Commission on Higher Education, 2017). This entails students from different health science programs to participate in a class or small group to learn with, from, and about each other's professional identity, shared goals, and teamwork towards improving health outcomes (Commission on Higher Education, 2017). With this goal in mind, students experience *interprofessional learning*. For instance, interprofessional learning occurs when students from two or more different programs (typically from physical therapy and speech-language therapy) are merged to attend a clinical course where they work together on a clinical case throughout a four-session span. This learning dynamics can also be done during the internship where students are given a shared patient with paraplegia to make an interprofessional plan and intervention; this is commonly called "co-management."

Apart from curricular activities, enrichment of learning also happens outside the curriculum, including being actively involved in organizations, whether on a professional, student, or socio-civic level. Within the university, students engage in extracurricular activities, such as those of university-based student organizations, professional organizations, volunteer work with professionals, and interest groups (e.g., choir, dance club, fitness group) to prepare for professional life. Almost all occupational therapy programs have a program-based occupational therapy society where students can also take leadership roles and be guided by an adviser who is a faculty member of the department. The student arm of the national professional organization is the Occupational Therapy Students Assembly (OTSA). Established and officially recognized in 2011, OTSA serves as an avenue for students to connect with fellow students within and outside the Philippines. OTSA closely collaborate with the PAOT in advocating for the profession, lead projects to support fellow students, and network with professionals who can also serve as their professional mentors (Sy et al., 2021; Francisco et al., 2017; see Figure 4.2). Through their engagement in the activities of these social groups, they further develop their inter-personal, communication, management, and leadership skills.

Throughout occupational therapy education and training, it is crucial that students are also trained to be globally competitive, equipped with academic knowledge, life skills, and cultural competence. To ensure that students become competent healthcare professionals within the ever-changing landscape of health and social care, it is imperative that occupational therapy educational programs are tailored to local and global needs and demands. Opportunities for cross-cultural learning have become available to occupational therapy students through student exchanges, international conferences, and online student forums (Katigbak & Sy, 2017; Cabatan & Grajo, 2017). Fieldwork placement activities, cultural immersion experiences, and reflective discussions with a mentor in an international fieldwork education (i.e., Filipino students attending courses in Sweden, and Swedish students attending courses in the Philippines) could foster the development of cultural competence (Panotes et al., 2015).

A critique of contemporary occupational therapy education and training in the Philippines

Now that we have outlined pertinent information on the contemporary occupational therapy education and training in the Philippines, it is important to take a step back, and engage in critical reflection and reflexivity

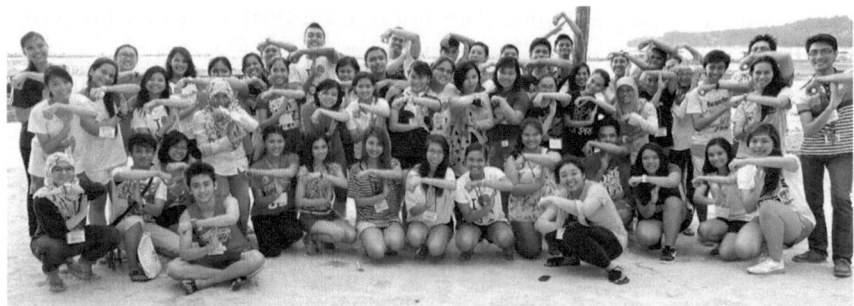

Figure 4.2 A group photo of the Occupational Therapy Students Assembly during a team-building activity in 2013; the students here are gesturing the "OT Pose"

processes (Robertson et al., 2015; Laliberte-Rudman, 2021). In the past decade, occupational therapy education in the Philippines has been purposely built on an outcomes-based education approach. This approach was perceived to be an educational reform especially in medical and health sciences curricula in the Philippines with the promise to match higher education with actual employment (Sana et al., 2015). The World Federation of Occupational Therapists (2017) minimum standards for education promotes a more competency-based than an outcomes-based education approach. In comparison to outcomes-based, a competency-based education emphasizes the development of essential competencies to be able to qualify for practice. A competency is the constellation of knowledge, skills, abilities, and behaviors that is performed efficiently, safely, and in a timely manner by an individual. Implementing any educational approach without critical examination may derail schools from actuating their primary role of producing competent health care professionals to meet local needs.

Outcomes-based education has been sponsored largely by the government and the approach is seldom questioned, especially by local occupational therapy educators. This could be because the educators would be inclined to adhere to local standards in exchange for national accreditation and recognition, which is reinforced by the fact that most occupational therapy programs are run by consumer-driven, private institutions. In one research forum on education, a Filipino philosophy professor, Paolo Bolaños, said, "An *obsession* with outcomes is not really centered on students, but instead reduces them to marketable employees" (The Varsitarian, 2018). He went on to argue that outcomes-based education was not learner-oriented, but rather a convenient way to quantify students so that they could be packaged and marketed in the world of work. While there is truth in ensuring that students obtain gainful employment after graduation, outcomes-based education has been critiqued to reduce education to a list of quantifiable and behavioristic units of statements that students need to tick off (Brady, 1996), which neglects competencies that are more implicit in nature, such as caring attitudes and occupation-focused knowledge and skills (Battaglia, 2016; Fisher, 2013).

To date, there has been no evaluation in local occupational therapy education that ascertains the effectiveness of outcomes-based education in making programs more responsive in meeting local health and social needs. Thomas and Penman (2019) asked if the 1,000 hours is informed by evidence or tradition? In their editorial piece, they were convinced that it was informed more by tradition and history when occupational therapy education was largely focused on providing one-on-one patient care to people in large mental health institutions and rehabilitation hospitals. At that time, occupational therapy practice was largely encroached upon by the biomedical paradigm where individualized supervision of occupational therapy students was widely practiced, which required the 1,000 hours of training. With the advancement of occupational therapy in the past ten years, expanding our services to working in organizations and populations, do we still need to require students to clock 1,000 hours for clinical placements? The question as to whether this practice is done based on evidence, tradition, or a business opportunity remains unanswered. If we intend to anchor our occupational therapy education and training towards achieving entry-level competencies rather than metrics that do not have direct translatable use in the modern world of work, then we need to reimagine the future of credentialing occupational therapists by actively benchmarking with other countries and by being more sensitive to our local health and social care needs.

Conclusion

The chapter provides an overview of being an occupational therapy student in the Philippines. Having around 20 occupational therapy schools available, it has become more available not only to senior high school graduates, but also to those who wanted to shift careers. Considering that the bachelor's program in the Philippines is the first one established in Asia, it has a long tradition of generating not only highly qualified occupational therapists, but also leaders and advocates of the profession then and now. However, to continuously advance the profession, it is important to intentionally revisit traditions and cultivate critical reflection, resulting in questioning the relevance of tradition and inviting emerging educational opportunities for students. This includes interprofessional learning, exchange programs abroad, and involvement in socio-civic organizations. Lastly, we also discussed the characteristics of Filipino occupational therapy students, specifically explaining the relevance of gender as a social construction, the importance of culture and language, and the consciousness of privilege as part of occupational therapy education and training.

Reflective activities

1   Occupational therapy education and training in the Philippines tend to reproduce values that promote classist (middle-class), ableist, and colonialist (Westernized) perspectives. First, you can discuss examples in your past and present experiences on how these perspectives are (re) produced in your class, internship, or practice. Second, what possibilities can be done to then produce occupational therapy content and practice that are indigenous (more Filipino), inclusive, and occupation-focused?

2   The question as to whether the 1,000 hours of internship is too short or too long remains unresolved. Regardless of the number of hours dedicated to complete internship hours within an entry-level occupational therapy curriculum, what opportunities and experiences could be integrated in the internship to ensure that students complete the program with confidence to practice the profession?

3   Licensure examination is not a prerequisite for OT registration in other countries. Research the requirements needed to be a registered occupational therapist in another country that does not require a licensure examination. First, what are the differences in terms of requirements in the Philippines? Second, why do you think it is not necessary for other countries to require a licensure examination?

References

Battaglia, J. (2016). Toward a caring curriculum: Can occupational therapy be taught in a caring context? *International Journal of Teaching and Learning in Higher Education*, 28(2), 265–270. https://files.eric.ed.gov/fulltext/EJ1111119.pdf.

Beagan B. L. (2007). Experiences of social class: Learning from occupational therapy students. *Canadian Journal of Occupational Therapy. Revue canadienne d'ergotherapie*, 74(2), 125–133. doi:10.2182/cjot.06.012x.

Bondoc, S. (2005). Occupational therapy in the Philippines: From founding years to the present. *Philippine Journal of Occupational Therapy*, 1(1), 9–22.

Brady, L. (1996). Outcome-based education: A critique. *The Curriculum Journal*, 7(1), 5–16. doi:10.1080/0958517960070102.

Bulan, P. M. P., Valleser, J. K. B., & Rojas, J. A. (2024). Perceived barriers to online learning amid COVID-19 pandemic: A national survey of occupational therapy students in the Philippines. *Philippine Journal of Health Research and Development*, 28(2), 1–7.

Cabatan, M. C., & Duque, R. L. (2020). Perspectives on occupational therapy education in Southeast Asia. In S. Taff, L. C. Grajo, & B. R. Hooper (Eds.), *Perspectives on occupational therapy education: Past, present, and future* (pp. 143–151). SLACK.

Cabatan, M. C., & Grajo, L. C. (2017). Internalization in an occupational therapy curriculum: A Philippine-American pilot collaboration. *The American Journal of Occupational Therapy*, 71(6), 1–9. doi:10.5014/ajot.2017.024653.

Carandang, K. A., & Delos Reyes, R. C. (2018). *Workforce survey 2017: Working conditions and salary structure of occupational therapists working in the Philippines survey.* Philippine Academy of Occupational Therapists.

Catabijan, C. G., Canal, J. P. A., Ignacio, S. D., & Rivera, A. (2016). Academic performance profile of the students of the UP College of Medicine: Lateral entrants from class 1990 to class 2013. *Philippine Journal of Health Research and Development*, 20(2), 30–41. https://pjhrd.upm.edu.ph/index.php/main/article/view/106.

Commission on Higher Education. (2017). CMO No. 52, s. 2017. Policies, Standards and Guidelines for the Bachelor of Science in Occupational Therapy Education (BSOT) Program. https://ched.gov.ph/wp-content/uploads/2018/04/CMO-No.-52-Series-of-2017-Policies-Standards-and-Guidelines-for-the-Bachelor-of-Science-in-Occupational-Therapy-Education-BSOT-Program.pdf.

Dela Cruz, F. Y. (2022). On the status of English in the Philippines. *UP Working Papers in Linguistics*, 1, 204–206, https://linguistics.upd.edu.ph/wp-content/uploads/2022/08/24-On-the-Status-of-English-in-the-Philippines.pdf.

Fisher A. G. (2013). Occupation-centred, occupation-based, occupation-focused: Same, same or different? *Scandinavian Journal of Occupational Therapy*, 20(3), 162–173. doi:10.3109/11038128.2012.754492.

Francisco, C. M. R., Guevarra, C. A. L., Viray, R. E. T., Panotes, A., & Sy, M. P. (2017, October 20–22). *Occupational therapy students assembly: Preparing students for professional life* [Paper presentation]. 1st Asia Pacific Occupational Therapy Symposium: Contextualizing Occupational Therapy Research, Practice, and Education, Taoyuan, Taiwan.

Hammell, K. W. (2011). Resisting Theoretical imperialism in the disciplines of occupational science and occupational therapy. *British Journal of Occupational Therapy*, 74(1), 27–33. doi:10.4276/030802211X12947686093602.

Karaba Bäckström, M., Luiz Moura de Castro, A., Eakman, A. M., Ikiugu, M. N., Gribble, N., Asaba, E., Kottorp, A., Falkmer, O., Eklund, M., Ness, N. E., Balogh, S., Hynes, P., & Falkmer, T. (2023). Occupational therapy gender imbalance; revisiting a lingering issue. *Scandinavian Journal of Occupational Therapy*, 30(7), 1113–1121. doi:10.1080/11038128.2023.2220912.

Katigbak, B., & Sy, M. P. (2017). *The occupational therapy internship exchange of Angeles University Foundation, Philippines and Chiang Mai University, Thailand: A qualitative study* [Paper presentation]. 1st Asia Pacific Occupational Therapy Symposium: Contextualizing Occupational Therapy Research, Practice, and Education, Taoyuan, Taiwan.

Laliberte-Rudman, D. (2021). Informing social occupational therapy: Unpacking the "social" using critical social theory. In R. E. Lopes & A. P. S. Malfitano (Eds.), *Social Occupational Therapy: Theoretical and Practical Designs* (pp. 141–149). Elsevier.

Lima, E. M. F. A. (2021). Occupational therapy: A feminine or feminist profession? *Brazilian Journal of Occupational Therapy*, 45(1), 154–167. doi:10.1590/0103-11042021E112.

Martin, I. P. (2020). Philippine English. In K. Bolton, W. Botha, & A. Kirkpatrick (Eds.), *The handbook of Asian Englishes* (pp. 479–500). Wiley Blackwell.

National Board for Certification in Occupational Therapy. (2023). Study pack. https://www.nbcot.org/products/studypack.

Newfield, N., Bartlett, L., Murray, E., Park, T., Chambers, K., Hameed, F., & Cockburn, L. (2019). Perceptions of low income by Canadian student occupational therapists. *Journal of Occupational Therapy Education*, 3(2). doi:10.26681/jote.2019.030203.

Overton, A., Clark, M., & Thomas, Y. (2009). A review of non-traditional occupational therapy practice placement education: A focus on role-emerging and project placements. *The British Journal of Occupational Therapy*, 72(7), 294–301. doi:10.1177/030802260907200704.

Panotes, A., Villon, J., & Fischl, C. (2015, November 26). *Combined clinical training and role-emerging settings as international fieldwork placements: Student and teacher perspectives* [Paper presentation]. Philippine Academy of Occupational Therapists Inc. 50th Anniversary Convention: Celebrating Occupation, Celebrating Life, Manila, Philippines.

Panotes, A., Villon, J., & Fischl, C. (2016, June 15–19). *Developing cultural competence based on reflections in international fieldwork education: Student and teacher perspectives* [Paper presentation]. 2016 COTEC- ENOTHE Congress:

COTEC and ENOTHE Connecting Education, Practice, Research, Policy, Galway, Ireland.

Pineda R. C., Abad-Pinlac B., Yao, D. P. G., Toribio, F. N. R. B., Josephsson, S., & Sy, M. P. (2023). Unraveling the "greener pastures" concept: The phenomenology of internationally educated occupational therapists. *OTJR: Occupational Therapy Journal of Research.* doi:10.1177/15394492231205885.

Robertson, D., Warrender, F., & Barnard, S. (2015). The critical occupational therapy practitioner: How to define expertise? *Australian Occupational Therapy Journal*, 62(1), 68–71. doi:10.1111/1440-1630.12157.

Sana, E. A., Roxas, A. B., & Reyes, A. L. T. (2015). Introduction of outcomes-based education in Philippine Health Professions Education setting. *Philippine Journal of Health Research and Development*, 19(1). https://pjhrd.upm.edu.ph/index.php/main/article/view/28.

Sy, M. P., Yao, D. P., Panotes, A., Kaw, J., & Mendoza, T. (2021). Contemporary history: Progress and resilience of occupational therapy in the Philippines (2004–2020). *World Federation of Occupational Therapists Bulletin*, 79(1), 80–93. doi:10.1080/14473828.2021.1995226.

The Varsitarian. (2018, February 24). Philosophy profs hit "outcomes-based education" in research forum. *The Varsitarian.* https://varsitarian.net/news/20180224/philosophy-profs-hit-outcomes-based-education-in-research-forum.

Thew, M., Thomas, Y., & Briggs, M. (2018). The impact of a role emerging placement while a student occupational therapist, on subsequent qualified employability, practice and career path. *Australian Occupational Therapy Journal*, 65. 198–207. doi:10.1111/1440-1630.12463.

Thomas, Y., & Penman, M. (2019). World Federation of Occupational Therapists (WFOT) Standard for 1000 hours of practice placement: Informed by tradition or evidence? *British Journal of Occupational Therapy*, 82(1), 3–4. doi:10.1177/0308022618788785.

Turcotte, P. L., & Holmes, D. (2023). From domestication to imperial patronage: Deconstructing the biomedicalisation of occupational therapy. *Health (London, England: 1997)*, 27(5), 719–737. doi:10.1177/13634593211067891.

Uy, S. J. (2019). Infusing service-learning into allied health profession curriculum: Perceived enablers and barriers. *Metropolitan Universities*, 30(3), 36–52. doi:10.18060/23195.

van Rensburg, V. J. (2011). Doing, being and becoming a first year occupational therapy student. *South African Journal of Occupational Therapy*, 41(2), 8–13. http://www.scielo.org.za/scielo.php?script=sci_arttext&pid=S2310-38332011000200003&lng=en&tlng=en.

World Economic Forum. (2023). *The Global Gender Gap Report 2023: Country Profiles.* https://www.weforum.org/reports/global-gender-gap-report-2023/economy-profiles-5932ef6d39.

World Federation of Occupational Therapists. (2017). *Minimum Standards for the Education of Occupational Therapists 2016.* https://wfot.org/resources/new-minimum-standards-for-the-education-of-occupational-therapists-2016-e-copy.

World Federation of Occupational Therapists. (2020). *WFOT Human Resources Project 2020.* https://wfot.org/resources/occupational-therapy-human-resources-project-2020-alphabetical.

World Federation of Occupational Therapists. (2022). *Human Resources Project 2022*. https://wfot.org/resources/occupational-therapy-human-resources-project-2022-numerical.

World Federation of Occupational Therapists. (2024, March 1). *WFOT Approved Education Programmes*. https://wfot.org/programmes/education/wfot-approved-education-programmes.

Zialcita, S. (2020). *Explainer: Who are the Filipino middle class?*https://pidswebs.pids.gov.ph/CDN/NEWS/04_25_cnn.pdf.

Chapter 5

Lifelong learning and continuing professional development

Icy Fresno Anabo and Caroline Fischl

Chapter objectives

1 Describe lifelong learning and continuing professional development in relation to the practice of occupational therapy in the Philippines
2 Identify national requirements and pathways for professional development for Filipino occupational therapists
3 Discuss reflective practice and the benefits of reflection
4 "Storytell" experiences of Filipino occupational therapists on lifelong learning
5 Describe activities that support lifelong learning and continuing professional development

There is a widespread consensus that continuous learning across various life stages and contexts serves as a means for society to equip itself and address technological, social, demographic, economic, and environmental challenges (UNESCO Institute for Lifelong Learning, 2022). Embraced by governments, higher education institutions (HEIs), and individuals worldwide, lifelong learning stands as a central concept in addressing these challenges. Moreover, lifelong learning is recognized for its broader impact on personal development, social justice, global solidarity, and collective responsibility toward a sustainable future (UNESCO, 2015). This wider perspective has gained momentum in recent years, reinforced by its endorsement in global agendas, such as the United Nations 2030 Agenda on Sustainable Development Goals. Within this agenda, there is a global commitment to ensuring "quality and inclusive lifelong learning for all," as stipulated in Sustainable Development Goal 4 (UNESCO, 2016).

For Filipino occupational therapists, lifelong learning is integral to their professional development. After earning a bachelor's degree in occupational therapy and passing the national occupational therapy licensure exams administered by the Professional Regulations Commission (PRC), entry-level occupational therapists are mandated to participate in continuing professional development (CPD) activities (Philippine

DOI: 10.4324/9781003321217-5

Occupational Therapy Law of 2018, 2019). This requirement ensures that occupational therapists remain well equipped with the knowledge, skills, and attitudes for safe, up-to-date, and effective practice. Furthermore, continuous engagement in learning activities enables occupational therapists to advance their careers and continuously improve their professional competences.

In the Philippines, occupational therapists should be able to perform various roles, including clinician, educator, manager, researcher, advocate, and community-based practitioner (Commission on Higher Education [CHED], 2006, 2017). Occupational therapists working in clinical and community settings often take on the responsibility of supervising occupational therapy students. Filipino occupational therapy clinicians work with clients of all ages, including persons with psychiatric, neurodevelopmental, degenerative, and neurologic conditions. However, a clear typology and roadmap of occupational therapy specializations in the Philippines are still being developed by the PRC and the Professional Regulatory Board (PRB) in the form of the Career Progression and Specialization Program and Credit Accumulation and Transfer System (CPSP-CATS) for the regulated profession. Career progression refers to the "process of developing or moving towards a more advanced state in a person's qualifications, job, title, position, or profession" (PRC, 2022, p. 2), while specialization is "the field of practice of a profession for a particular area of knowledge or the process of becoming an expert in a particular field of professional practice" (PRC, 2022, p. 4). This initiative is part of CPD and aims to enhance professional mobility and align domestic qualifications with international competence frameworks. The CPSP for Occupational Therapy is not yet available. Nevertheless, the Philippine Academy of Occupational Therapists (PAOT) is making progress by encouraging the establishment of Special Interest Groups, which would support the implementation of CPD activities within specialized areas (PAOT, 2020, n.d.). Despite this ongoing process, participation in lifelong learning and professional development activities enables occupational therapists to accumulate credits toward recognized formal qualifications, continually acquire knowledge and skills, and advance in their careers.

Principles in lifelong learning

Lifelong learning mainly involves "all learning activities undertaken throughout life, which result in improving knowledge, know-how, skills, competences and/or qualifications for personal, social, and/or professional reasons" (European Centre for the Development of Vocational Training [CEDEFOP], 2011, p. 105). Relevant literature on the topic commonly alludes to three forms of learning: formal, non-formal, and informal learning.

Formal learning typically takes place within structured environments such as HEIs or training facilities. It follows an organized approach with clearly defined objectives, a timeframe, and resources, often resulting in formal qualification or certification (CEDEFOP, 2011), including undergraduate and graduate university studies. In contrast, non-formal learning occurs within planned activities that are not explicitly labeled as learning but may still adopt a structured approach and lead to formal qualifications (CEDEFOP, 2011). Examples include professional conferences, seminars, and CPD courses. Both formal and non-formal learning are deliberate from the learner's perspective. Informal learning, on the other hand, emerges from participation in daily activities at work, at home, or during leisure time. This form of learning is usually referred to as "experiential learning," which is often unstructured and unplanned (CEDEFOP, 2011).

In the Philippines, formal, non-formal, and informal learning are integrated in CPD for the continued practice of occupational therapy, as mandated by the Continuing Professional Development (CPD) Act of 2016 and the Philippine Occupational Therapy Law of 2018 (section 29). The PRC[1] will publish guidelines on the creation of a CPSP for occupational therapy once they are drafted by the Philippine Regulatory Board for Occupational Therapy.

Formal learning

For Filipino learners, including occupational therapists, formal learning pathways are defined in the Philippine Qualifications Framework (PQF),[2] which was launched in 2012 through Executive Order No. 83. The PQF serves as "the national system for the development, recognition and award of qualifications based on standards of knowledge, skills and values acquired in different ways and methods by learners and workers of the country."[3] It was collaboratively developed by the Department of Education (DepEd), Technical Education and Skills Development Authority (TESDA), Commission on Higher Education (CHED), Professional Regulation Commission (PRC), and the Department of Labor and Employment (DOLE) to allow learners to move easily between education and training sectors. It also aligns domestic standards with international frameworks, thereby enhancing comparability and supporting Filipino students' and workers' mobility. It consists of eight qualification levels distinguished from each other by a set of descriptions and learning outcomes in terms of knowledge, skills, and values; application; and degree of independence. Within the PQF, qualification levels 6, 7, and 8 correspond to bachelor's, master's, and doctoral studies, respectively (see Figure 5.1).

In the Philippines, occupational therapists make their way into the profession by completing an undergraduate (also called bachelor or baccalaureate) program equivalent to PQF Level 6 from a recognized HEI.

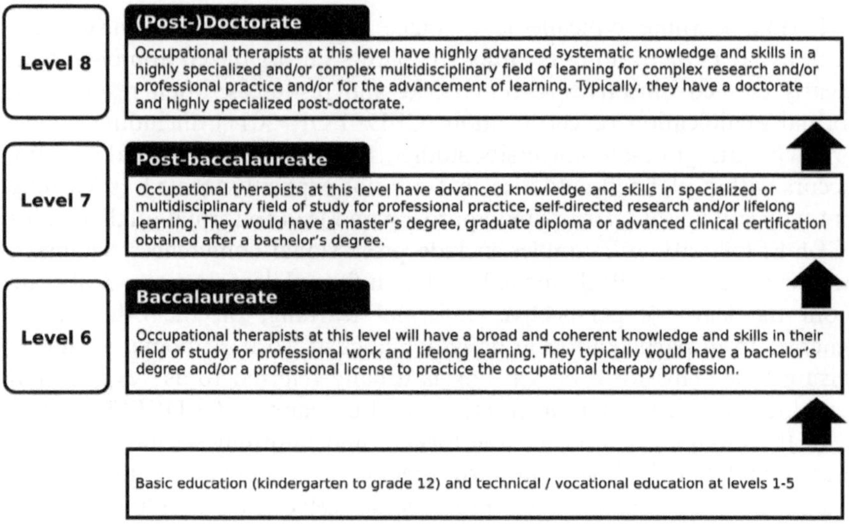

Level 8

(Post-)Doctorate

Occupational therapists at this level have highly advanced systematic knowledge and skills in a highly specialized and/or complex multidisciplinary field of learning for complex research and/or professional practice and/or for the advancement of learning. Typically, they have a doctorate and highly specialized post-doctorate.

Level 7

Post-baccalaureate

Occupational therapists at this level have advanced knowledge and skills in specialized or multidisciplinary field of study for professional practice, self-directed research and/or lifelong learning. They would have a master's degree, graduate diploma or advanced clinical certification obtained after a bachelor's degree.

Level 6

Baccalaureate

Occupational therapists at this level will have a broad and coherent knowledge and skills in their field of study for professional work and lifelong learning. They typically would have a bachelor's degree and/or a professional license to practice the occupational therapy profession.

Basic education (kindergarten to grade 12) and technical / vocational education at levels 1-5

Figure 5.1 Qualification levels adapted from the Philippine Qualifications Framework

Presently, there are five Bachelor of Science programs in Occupational Therapy approved by the World Federation of Occupational Therapists (WFOT).[4] These programs are offered by Cebu Doctors' University, Emilio Aguinaldo College, University of Santo Tomas College of Rehabilitation Sciences, University of the Philippines Manila, and Velez College. Through elective, short-term student exchange in foreign HEIs, study credits leading up to formal university qualifications may be accumulated. In this scenario, bilateral agreements between HEIs may include waived registration fees, which allows Filipino students to take otherwise costly courses at foreign HEIs. As a regulated profession, graduates of occupational therapy must also pass the national licensure examination for occupational therapists to be issued a professional license, thereby demonstrating their competence for the independent practice of the profession.

Beyond an undergraduate degree, occupational therapists in the Philippines may wish to pursue graduate education and gain higher competences in research, teaching, and professional practice (CHED, 2019). Graduate degrees in the Philippines include master's and doctoral programs, which correspond to PQF Levels 7 and 8, respectively. These levels require more advanced and specialized knowledge and skills in the field as well as a high degree of independence in conducting research. According to CHED (2019), graduate programs in the Philippines usually involve an Academic or Research Track on the one hand and a Professional Track on the other. However, the Academic Track, which is based on coursework combined with a thesis or dissertation, remains prevalent. Currently, Cebu

Doctors' University and the University of Santo Tomas offer Master of Arts in Occupational Therapy and Master of Science in Occupational Therapy programs, respectively. Other local programs for both master's and doctoral studies open to occupational therapy professionals include degrees in rehabilitation sciences, health professions education, special education, international health, business and health, community development, psychology, counseling, and public health, to name a few.

Overall, participation in graduate programs remains limited among Filipino Occupational therapists. According to PAOT's Workforce Survey (Carandang & Delos Reyes, 2018), only 5% of the surveyed population have completed graduate programs, mainly specializing in special education, rehabilitation science, and guidance counseling. This severely limits the engagement of Filipino occupational therapists in educator and researcher roles and potentially slows down the advancement of occupational therapy education and research in the country.

Non-formal learning

Currently, CPD programs are integrated into the Philippine Education and Training System as a form of non-formal learning in higher education alongside extension programs and certificate courses. According to the PRC (2017), CPD refers to "the inculcation of advanced knowledge, skills, and ethical values in a post-licensure specialization or an inter- or multidisciplinary field of study, for assimilation into professional practice, self-directed research and/or lifelong learning" (p. 2). In other countries, CPD is also referred to as continuing education and/or professional development and is viewed as a crucial component for the employability of individuals (CEDEFOP, 2011).

In the Philippines, only accredited providers can offer CPD courses for which CPD units may be awarded (see section 7.7 under additional resources to access the list of accredited CPD programs for occupational therapists). A minimum of 15 CPD units is required for the renewal of the professional license, which is set to be re-issued every three years (PAOT, 2019). Participants of accredited CPD programs are awarded CPD credit units, which can be accumulated towards a formal qualification in the future, including graduate programs (CHED, 2019).

While limited, some occupational therapists also specialize by attending certification courses. Based on PAOT's Workforce Survey (Carandang & Delos Reyes, 2018) with 268 respondents, 15% have completed certification courses, mainly in cognitive behavioral therapy, neuromuscular reflex integration, wheelchair training, and sensory integration. The survey also noted that such certification courses are commonly organized by the national association or local universities in the country, and rarely do the respondents become certified through programs not endorsed by the aforementioned institutions.

Informal learning

Learning experienced in daily life is integrated into the concept of CPD in the Philippines. During the COVID-19 pandemic, this mode of learning became particularly salient. According to the PRC (2021), informal learning, including professional work experience and other self-initiated activities, could be evaluated and granted CPD credit units. Examples of these activities include the following:

1   Self-study, which may include reading books, journal articles, magazines, or similar materials and viewing educational videos
2   Online learning activities (e.g., webinars, online courses)
3   Critically appraising journal articles as they relate to one's practice
4   Mentored experience
5   Provision of services to clients
6   Serving as a resource person for activities like public education
7   Participation in symposia and fora related to practice issues
8   Participation in socio-civic activities aimed at assisting efforts related to the public health emergency
9   Engagement in research either as investigator/author or as participant
10 Reviewer/evaluator of research/research proposals or projects

Beyond credit-bearing informal learning activities, social and reflective forms of learning are seen as an integral part of professional development. As for the former, *communities of practice*[5] (CoP) are widely viewed as means for learning and competence development. They have been defined as "groups of people who share a concern, a set of problems, a passion about a topic, and who deepen their knowledge and expertise in this area by interacting on an ongoing basis" (Wenger et al., 2002, p. 4). CoP has been reported by Barry and colleagues (2017) to be a source of knowledge and support for knowledge translation, i.e., application of knowledge in real-life situations. It also provides opportunities to engage in reflection on action with other professionals. Professional development could occur through interactions with occupational therapists and other professionals in other settings, roles, institutions, countries, and cultures. The concept and application of CoP flourished with the popularity of social media and other digital fora, facilitated by access to other professionals and both synchronous and asynchronous discussions over borders.

Reflection

Reflection plays a crucial role in all forms of learning, whether formal, non-formal, or informal. According to WFOT's Revised Minimum Standards for the Education of Occupational Therapists (2016), it is an essential aspect of competent occupational therapy practice. The document emphasizes the importance of "attitudes toward the need to update knowledge, skills, and attitudes throughout one's professional life through embracing life-long learning and reflection" (2016, p. 40). Reflective practice means "systematically, routinely, and critically thinking about [one's] practice, in order to maximize learning from experience" (WFOT, 2016, p. 71).

Occupational therapy graduates of WFOT-accredited entry-level programs are expected to have knowledge of reflective practice theories, skills in "systematically reflecting on the quality of all aspects of one's practice, both prior, during and after performance" (p. 40), and attitudes that view reflection on the effectiveness and consequences of one's actions as important for development (WFOT, 2016). As it is part of their basic education, occupational therapists should be aware of models related to reflection, such as Kolb's Experiential Learning Cycle (Kolb, 1984; Morris, 2020), Gibbs' Reflective Cycle (Gibbs, 1988), and the What model (Borton, 1970; Driscoll, 2006). Unfortunately, it has been reported that some practitioners are unaware of and do not use reflection models (e.g., Guy et al., 2020; Knightbridge, 2019). More information about these models can be read elsewhere, but we summarize them here. Kolb's cycle (1984; Morris, 2020) proposes four stages for one's learning:

1   Concrete experience: having the actual experience
2   Reflective observation: critically reflecting on the experience
3   Abstract conceptualization: conceptualizing the meaning of that experience (and thus learning from it)
4   Active experimentation: testing the learning on new situations

Gibbs' model (1988) provides a cyclical structure to understanding and learning from a specific experience or situation:

1   Description: describe the experience itself
2   Feelings: describe feelings and thoughts during the experience
3   Evaluation: evaluate what went well and not so well with the experience
4   Analysis: analyze why the experience turned out well or not so well
5   Conclusion: make conclusions about the experience and your learning from the experience
6   Action plan: Plan for how you would respond in a similar situation

On the other hand, the What model (Borton, 1970; Driscoll, 2006) poses three questions to guide reflection:

1   What? Describe the experience (or situation)
2   So what? Analyze the experience. That is, why was it important? What have you learned from it?
3   Now what? Apply the learning about this experience to a new situation

Some authors (e.g., Ghaye & Lillyman, 2010; Wong et al., 2016) have raised the concern that using reflective cycles often results in procedural thinking rather than reflection. It is important to avoid superficial responses to questions posed in these models, and instead objectively analyze aspects of the experience, relate to previous experiences, and identify gaps in knowledge in order to open oneself to new perspectives. Reflection is intended to enhance one's practice; hence, learning resulting from reflection should be applied when similar situations arise or when opportunity comes. Furthermore, as reflection could be triggered by challenges in practice situations (e.g., Krueger et al., 2020), practitioners often reflect on negative experiences and what they can do better next time (Wong et al., 2016). Dewey (1933) and Schön (1983), for example, focus on some negative state or problem that prompts reflection. If reflection is intended to "develop professional identity and artistry" (Johns, 2017), then it would be important to reflect on positive experiences to reinforce what one does sufficiently as well as augment implicit knowledge or "tacit recognitions, judgments and skillful performances" (Schön, 1983, p. 50). Instead of always reflecting on problems, Ghaye and Lillyman (2010) advocate engaging in "appreciative reflection," which emphasizes an appreciative intent towards knowing, relating, action, and organizing (p. 33). It is about "valuing and building upon what works, what makes us feel good, what we perceive as positive, and what gives us a sense of strength and well-being in the work we do" (Marchi, 2011, p. 181). Through appreciative reflection, practitioners could develop a more positive vision of practice and strive towards it. Strengths-based questions could also develop positive language, empower people to communicate, and foster a sense of community. Ghaye and Lillyman (2010, p. 37) suggest these core questions to facilitate strengths-based reflective practice:

1   What is currently working well and why?
2   What needs changing and how?
3   What are you/we learning and so what do we do next?
4   Where do you/we go from here and what are its implications?

Reflection serves as an essential tool for individuals, including occupational therapists, enabling them to gain insights into their practice and identify learning needs necessary for adapting to changing circumstances and challenges. By embracing reflection, occupational therapists can continuously improve their skills and knowledge throughout their careers, making reflection a cornerstone of lifelong learning.

After developing a reflective practice, it is crucial to move beyond it and engage in critical reflection. According to Mezirow (1990), critical reflection "involves a critique of the presuppositions on which our beliefs have been built" (p. 1). Filipino occupational therapists should not only reflect on their actions and experiences to determine what should be done next, but also start questioning the basis of their thinking and how they address these experiences. This means challenging established assumptions and understandings surrounding their occupational therapy practice and the issues they encounter, and opening themselves up to new perspectives that reorient their thinking.

Engaging in formal learning activities provides structured opportunities for occupational therapists to reassess how they have defined and addressed problems and to reevaluate their own pre-understandings, perceptions, and attitudes over a prolonged period. Additionally, participating in non-formal and informal learning activities outside of one's main field of study or specialization can expose occupational therapists to new views and perspectives, potentially challenging existing assumptions about occupational therapy. On a micro level, reflection and critical reflection empower occupational therapists to refine their skills and knowledge through self-evaluation and ongoing learning. On a macro level, lifelong learning fosters the reskilling and upskilling of individuals, thereby promoting economic growth and societal advancement.

Filipino occupational therapists' lifelong learning stories

This section presents four occupational therapists' experiences of formal, non-formal, and informal learning. Their stories demonstrate the potential of these modalities to reinforce each other and how they enhance not just the professional but also the personal lives of the learners.

Aaron and Maria were both doing their internship for their undergraduate program when they learned about the three-month student exchange program in Sweden. Maria was interested in being immersed in an international community as well as learning about different practice areas such as hand therapy, user interaction and knowledge modeling. Meanwhile, Aaron wanted to widen his perspective of the profession and experience the similarities and differences between his practice in the Philippines and in a foreign country. Both Maria and Aaron had high hopes when they embarked on their learning journey. Maria was looking to apply what she would learn in her practice in the Philippines, while Aaron imagined himself as being less afraid to try out new things, being more culturally competent, and gaining an international experience that could give him a competitive edge in the labor market.

Maria and Aaron's exchange program involved a clinical rotation at the hand and surgery clinic of the host's university hospital. They also spent time in a role-emerging setting doing collaborative work with the computing sciences department on assistive technology, with the goal of developing content that can guide clients with cognitive impairments in a chosen activity. Their duties would start from 9 AM to 3 PM from Mondays to Thursdays, and they had the chance to see many clients due to shorter sessions of 15 to 30 minutes. Besides their coursework, they also engaged with the local community. Maria would hang out with her buddy group in the afternoon, while Aaron dined out and had field trips with other international students during weekends. At a personal level, Aaron appreciated being able to maintain a balance between work and leisure and aimed to sustain his professional practice by nurturing these aspects of his life.

Beyond the personal benefits, the formal learning space provided by the study exchange program allowed both Maria and Aaron to grow as healthcare practitioners. Maria identified becoming more adaptable, culturally competent, and confident as a result. As she shares:

> I think being in a new country challenged me to adapt to a lot of things, [including] differences in climate and culture ... This facilitated my personal development which also positively influenced my professional self. I developed cultural competence. I was more confident in expressing my ideas and opinions. Before, I was usually too afraid to voice out my thoughts as I am afraid of what my professors will say about it, but the social environment in Sweden was so accepting of different perspectives and that encouraged me to speak.

Learning to become more open about his opinions was also one of the highlights of Aaron's study exchange experience, which he was then able to apply in his role as an instructor at a university:

> The educators and supervisors I met in Sweden were so approachable. I can freely ask questions and say my thoughts without being so nervous. I was used to being fearful of my mentors but my mentors in Sweden taught me how to be open and maintain professional relationships among students. That's why when I became an instructor in the university, I also made sure that my students could openly ask and discuss their ideas with me.

Additionally, Aaron was also given the freedom to plan his tasks, which enabled him to learn the value of independence and accountability for his role as an occupational therapist. As he shared:

> I was really surprised when we were trusted to create and follow our own timelines during our collaborative work with the Computing Sciences department ... I think the practice of creating and following our own timeline gives us more independence and forces us to be more accountable as budding professionals. In reality, when one becomes an occupational therapist, one must know how to be efficient in delivering tasks.

For Aaron, the study exchange program and the exposure to advanced economies triggered a reflective process that then led him to adopt a systemic view in his professional practice:

> Seeing how things work in a developed country makes me want to always think of ways on how I can improve things in my current workplace here in the Philippines. I appreciate how I was wired to be hardworking, resourceful, and creative; but as an occupational therapist and with this exchange student experience, I realized that we can also look at the system, process, and the environment so we can be more efficient and effective. Just like how we analyze the PEO (person-environment-occupation) factors of our clients—no need to always focus on the P aspect alone.

Meanwhile, Maria also alluded to the outcome of the study exchange in making her realize the value of developing herself professionally and resulted in an expansion of her career horizons beyond being a clinician. In her words:

> The exchange program opened up my interest in research and the value of professional development. It gave me the realization that learning will continue after graduation and that there are a lot of opportunities for me to grow within the profession—that it is not only about being a clinician, and that there are a lot of practice areas to explore. It was during the exchange program that I realized that I will direct my own learning after I leave the university... that it is my action to develop my own personal learning objectives and engage in activities to achieve them, such as attending seminars and conferences, looking for mentors ...

For Julia and Cha, embarking on the journey of doing a graduate study was a worthwhile goal to pursue. Julia was a full-time faculty member then at a university in the Philippines, while Cha was working as an occupational therapist in private clinics. Julia felt that a master's degree would allow her to advance her career and to achieve her dream of having a doctorate degree, so she enrolled part-time in a Master of Science in Occupational Therapy program at a Manila-based university. Cha, whose desire to pursue higher studies abroad was sparked by her exchange experience as an intern, decided to attend a similar program in Edinburgh, UK as a full-time student. In both cases, the experience enhanced their motivation to pursue continuing education. Julia also developed a greater appreciation of the importance of research in the profession, while the self-directed learning approach in Cha's program allowed her to more deeply engage with occupational science, an area of interest but a topic that she previously had limited knowledge of. She was also grateful for the mentorship she received during the program, which gave her the valuable opportunity to discuss and work alongside experts in her field. Julia is currently enrolled in a doctoral program while Cha is able to incorporate what she had learned about research and occupational science into her work as a university instructor.

The experiences of Maria, Aaron, Julia, and Cha point to the value of lifelong learning for occupational therapists and the synergies that occur between formal (coursework), non-formal (mentoring), and informal (community) learning spaces. Despite the relatively short time spent by Maria and Aaron as exchange students, their experience yielded important benefits not just in the form of professional competences (such as cultural competence, systems thinking, independence, self-directed learning, and adaptability) but also expanded imaginings for their career and learning goals. Meanwhile, Julia and Cha's pursuit of graduate studies reinforced their interest in and capacities for doing research, which could have wider effects to build the capacity of future occupational therapists in engaging with scholarship and evidence-informed practice.

Conclusion

Lifelong learning, recognized globally for its role in personal and societal development, is particularly crucial for Filipino occupational therapists to maintain professional competences and adapt to evolving practice demands. Formal learning, such as university education and specialized training, is supplemented by non-formal activities like CPD courses and certification programs. Additionally, informal learning includes self-initiated activities such as on-the-job experiences and self-directed study. Reflection, a key component across all these learning forms, enables occupational therapists to critically evaluate their practice, identify areas for improvement, and contribute to their ongoing professional development. Overall, lifelong learning empowers occupational therapists to enhance their skills, advance their careers, and ultimately contribute to both personal growth and societal progress.

Questions for reflection and suggestions for action

1 What makes you happy and fulfilled in your work? How do you envision yourself in 5, 10, or 20 years? What are your priorities right now? How do your priorities fit into your vision? Draft a career development plan. In this document, include a vision statement about how you envision your career, goals to bring you closer to your vision, what skills you have now and what skills you need, and an action plan.

2   What are the formal, non-formal, and informal learning pathways needed to pursue your personal and professional goals? What are the barriers to engaging in these activities and what types of support can you seek to overcome them? Plan and record your CPD activities. Identify certified CPD providers and identify ways to get regularly updated about their CPD course offerings. If they are on social media, you can follow them. Maintain a system for documenting the CPD activities you have participated in.

3   For what purpose would you develop and maintain a professional portfolio? What elements do you think are important to include in a portfolio? Draft an ePortfolio. An ePortfolio is a digital collection of artifacts documenting your various experiences from formal, non-formal, and informal learning. It can include certificates, reports, project ideas and proposals, notes from self-study, research and teaching activities, practice, and civic and other professional activities. Most importantly, it should include personal reflections on these learning experiences, which distinguishes it from a curriculum vitae where one's merits are listed. Depending on the purpose of your portfolio, you can decide to open or restrict access to others.

Notes

1   https://www.prc.gov.ph/guidelines-creation-career-progression-and-specialization-program
2   URL: https://pqf.gov.ph/
3   What is PQF? (n.d.). Retrieved 17 December 2022 from https://pqf.gov.ph/Home/Details/3
4   https://www.wfot.org/programmes/education/wfot-approved-education-programmes
5   https://www.wenger-trayner.com/introduction-to-communities-of-practice/

References

Barry, M., Kuijer, W., Nieuwenhuis, A. F., & Scherpbier, N. (2017). Communities of Practice: a means to support occupational therapists' continuing professional development. A literature review. *Australian Occupational Therapy Journal*, 64(2), 185–193. doi:10.1111/1440-1630.12334.

Borton, T. (1970). *Reach, touch, and teach*. McGraw-Hill.

Carandang, K. A., & Delos Reyes, R. C. (2018). *Workforce survey 2017: Working conditions and salary structure of occupational therapists working in the Philippines survey*. Philippine Academy of Occupational Therapists. Retrieved from https://paot.org.ph/pdf/other/Workforce%20Survey%202017%20Technical%20Report.pdf.

CEDEFOP. (2011). *Glossary: Quality in education and training*. Office of the European Union. Retrieved December 17, 2022, from https://www.cedefop.europa.eu/files/4106_en.pdf.

CHED. (2006). *CHED Memorandum No. 24 Series of 2006. Policies, standards, and guidelines for Physical Therapy and Occupational Therapy education.* Retrieved December 31, 2022, from https://paot.org.ph/pdf/education/CHED% 20Memo%20No.24%20(2006).pdf.

CHED. (2017). *Memorandum Order 52, Series of 2017. Policies, standards and guidelines for the Bachelor of Science in Occupational Therapy (BSOT) education program.* https://ched.gov.ph/wp-content/uploads/2018/04/CMO-No.-52-Ser ies-of-2017-Policies-Standards-and-Guidelines-for-the-Bachelor- of-Science-in-Occupational-Therapy-Education-BSOT-Program.pdf.

CHED. (2019). *AQRF referencing report of the Philippines.* May 28, 2019. Retrieved October 12, 2022, from https://asean.org/wp-content/uploads/2017/03/ AQRF-Referencing-Report-of-the-Philippines-22-May-2019_FINAL2.pdf.

Dewey, J. (1933). *How we think: A restatement of the relation of reflective thinking to the educative process.* D.C. Heath & Co Publishers.

Driscoll, J. (2006). *Practising clinical supervision: A reflective approach for health-care professionals* (2nd ed.). Bailliere Tindall Elsevier.

Ghaye, T., & Lillyman, S. (2010). *Reflection: Principles and practices for heathcare professionals* (2nd ed.). MA Healthcare Limited.

Gibbs, G. (1988). *Learning by doing: A guide to teaching and learning methods.* Oxford Brookes University.

Guy, L., Cranwell, K., Hitch, D., & McKinstry, C. (2020). Reflective practice facilitation within occupational therapy supervision processes: A mixed method study. *Australian Occupational Therapy Journal*, 67(4), 320–329. doi:10.1111/ 1440-1630.12660.

Johns, C. M. (2017). Imagining reflective practice. In C. Johns (Ed.), *Becoming a reflective practitioner* (5th ed., pp. 1–20). John Wiley & Sons.

Knightbridge, L. (2019). Reflection-in-practice: A survey of Australian occupa-tional therapists. *Australian Occupational Therapy Journal*, 66(3), 337–346. doi:10.1111/1440-1630.12559.

Kolb, D. A. (1984). *Experiential learning: Experience as the result of learning and development.* Prentice Hall.

Krueger, R. B., Sweetman, M. M., Martin, M., & Cappaert, T. A. (2020). Self-reflection as a support to evidence-based practice: A grounded theory explora-tion. *Occupational Therapy in Health Care*, 34(4), 320–350. doi:10.1080/ 07380577.2020.1815929.

Marchi, S. (2011). Co-constructing an appreciative and collective eye: Appreciative reflection in action in lifelong career guidance. *Reflective Practice*, 12(2), 179–194. doi:10.1080/14623943.2011.561530.

Mezirow, J. (1990). *Fostering critical reflection in adulthood.* Jossey-Bass Publishers.

Morris, T. H. (2020). Experiential learning—A systematic review and revision of Kolb's model. *Interactive Learning Environments*, 28(8), 1064–1077. doi:10.1080/ 10494820.2019.1570279.

PAOT. (n.d.). Position Statement on Special Interest Groups. Retrieved July 3, 2024, from https://paot.org.ph/downloads.html.

PAOT. (2019). *Essential features of Republic Act No. 11241: The Philippine Occu-pational Therapy Law of 2018.* Retrieved December 7, 2022, from http://paot.org. ph/pdf/otlaw/Essential%20Features%20of%20the%20Philippine%20OT%20Law% 20of%202018%20(RA%2011241).pdf.

PAOT. (2020). Guidelines on the Institutionalization and Governance of Special Interest Groups (Board Resolution No. 2020–2003). Retrieved July 3, 2024, from https://paot.org.ph/downloads.html.

Philippine Occupational Therapy Law of 2018. (2019). Senate of the Philippines Legislative Reference Bureau. Retrieved December 31, 2022, from https://issua nces-library.senate.gov.ph/subject/philippine-occupational-therapy-law-of-2018.

PRC. (2017). *Implementing rules and regulations (IRR) of Republic Act No. 10912, known as the "Continuing Professional Development (CPD) Act of 2016."* Retrieved December 30, 2022, from https://www.prc.gov.ph/sites/default/files/ CPD_IRR_p%202016.pdf.

PRC. (2021). *Continuing Professional Development Council of Occupational Therapy, Resolution No. 02 Series of 2021. Guidelines on the evaluation and granting of CPD credit units to activities under informal learning and professional work experience including activities undertaken during the state of public health emergency due to COVID-19 crisis that may earn CPD credit units.* Retrieved December 7, 2022, from https://www.prc.gov.ph/sites/default/files/2021-02CPD%20OT.pdf.

PRC. (2022). *Resolution No. 1591 Series of 2022. Guideline on the accreditation of specialty society/organization and other specialty categories providing structured training programs for professionals.* Retrieved July 3, 2024, from https://www.prc. gov.ph/sites/default/files/2022-1591%20published.pdf.

Schön, D. A. (1983). *The reflective practitioner: How professionals think in action.* Basic Books.

UNESCO. (2015). *Rethinking education—Towards a global common good?* Retrieved December 31, 2022, from http://unesdoc.unesco.org/images/0023/ 002325/232555e.pdf.

UNESCO. (2016). *Education 2030: Incheon Declaration and Framework for Action for the implementation of Sustainable Development Goal 4.* Retrieved December 17, 2022, from https://unesdoc.unesco.org/ark:/48223/pf0000245656.

UNESCO Institute for Lifelong Learning. (2022). *UIL Policy Brief 14: Transforming higher education institutions into lifelong learning institutions.* Retrieved October 26, 2024, from https://unesdoc.unesco.org/ark:/48223/pf0000382491.locale=en.

Wenger, E., McDermott, R. A., & Snyder, W. (2002). *Cultivating communities of practice: A guide to managing knowledge.* Harvard Business Press.

WFOT. (2016). *Minimum standards for the education of occupational therapists - Revised 2016.* Retrieved August 12, 2022, from https://wfot.org/resources/new-m inimum-standards-for-the-education-of-occupational-therapists-2016-e-copy.

Wong, K. Y., Whitcombe, S. W., & Boniface, G. (2016). Teaching and learning the esoteric: An insight into how reflection may be internalised with reference to the occupational therapy profession. *Reflective Practice,* 17(4), 472–482. doi:10.1080/14623943.2016.1175341.

Chapter 6

Becoming a Filipino occupational therapy educator

Michael Sy, Chamaine Kristabel De Vera-Fevidal and Maria Elizabeth Grageda

Chapter objectives

1 Discuss the process of transforming occupational therapy education and training through cultivating a systems-based curriculum, occupation-focused instruction, and transformative learning experiences

2 Describe the Technological-Pedagogical and Content Knowledge (TPaCK) model as a guide in designing and developing occupational therapy teaching-learning opportunities for students.

3 Outline the process of becoming an occupational therapy education as a career pathway

4 Narrate the experiences of an occupational therapist who transitioned to an educator role

Becoming is the process of redefining values and rethinking priorities to prepare for a new life role. After some time of studying, training, and practicing, some occupational therapists would see themselves transitioning from a clinical to an educator role. An educator working in a university is primarily responsible for teaching content, training competencies, and supervising practice to aid the qualification of the next generation of occupational therapists. However, occupational therapy educators of today must be cognizant that educating students today is different from how the educators were taught and trained. This compels occupational therapy educators to be continuously attuned to the local needs and be critical towards dominant approaches from both practice and education to transform the occupational therapy curriculum, training, and continuing professional development activities. This chapter will discuss the expectation from educators to bring forward systems-based educational approaches, entailing the need to outline the intersection between core, profession-centric, and interprofessional competencies for occupational therapy students today. To do that, educators in occupational therapy programs must have expertise in occupational therapy epistemologies, teaching and learning methodologies, and technological utility via the

DOI: 10.4324/9781003321217-6

Technological, Pedagogical and Content Knowledge (TPaCK) model by Mishra and Koehler (2006). We then outline the process of becoming an occupational therapy educator in the Philippines. This chapter ends with a story related by one of the authors about her personal journey from being a clinician to becoming an occupational therapy educator.

Transforming occupational therapy education

The educational process within the occupational therapy profession is attempting to evolve from a biomedical to a more occupation-focused approach to curriculum, instruction, and training. This intentional shift should not be surprising as this indicates how occupational therapy education and training today are becoming more conscious of its history rooted in the therapeutic power of occupations towards health (Turcotte & Holmes, 2021). If we would describe this shift as transformational, then there needs to be a permanent and irreversible change in terms of how occupational therapists think, feel, and act today. But what change do these shifts in education and training entail? If we are referring to Mezirow's theory on transformative learning (Mezirow, 1978, 1991), this change denotes a change in how adult learners behave, think, and act during and after engaging in learning experiences and critical dialoguing with the self and fellow learners. In other words, transformative education entails a shift in worldview and a permanent and irreversible change in behavior, both resulting in an expansion of the self and a contribution to praxis change. Otherwise, the concept "transformative" remains a buzzword that occupational therapy educators use out of trend, rather than an educational approach that intentionally produces significant change in thinking, feeling, and interacting of learners towards social change (Hoggan, 2016).

At the turn of the twenty-first century, when the world had seen global health crises and more complex health conditions of people and populations, health professionals required education and training about the health system, as well as seeing the system's parts and seeing it as a whole. They called this third-generation educational reform "systems-based curriculum" (Frenk et al., 2010). Embracing a systems-based curriculum requires an expansion from science-based (first-generation) and problem-based (second-generation) health professions education. This means that health profession students, including occupational therapy students, must learn that people and populations' health are not merely affected by bodily diseases but are equally influenced by systems constituted by physical environments and societal structures. Shifting the focus of learning on the systems level thus requires the development of not only profession-specific (e.g., occupational therapy assessment skills), but also core professional (e.g., use of technology, analytical and problem-solving skills), and interprofessional competencies (i.e., teamwork, conflict resolution).

For occupational therapy education to be transformative, it is important that occupational therapy educators cultivate teaching practices that encourage critical questioning of dominant worldviews about health and disability, develop knowledge and skills that are translated into different contexts and settings, and welcome pluralistic perspectives and conceptualizations on the meaning of occupation to diverse groups of people (Zafran, 2020). One way of cultivating transformative learning for occupational therapy students is by providing instruction that foregrounds occupation as a concept. Fisher (2013) coined the terms: occupation-centered, occupation-based, and occupation-focused. While these terms differ in how and where they are used, they share a common value of putting occupation at the core of occupational therapy research, education, and practice. For instance, an occupation-focused curriculum will be designed based on areas of occupation (e.g., self-care, work, leisure, and play) rather than diseases and medical pathologies. As a result, occupational therapy students will not be limited in becoming competent clinicians, but also competent practitioners who are taught to navigate the ever-changing needs of contemporary societies beyond clinical practice.

Occupational therapy educational programs in the Philippines have constantly been revised according to WFOT and local standards (Cabatan & Duque, 2020), yet remnants of the biomedical paradigm continue to dominate and silence the movement towards becoming more occupation-centered (Turcotte & Holmes, 2023). Concretely, this situation can be attributed to the fact that many occupational therapy educational programs are still closely linked with the medical school and teaching hospital within universities. Although this allows for better access and linkage with the health and medical aspects of teaching, learning, and training occupational therapy, it can somehow limit opportunities for students to learn about and think about occupational therapy as a profession beyond clinical practice. For example, when occupational therapy programs are isolated from social work programs, it could reduce opportunities to learn about social policy work in relation to health, community development, and public social service work. Hence, it is crucial that occupational therapy educators seek opportunities to take advantage of technology, learn about different ways of teaching, and collaborate with other disciplines and professions beyond the biomedical field to inform occupational therapy education. Chapter 4 discusses the undergraduate program for occupational therapy in the Philippines.

TPaCK: An instructional model to enact transformative education

Keeping in mind the perspective of Mezirow's transformative learning theory, this chapter will be highlighting the Technological, Pedagogical and Content Knowledge (TPaCK) model by Mishra and Koehler (2006) as a guide in instructional and curricular designing in occupational therapy education and training. While we are aware that other instructional models are being used by other occupational therapy educators, we will be using the TPaCK to pay greater attention in guiding our readers to use technology effectively (Saubern et al., 2020) in occupational therapy teaching and learning.

In this section, we describe the TPaCK model and its components in relation to occupational therapy education (see Figure 6.1). This will be followed by a discussion of how we can integrate these conceptual components in designing occupational therapy teaching and learning sessions in the classroom and clinical placements. We begin by describing Content Knowledge, Pedagogical Knowledge, and Technological Knowledge. Then, we move to describing the intersections of these knowledges: Pedagogical Content Knowledge, Technological Pedagogical Knowledge, and Technological Content Knowledge.

We start with Content Knowledge (CK), which pertains to "what" is being taught. They can be knowledge of facts, concepts, and theories. For example, CK can be facts about local occupational therapy history, definitions of occupational therapy terms such as "occupational justice," and theories like the Model of Human Occupation by Gary Kielhofner and the Kawa Model by Michael Iwama. However, CK alone is not an assurance that occupational therapy students will effectively learn; teachers need Pedagogical Knowledge (PK) to know how to teach this CK.

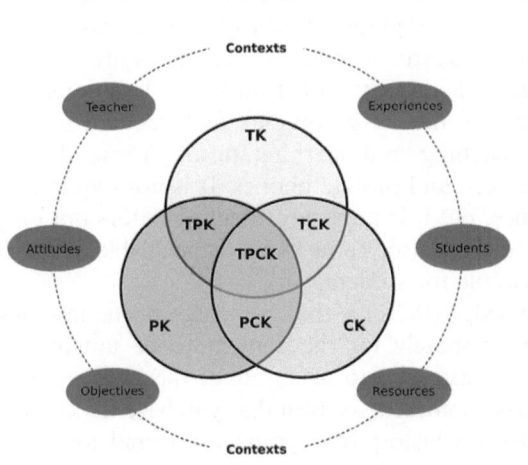

Content Knowledge (CK)
What is to be taught?
Examples: local occupational therapy history; definition, terms, and theories in occupational therapy

Pedagogical Knowledge (PK)
What teaching model is used?
Examples: learning theories and their application, strategies for teaching, and assessment of learning

Technological Knowledge (TK)
What technology(s) is/are available for teaching and learning?
Example: different types of technologies, i.e., low-, mid-, and high-technologies in education

Pedagogical Content Knowledge (PCK)
How do we teach and facilitate learning in this specific content effectively?
Example: using advanced reading assignments and group work to teach history in occupational therapy

Technological Pedagogical Knowledge (TPK)
How do we adapt our teaching and learning facilitation using technology?
Examples: using online databases, recorded videos online, archives from libraries, interviewing key people

Technological Content Knowledge (TCK)
How do we improve the content through the application of technology?
Example: invite key personalities to join your class via videoconferencing to give a talk about historical events in occupational therapy

Figure 6.1 The TPaCK Model by Mishra and Koehler (2006) with examples as applied in occupational therapy teaching and learning processes

PK entails knowledge of learning theories, methods of teaching, assessment of learning, and designing a teaching and learning plan. For example, PK can include Mastery Learning by Benjamin Bloom or critical pedagogy by Paulo Freire. Knowing these learning theories can inform how you design your modules or syllabi. When using Mastery Learning, you are conscious that your modules begin by introducing basic principles (e.g., defining the concept of occupation), and then move towards building more complex principles (e.g., critiquing the conceptualization of occupation from different perspectives) in occupational therapy as they move along the next modules. When framing your syllabi from Critical Pedagogy, you will be designing your classes with a lot of dialogical sessions wherein both teacher and students discuss their lived experiences in terms of social realities, oppressive experiences, and politics. The classes are not limited to the classroom because, as a teacher, you will be exposing your students to the real world where they can get information about social realities through note taking, taking photos, and journaling. These snippets of information are then brought back into your class, whether online or on campus, for a dialogical session. The session will then end up identifying themes that can be used to inform the next sessions or the final assignment.

Technological Knowledge (TK) entails knowledge about standard technological tools for teaching and acquiring content for learning. TK also involves knowledge in the operation and use of these technologies to facilitate teaching and learning. There are three types of technologies used for teaching and learning: low-tech, mid-tech, and high-tech. Low-tech devices are inexpensive, simple, and do not require batteries or electricity. They include chalk, rulers, and highlighters. Mid-tech devices are digital and require batteries or a power source to operate. Examples are calculators, audiobooks, and a digital dictionary with translation functions. Hi-tech devices are computer-based and have complex features that can be adapted based on specific teaching and learning needs. These devices include laptop computers, tablets, and mobile phones. It is not required to use all these devices all at once, but it is important that educators not only know these types of devices, but also know what is available in their institutions and what is accessible for students.

Pedagogical Content Knowledge (PCK) is the knowledge of the teaching method to be used most appropriately for the content to be taught and learned. For instance, you were assigned to teach about the local occupational therapy history for first-year students. Given that you have the content knowledge of occupational therapy history from your own formal education and continuing learning, you are now challenged to teach it effectively to your students. The question is: how are you going to teach it? Of course, with academic freedom in mind, you are free to teach it either the way you were taught or differently. But when you become more conscientious about your PCK, considering that your students now are from a different generation, you may want to be more intentional in your lesson planning. For instance, you may include the integration of advanced reading assignment (PK) of records pertaining to the local occupational therapy history (CK) as well as group work (PK), where each group will generate a timeline with historical milestones (CK) of an assigned historical period.

Technological Pedagogical Knowledge (TPK) will now have to be in place to further improve teaching your course. TPK is your knowledge of how teaching can be adapted based on the technologies you know are available for teaching and learning. Going back to our example above, your advanced reading assignment can also include readings and records that come from online databases, YouTube videos, archives from the library and museums, and interviewing historical figures via a video conferencing application. To enhance the group work activity, you may also ask the students to create timelines through an infographic. Since you are aware of low-tech and hi-tech devices, you will give them the freedom to create the infographic using an A1-sized easel paper with drawing materials or using digital design software.

Technological Content Knowledge (TCK) is the knowledge on how technology and content are interrelated. In other words, this domain expects teachers to know how the subject matter can be changed or adapted with the application of technology. Referring to our example, you will think that it is challenging to change the history of occupational therapy as a subject matter (CK). While it makes no sense changing the dates and key information about history in general, what TCK intends to contribute to the TPaCK model is to acknowledge the ability of the teacher to raise the way learners think from simple to more complex processes with the aid of technology. For example, provided that your students were already tasked to do advanced reading assignments and group work activities, you may then maximize technological infrastructure in an institution to invite a historical figure into your class through a videoconferencing platform to facilitate an online interview (TK) in a talk show format with the whole class. Using this hi-tech arrangement can enrich your students' current knowledge on the subject matter by acquiring undocumented stories and information from a primary source.

We have just provided you with some approaches, with specific examples, on how to design your instruction guided by the TPaCK model. Considering the shift to a more hybridized arrangement of occupational therapy educational programs today, it is inevitable not to foreground the use of technology as part of the teaching and learning process.

Becoming an occupational therapy educator

Entry-level occupational therapists are usually expected to work in clinics to practice as healthcare providers for people of all ages in different settings. Although numerous clinical pathways are available for occupational therapists, our professional competencies afford us the flexibility to carve out our own career paths beyond clinical practice. One of the narrow yet worthwhile career paths Filipino occupational therapists go into is higher education (Cabatan et al., 2020). The latest survey from the national association revealed that approximately 30 occupational therapists work as an occupational therapy educator (Carandang & Delos Reyes, 2018). In this career path, a range of roles are expected, such as teaching, assessing student learning, supervising clinical interns, selecting students for admission, facilitating administrative work, leading research groups, engaging in community service, and publishing scholarly works (Cabatan et al., 2020).

To begin a career in academia, a Filipino occupational therapist (the "aspirant") typically would take a part-time or full-time instructor or clinical supervisor job in any academic institution or teaching hospital. Full-time work in higher education entails five days (40 hours) of workload in a week, whereas a part-time work arrangement would require fewer hours. Anyone who would work as an educator typically has to fulfill the requisites outlined in Table 6.1.

Among the master's degree programs available locally and internationally, the occupational therapy track is the most common path that aspirants take to assume academic posts according to the memorandum (CHED, 2017). Similarly, taking advanced degrees in education or educational sciences

Table 6.1 Minimum requirements to be fulfilled to become an occupational therapy educator

World Federation of Occupational Therapists (2017)	*Commission on Higher Education (CHED, 2017)*
• Graduate from an occupational therapy education program approved by WFOT	• Must possess a bachelor's degree in occupational therapy
• Possession of a higher qualification than the education program will offer, or a commitment for obtaining the qualification	• Registered and licensed occupational therapist in the Philippines (if licensed abroad, must be recognized by the Professional Regulations Commission)
• Varied clinical, teaching, and leadership experience	• Have at least one year of clinical experience
• Understanding the local culture	• Have completed a master's degree aligned with, or allied to, occupational therapy
• Fluency in the language of the country	• Must be a member of the accredited professional organization
	• Minimum of 20 hours of training in outcomes-based education

Note: For the lead, a full-time contract is a requirement. For faculty members, they should also have a mix of professional backgrounds, qualifications, and experiences.

would equip aspirants with competencies that are more focused on acquiring pedagogical competencies. For instance, taking a Master of Health Professions Education entails taking formal courses on educational philosophy, instructional and curriculum design, test construction, program evaluation, educational administration, education research, and electives that equip pedagogical competencies specific to health sciences. Other professional development activities towards becoming a more competent educator and occupational therapist are discussed in Chapter 5.

Following the American academic ranking system, a Filipino occupational therapy educator typically begins at the entry-level position called "instructor" (Sy Su, 2015) whose main duty is to teach undergraduate courses, assist laboratory sessions, mark and grade assignments and outputs, and attend to committee work. Once the aspirant obtains a recognized master's degree, a promotion is given towards becoming an assistant professor. Aside from the roles of an instructor, an *assistant professor* is given more research and administrative duties while potentially working towards obtaining a Ph.D. Completing a Ph.D. with a reasonable number of reputable publications allows the aspirant to be promoted to *associate professor* with tenure. At this point, the aspirant becomes a recognized occupational therapy academic. In a research-intensive university, obtaining the title *professor* means long-term commitment to do more research, obtain grants, and develop new courses for both undergraduate and graduate programs. In the Philippine context, this academic trajectory is uncommon since there are only a few occupational therapists who have obtained the "professor" title. While this trajectory may not be applicable to all, these titles and associated roles can be adjusted based on the type of institution, country, and context. In certain occassions, someone without a Ph.D. can still become a professor.

Expanding educator opportunities

Not all occupational therapy programs in the Philippines are designated research universities. Some are operating under a community college or a professional institute. These institutions typically hire occupational therapists who could mainly teach courses for entry-level occupational therapy students who would become part of the workforce. Aspirants who would apply to these institutions are designated instructor or clinical instructor positions with limited opportunities to do research. It is, however, equally important to emphasize that some occupational therapists desire to primarily engage in teaching through supervisorship and mentorship.

Clinical supervisors are typically based in affiliated institutions which can be a community clinic, hospital, or a non-profit institution where occupational services are rendered (CHED, 2017). Their main role is to supervise occupational therapy students during their clinical placements.

While only affiliated to the academic institutions, supervisors are responsible for ascertaining the completion of the 1,200 internship hours required for occupational therapy students to complete the occupational therapy program and consequently take the licensure exam (CHED, 2017). A mentor could come from any institution or facility and be willing to provide support to young occupational therapists in terms of their professional and career development and personal growth. Mentorship is encapsulated in a partnership between the mentor (or group of mentors) and the mentee. The one receiving mentorship or support is commonly younger than the mentor in terms of age and experience (Gutierrez, 2016). To initiate this partnership, a mentee usually selects a mentor based on expertise, experience, and trust. Unlike supervision, which is more structured in nature with a definitive timeline, mentorship typically constitutes structured and unstructured arrangements between the mentor and the mentee, bounded by short- and long-term goals for personal and professional development.

Other career paths await an aspirant in case he or she does not want to engage in research-heavy and teaching-intensive workloads. They could opt to choose an administrative path by becoming a program lead, a department chair, or a dean of a faculty or college. One can also become an evaluator after obtaining years of experience in academia and work with accrediting institutions to do auditing and tuning roles. Moreover, other pathways can include working in policymaking where the aspirant can merge one's scholarship into governmental engagements as well as community service where one can focus on providing expertise in service provisions for the university and other partner institutions across varied sectors.

Becoming an educator is not all about teaching. It is also about being able to generate what you will teach. Becoming an educator entails learning about various fields and perspectives, not only for use in practice but also for use in the creation of new knowledge. Educators are expected to juxtapose, intersect, and critique past, present, and future knowledge, creating new ones to be passed on to the next generation of occupational therapists through educational opportunities. For instance, it is valuable to have members of the faculty who are not just occupational therapists but also those with advanced degrees in occupational science, assistive technology, sociology, architecture, medical rehabilitation, social work, community development, and other fields that are related to occupational therapy. Having a team of educators who can bring in their varied expertise in designing a course or a whole curriculum will not only make the teaching and learning experiences of the students interdisciplinary but also expansive and future-proof.

The outcome of Mezirow's transformative learning perspective is expansive learning, which entails the ability to understand knowledge from pluralistic perspectives, question it, identify the problem, develop solutions, reflect on the process, and learn something new. Allowing our students to develop this way of thinking orients our students to think about the future. Educators of today need to learn not only about teaching and developing competencies that are relevant today but those that will be useful in the next five to ten years. Hence, wise educators will be integrating future-focused outcomes to develop competencies that will be useful to occupational therapy such as using artificial intelligence, data analytics, content creation, entrepreneurship, digital designing, computer programming, robotics, learning different languages and cultures; the list goes on.

From the hospital to the university: Chronicling an educator's journey

To conclude this chapter, we would like to share with you a story by one of the chapter authors about her journey toward becoming an educator. Charmaine considers herself to have experienced broad educational opportunities as an occupational therapist in the Philippines.

When I was studying for my undergraduate degree, being an educator never really crossed my mind. At that time, our curriculum was heavily focused on developing our clinical skills to prepare us to become practitioners. Now that I am aware of the prescribed occupational therapy curriculum, professional competencies to become an educator are stated in the minimum standards. However, specific activities to achieve knowledge, skills, and attitudes to become a teacher were not employed in my institution at that time. I reckon that this could be due to the unintended pressure for schools to prepare their occupational therapy students for the licensure examination; hence competencies towards other professional roles were not emphasized.

Soon after I got my license to practice occupational therapy, I applied to a public training hospital focused on pediatric care. Apart from providing clinical services for patients in the hospital, my role in the training hospital involved being a clinical supervisor for occupational therapy interns (those in their final years). As clinical supervisors, we had to undergo a course on clinical teaching and evaluation to ensure that we had the basic competencies in clinical teaching. Apart from supervising occupational therapy interns, I also had the opportunity to supervise physical therapy and speech therapy interns in our training hospital. As a novice clinician at that time, I was encouraged to enroll in advanced training to upskill myself both as a clinician and a supervisor. One of the most challenging moments as a supervisor was the interprofessional case conferences. We assigned our interns a shared client, who they would evaluate, plan for an intervention, and treat not as individual interns but as a healthcare team. This was special for me because the students not only built profession-specific competencies, but also core and interprofessional competencies, which are very useful in actual practice.

Acknowledging that I did not have any formal education in teaching or supervising interns, I questioned my competence in my clinical supervisor role. I reflected and thought of applying for graduate studies that offered a master's program in occupational therapy. I applied and got in. While doing clinical practice and supervision in the same training hospital, I went back to school to develop advanced skills and expand my competencies beyond those of an occupational therapy clinician. My graduate program had a course entitled "Educational Strategies for Health Professionals" where we studied the basic principles of learning, teaching, instructional designing, and assessment of learning. This course inspired me to do a master's thesis related to teaching and training pediatric occupational therapists. In particular, my master's thesis aimed to examine the process of achieving entry-level clinical competencies for the pediatric practice of current occupational therapy training programs in the Philippines.

The process of developing my thesis idea allowed me to go beyond my comfort zone. Aside from reading literature and reviewing my notes from my coursework, I reached out to more established occupational therapy educators at that time to seek mentorship in relation to my thesis. I sought someone who was not only an occupational therapy educator, but someone with an advanced degree in health professions education, and, most importantly, someone I trust. While working on my thesis, one of the mentors I reached out to invited me to work part-time as an instructor in one of the newly developed occupational therapy programs in the country at that time.

Upon accepting my first academic job as a part-time instructor, I was assigned to teach clinical courses focused on children's care, a topic I was familiar with due to my clinical practice and supervisory experiences. My first months were considered an adjustment period. I was not only adjusting to the teaching role, but also navigating a new workplace with new responsibilities such as administrative duties, research, and attending continuing professional activities related

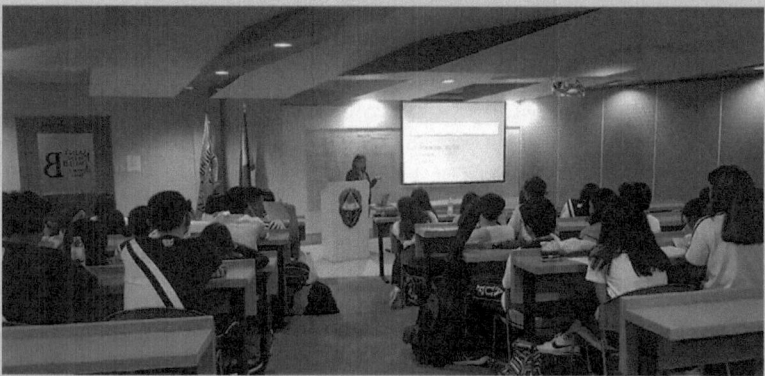

Figure 6.2 Charmaine De Vera-Fevidal providing a lecture to a cohort of occupational therapy students

to teaching and learning. After a year of doing part-time teaching, our program chair then had to leave the position for another opportunity. While I did not feel good about colleagues leaving, it became an opening for others to step up. At that time, the dean of the college called me into a closed-door meeting to discuss the vacant position. I was just starting my teaching stint and learning a lot from the experiences, but the role being offered to me now entailed not only teaching but also managing the whole department (see Figure 6.2).

At that time, I thought that the job offer was too big for me to handle. But opportunities like these do not come by very often. After giving it some thought, I went back to talk to my dean and sought advice about whether going for a formal education in health professions education would help me in assuming the program chair position. She supported the idea. In the middle of this crossroad, I decided to enroll again and go back to school, this time to take a Doctor of Health Professions Education program.

One of the thrusts of the doctoral program is to bridge the gap between what is taught through the curriculum and the goals of Universal Health Care; hence, I recognized the pressing need to integrate the principles of universal healthcare into the OT curriculum. With healthcare disparities widening and access to quality care becoming increasingly challenging for marginalized populations, it is important to infuse our courses with a focus on equitable healthcare delivery. To bring this to fruition, educators need to collaborate with colleagues from various health sectors and draw upon the latest research and best practices. To redesign the curriculum to include health equity, cultural competence, and social determinants of health, I also applied to an Evidence-Based Healthcare Fellowship program by the University of the Philippines-National Institutes of Health and the Department of Health. As a fellow, my understanding of evidence-based approaches deepened the experience, provided hands-on training in research methodologies, and connected me with health leaders in the field.

As I continue to navigate through my ever-changing roles as an educator, an occupational therapist, and both a human and occupational being, one of the challenges that I face is the reality of the inequities surrounding women in higher education. Being newly married and having my firstborn, I am pressured to deal with the constant struggle of choosing priorities and dividing my time between work and family lives, while sustaining a career. Living in a traditional and family-orientated country with delineated gender roles, women in higher education could still have limited opportunities to get promoted, sustain academic productivity, and assume leadership positions.

Despite these realities, I am still convinced that women in higher education have a place and space to contribute to the transformation that we envision in occupational therapy education and training. The constellation of my experiences, including transitions, is a testament to my commitment to pursue educating the next generation of occupational therapists.

Conclusion

This chapter discussed the value of transformative learning within the space of occupational therapy education in the Philippines. Drawing from global and local knowledge, praxis, and perspectives, the chapter provided a discussion on transformative learning and how this translates to teaching and training future generations of Filipino occupational therapists. We specifically used the TPaCK model as a guide for educators in designing contemporary instructions and curricula in occupational therapy, consequently challenging them to be mindful of the profession-centric competencies that need to be built as proposed by the WFOT. These themes encouraged foregrounding teaching and learning contents that are occupation-centered, systems-based, population-focused, and cognizant of sustainability. The chapter also described the process of becoming an occupational therapy educator in the Philippines, highlighting the diverse roles of educators and the requisites to be considered to secure a job in academia. The chapter ends with a story from one of the authors who shared her career journey and is drawn from her lived experience as an occupational therapy educator.

Reflective actions and questions

1   In one of your faculty meetings, facilitate a dialogue about the idea of having Ph.D. as a minimum educational qualification for educators in higher education. While this is not yet a reality in some contexts, this could be a possibility in the following years to upscale the quality of faculty members in universities.

2   If you are a clinician who wants to transition towards becoming an educator, reflect on the following questions: What are your apprehensions in making this career transition? What support do you think you might be needing to make this transition as smooth as possible?

3   Academics are typically seen to have privileges afforded to them because of their educational attainment, social status, and resources. However, there are a growing number of academics and educators who are experiencing marginalization and disadvantages because of their intersecting identities. In your institution, what are the reasons for these disadvantages for academics, and how do you think we can address them concretely?

References

Cabatan, M. C., & Duque, R. L. (2020). Perspectives on occupational therapy education in Southeast Asia. In S. Taff, L. C. Grajo, & B. R. Hooper (Eds.), *Perspectives on occupational therapy education: Past, present, and future* (pp. 143–151). SLACK Incorporated.

Cabatan, M. C., Grajo, L. C., & Sana, E. A. (2020) Occupational adaptation as a lived experience: The case of Filipino occupational therapy academic educators. *Journal of Occupational Science*, 27:4, 510–524. doi:10.1080/14427591.2020.1741020.

Carandang, K. A., & Delos Reyes, R. C. (2018). *Workforce survey 2017: Working conditions and salary structure of occupational therapists working in the Philippines survey.* Philippines Academic of Occupational Therapists. https://paot.org.ph/pdf/other/Workforce%20Survey%202017%20Technical%20Report.pdf.

CHED. (2017). *Policies, standards, and guidelines for the Bachelor of Science in Occupational Therapy Education (BSOT) program.* Retrieved from: https://ched.gov.ph/wp-content/uploads/2018/04/CMO-No.-52-Series-of-2017-Policies-Standards-and-Guidelines-for-the-Bachelor-of-Science-in-Occupational-Therapy-Education-BSOT-Program.pdf.

Fisher A. G. (2013). Occupation-centred, occupation-based, occupation-focused: same, same or different? *Scandinavian Journal of Occupational Therapy*, 20(3), 162–173. doi:10.3109/11038128.2012.754492.

Frenk, J., Chen L., Bhutta, Z., Cohen, J., Crisp, N., Evans, T., Fineberg, H., Garcia, P., Ke, Y., Kelley, P., Kistnasamy, B., Meleis, A., Naylor, D., Pablos-Mendez, A., Reddy, S., Scrimshaw, S., Sepulveda, J., Serwadda, D., Zurayk, H. (2010). Health professionals for the new century: Transforming education to strengthen health systems in an interdependent world. *The Lancet*, 376(9756), 1923–1958. doi:10.1016/S0140-6736(10)61854-5.

Gutierrez, M. M. (2016). Effectiveness of junior faculty mentoring relationships in the colleges of pharmacy in metro Manila, Philippines. *Journal of Asian Association of Schools of Pharmacy*, 5, 367–376. https://www.aaspjournal.org/uploads/155/5929_pdf.pdf.

Hoggan, C. D. (2016). Transformative learning as a metatheory: Definition, criteria, and typology. *Adult Education Quarterly*, 66(1), 57–75. doi:10.1177/0741713615611216.

Mezirow, J. (1978). *Education for perspective transformation: Women's re-entry programs in community colleges.* Teachers College, Columbia University.

Mezirow, J. (1991). *Transformative dimensions of adult learning.* Jossey-Bass.

Mishra, P., & Koehler, M. J. (2006). Technological pedagogical content knowledge: A Framework for teacher knowledge. *Teachers College Record*, 108(6), 1017–1054. doi:10.1111/j.1467-9620.2006.00684.x.

Saubern, R., Urbach, D., Koehler, M., & Phillips, M. (2020). Describing increasing proficiency in teachers' knowledge of the effective use of digital technology. *Computers & Education*, 147. doi:10.1016/j.compedu.2019.103784.

Sy Su, C. C. (2015). Tenure as a threat to sustainability in Philippine tertiary education institutions. *Jurnal Teknologi*, 77(26), 29–35. doi:10.11113/jt.v77.6856.

Turcotte, P. L., & Holmes, D. (2021). The (dis)obedient occupational therapist: A reflection on dissent against disciplinary propaganda. *Cadernos Brasileiros de Terapia Ocupacional*, 29, e2924. doi:10.1590/2526-8910.ctoARF2211.

Turcotte, P. L., & Holmes, D. (2023). From domestication to imperial patronage: Deconstructing the biomedicalisation of occupational therapy. *Health*, 27(5), 719–737. doi:10.1177/13634593211067891.

World Federation of Occupational Therapists. (2017). *Minimum standards for the education of occupational therapists 2016*. Retrieved from https://wfot.org/resources/new-minimum-standards-for-the-education-of-occupational-therapists-2016-e-copy.

Zafran H. (2020). A narrative phenomenological approach to transformative learning: Lessons from occupational therapy reasoning in educational practice. *The American Journal of Occupational Therapy*, 4(1), 7401347010p1–7401347010p6. doi:10.5014/ajot.2020.033100.

Chapter 7

Traditional occupational therapy practice settings

Roi Charles Pineda, Sally Jane Uy, Joel R. Guerrero, Constantine L. Yu Chua, Camille Anne L. Guevara, Christianne Marie Coronel-Andigan, Paulin Grace Morato-Espino and Daryl Patrick Yao

Chapter objectives

1   Describe the Philippine landscape of occupational therapy practice in four traditional practice settings, i.e., geriatrics, mental health, pediatrics, and physical rehabilitation
2   Analyze the forces influencing the direction of these practice settings
3   Using case examples, illustrate the typical occupational therapy roles and process as it is adapted for the local context
4   Reflect on strategies for current practice issues faced by the profession

Occupational therapists work in diverse practice areas or settings, demonstrating the range of clients from across the lifespan who can benefit from occupational therapy. Some of these practice areas are defined by the physical setting where occupational therapy is received (e.g., hospital-based, school-based, skilled nursing facility, and community-based) while other practice areas reflect the service-user's age (e.g., pediatrics and geriatrics) or impairment type (e.g., mental health and physical rehabilitation). As a dynamically evolving profession, non-traditional practice areas emerge in response to opportunities presented by the fluctuating needs and demands of occupational therapy service-users.

Many factors contribute to which practice settings have a demand for and are popular among occupational therapists. A country's demographics, health and disability profile, and healthcare system can strongly influence where occupational therapists are employed. Japan's aging population and robust universal healthcare, for example, reflect the orientation of Japanese practice towards physical rehabilitation and geriatric occupational therapy (Kondo, 2018). In contrast, representative of the Philippines' young population and out-of-pocket spending for healthcare, which accounts more than half of total healthcare expenditure (Dayrit et al., 2018), private pediatric practice is significantly far ahead of other practice areas in terms of number of occupational therapists based on the

DOI: 10.4324/9781003321217-7

most recent workforce survey of the Philippine Academy of Occupational Therapists (PAOT) (Carandang & Delos Reyes, 2018). This is a sharp departure from the historical link of occupational therapy in the Philippines to mental health and physical rehabilitation (for further reading, see Chapter 2), with funded positions in mental health settings in the Philippines even having a shortage of occupational therapists (World Federation of Occupational Therapists [WFOT], 2022).

In this chapter, we discuss four traditional occupational therapy practice settings in the Philippines, namely geriatrics, mental health, pediatrics, and physical rehabilitation. The cases of *Lola* [1] Puring, Juan, Carlo, and Anton provide examples for each practice and serve as a backdrop to describe the current practice landscape in the Philippines and the underlying factors that shape it. Practice issues are discussed, as well as some suggestions to address them.

Geriatric occupational therapy: Re-imagining aging-in-place

Box 7.1 The case of Lola Puring

Lola Puring is a 78-year-old impeccably well-groomed and dressed widow, currently living on her own. She spent most of her time rearing her seven children. She helped in her husband's business and served as a church volunteer. She loved dancing, shopping, and tending to her orchid garden. One day, her daughter, who is the only one living in the Philippines, observed an unsafe engagement during their daily activities. Lola Puring retorted, "*pagod lang ako kaya ako nakakalimot*" [I am just tired, that's why I forget] when the daughter pointed out her forgetfulness. Her daughter raised this concern with their family physician. Lola Puring was diagnosed with dementia and referred to occupational therapy.

Lola Puring is one of the 12 million older Filipinos aged 60 years and above, who are referred to as *senior citizens* (Philippine Statistics Authority, 2022). Corollary to the rapidly increasing growth rate of the senior citizen population is an alarming increase in economic and social costs to manage the progressive functional difficulties associated with aging. This is distinct from older persons' other health- (i.e., age-related disorders such as stroke) and societal-related issues (i.e., elder abuse and neglect). A prevalent problem among older Filipinos is dementia, with an estimated 16 per 1,000 incidence rate (Dominguez et al., 2021).

To address this rapid growth of the global aging population, aging-in-place, as a public policy framework guiding the creation of programs and services in which older persons can choose where they can live safely and independently, is widely adopted (UNFPA Asia-Pacific, 2017). In many developed countries, aging-in-place is exemplified by government-funded institutionalized care for older persons with dementia. In the Philippines, the Senior Citizens Act and its amendment provide discounted privileges for health and social services, including but not limited to medications, groceries, restaurants, public transportation, and recreational activities. While these modest entitlements reduce living costs for community-dwelling older persons and their family, there is a dearth of government-supported institutional care and community-based programs for older Filipinos with specialized care needs (Dominguez et al., 2021). Formal caregiving is likewise constrained due to issues like poverty, increasing cost of caregiving, and migration-related shortage in highly skilled practitioners (Antonio, 2015; Vega et al., 2018).

Members of a typical Filipino family commonly share the informal role of caregiving, which is possible because 60% of older Filipinos reside with at least one adult child (Cruz & Cruz, 2019). Taking care of one's older family members instead of placing them in institutionalized care is preferred in many cultures that value filial piety (Kadar et al., 2013; Miao et al., 2022), including Filipino. Informal caregiving is thus recognized as the pillar of dementia care for the Filipino aging population. With these issues in mind, how can occupational therapy support aging-in-place for older Filipinos?

Much can be gleaned from Clark and colleagues' (1997) Well Elderly study, whose central theme was "health through occupation" (p. 1322). Through didactic and practical teaching on a wide variety of activities, older people were taught how to select and perform activities that support a healthy and satisfying lifestyle. Their occupational therapy intervention showed benefits in older people's health, functional status, and quality-of-life. This highlights the role of occupational therapy in the care of older people.

Framed by the Person-Environment-Occupation (PEO) model (Law et al., 1996), occupational therapists typically construct the older person's occupational profile through an interview with the family and a review of medical history. The evaluation identifies the client and their family's goals and unveils person-, environment-, and task-factors that facilitate and hinder participation in valued daily activities, routines, and life roles.

Box 7.2 The case of Lola Puring (*continuation*)

When the family was asked for goals for occupational therapy, they stated, "para maging okey" ["to be okay"]. It lacked specificity and relied on the occupational therapy recommendations for her to be "better." Montreal Cognitive Assessment-Filipino (Dominguez et al., 2013) results indicated mild dementia. Functionally, Lola Puring is able to perform her basic activities of daily living (ADL) independently, although occasional supervision when bathing or toileting is needed. She sometimes forgets her doctor's appointments and *meryenda* [afternoon snack] and her *barkada* [friend group] often calls to remind her about their get-togethers. She continues attending Mass every 6:15 a.m. in the nearby church. Her communication and social interaction skills, like buying *pasalubong* [treats] for her 17 grandchildren and neighbors, are significantly reduced. At times, she fails to recognize her grandchildren or close friends. Lola Puring seems to be aware of these changes and has started to withdraw from social events. Her daughter describes that her mother, who once led a socially active life, may be depressed and experiencing social isolation.

The design of occupational therapy interventions for older persons relies on a comprehensive assessment in collaboration with the older person's family. Struckmeyer and Pickens (2016) emphasize the importance of learning about the client's environmental and social contexts as they offer an understanding of the living spaces and support system that sustain participation in occupations. From there, occupational therapists can recommend family and caregiver coaching in respect of assisting the older person, home and task modifications in response to declining function, and recreation of life routines around the living spaces that match their current level of participation.

Box 7.3 The case of Lola Puring (*continuation*)

Lola Puring joined the occupational therapy group sessions once a week in a private hospital-based dementia care facility. She is accompanied by her caregiver, who helps her with ADLs. Her weekly sessions include some form of dancing or light exercise, *meryenda* preparations, cognitive and communication activities, and are capped off with socialization with peers while eating their *meryenda*. Individual sessions, which are held with her caregivers, focus on fall prevention, home modification, and behavioral management to encourage participation in her valued occupations.

The Filipino social environment, comprising the family, caregivers, neighbors, *barkada*, and close-knit *kababayan* [compatriot], plays a dichotomous role in supporting the older person. On the one hand, a strong social environment promotes a sense of familiarity and trust, which is supportive of aging-in-place (and is typically missing in Westernized institutionalized care). This sense of familiarity and trust shared with family members and their neighborhood are highly valued among older Asian persons (Bhuyan et al., 2020; Tiraphat et al., 2017; Miao et al., 2022). On the other hand, this unique social environment may pose a hindrance in promoting their independence. For instance, older persons may resist the use of assistive devices and adapted techniques of doing occupations as they only draw attention to their declining function and are unnecessary when, culturally, family members or formal caregivers are expected to assist in all ADLs (Cruz & Cruz, 2019). Because the value of independence is low, safe ADL performance with the caregiver becomes a more suitable outcome.

Box 7.4 The case of Lola Puring (*continuation*)

When mobility issues arose because of her recent fall, Lola Puring had to use a wheelchair. Her OT recommended moving her bedroom to the first floor of the house, installing PVC-type grab bars in her relatively smaller bathroom, and re-arranging her antique furniture pieces to provide more space for her wheelchair. Her wheelchair use posed a challenge in entering the multiple-stepped church. Her caregivers had to carry her wheelchair so that she could continue attending her daily mass. "Online mass cannot substitute my physical presence inside the church," she says. The family subsequently built a makeshift ramp at the side entrance of the church, making it easier for the family to push her wheelchair to enter or exit the century-old cobblestoned church.

With the limited financial and physical resources of Filipino households, Quiambao et al. (2020) emphasize creativity in executing cost-effective home modification in the Philippines, such as improvised mobility options to suit the various terrain as well as locally sourced bathroom fixtures at home, as illustrated in Lola Puring's case.

These environmental and task modifications would allow continued occupational engagement among older persons and their continued engagement in chosen occupations highlights their meaningfulness. For many homemakers like Lola Puring, reminiscing and sharing family recipes bring happiness and uplift their overall sense of well-being. Research has posited that aging-in-place among older Asian women revolved around similar food-based occupations, where they continued their parenting role of providing food to their children and grandchildren (Park & Ko, 2020), re-established their "place" as homemaker, and transferred cultural food preparation practices from one generation to another (Hocking et al., 2002).

Another common occupation among older people is devotion to church activities, indicating a strong spiritual foundation of occupational participation among older Filipinos. Because the Filipino worldview on life (and death) is firmly anchored in spirituality (Ladrido-Ignacio, 2011), older Filipinos often speak about forgiveness, devotion, prayer, burden-bearing, and sharing as aspects of Filipino spirituality that are important in achieving *ginhawa* [ease of living, freedom from suffering]. Paz (2008) proposed *ginhawa* as a more powerful Filipino concept of well-being that integrates the physical, social, emotional, and spiritual dimensions of wellness (Strout et al., 2012). It is expressed in the body's vitality (*sigla*), ease in dealing with life (*gaan*), life potency (*gana*), and joy (*ligaya*).

As dementia progresses and an older Filipino's cognitive status declines, participation in meaningful daily activities should be sustained and, at times, re-discovered (Uy, 2011). This can be done by leveraging the inherent importance of social relationships that is central to Filipino culture. Through occupational therapy group sessions for older Filipinos with dementia, Uy (2013) reported improvement in well-being, rebuilt friendships, and re-engagement in occupations. These outcomes match Filipino well-being elements of *gana* and *gaan, sigla*, and *ligaya*, respectively. These elements underscore the culturally based outcomes of successful aging-in-place, alongside the safe and independent performance outcomes typically emphasized in standard occupational therapy practice.

Lola Puring's case exemplifies the valuable role of occupational therapy in maintaining a good person-environment fit for continued occupational engagement. Consequently, *ginhawa* in physical, social, and, more importantly, spiritual aspects can be achieved regardless of the older Filipino's socioeconomic, health, and disability status. Various factors challenging formal caregiving and weak community-based programs for older Filipinos amplify the caregiver role of the family. Occupational therapists working with older Filipinos should creatively design programs with Filipino culture (e.g., family orientation and spirituality) in mind. The unwavering Filipino's *malasakit* [care, concern] towards senior citizens enriches the role of occupational therapy in reminding people that there is *ginhawa*, even with dementia and other age-related health conditions. Occupational therapy, indeed, offers a broad yet innovative array of solutions to help re-imagine the crafting of independent occupational choices for older Filipinos to successfully age-in-place.

Mental health occupational therapy: Recovery and reintegration beyond stigma

Box 7.5 The case of Juan

Juan, a 22-year-old man, is the eldest of seven from a province adjacent to Metro Manila. Hardened but not broken by the poverty of life, he began working right after high school to supplement the meager income of his family. He juggled being a bagger in a supermarket in the daytime and taking passengers in a pedicab in the early hours of the morning.

Around six months into his job, his workmates noticed changes in Juan's behavior. He was described to be *tulala* [spaced out], causing him to make a lot of mistakes at work. He progressed to becoming *bugnutin* [hot-headed, irritable] a few weeks later and was observed mumbling to himself. He was terminated after an incident when he began dismantling the cash registers, claiming they were rigged with recording devices. He was called *praning* [paranoid]. At home, he was unable to sleep and was described as *balisa* [restless], claiming that his family members were replaced by impostors. His family brought him to an *albularyo* [faith healer]. This brought them some comfort, but symptoms persisted.

As weeks passed, he became progressively agitated, labile, and disorganized. The family locked him up in a make-shift cell outside their main residence. He would be given food on plasticware and hosed down (as a substitute for bathing). One day, while his place was being cleaned, a struggle broke out and he ended up hurting his mother. The local *barangay tanod* [peace and order enforcers] brought him to the emergency room of a tertiary hospital where he was seen by a psychiatrist for the first time in months. He was diagnosed with schizophrenia, advised admission, and started on medical treatment.

Acute psychiatric care and occupational therapy

Juan represents the common experience of Filipinos with a severe mental illness. Despite the mandate of the new Philippine Mental Health Act (RA 11036) that requires the integration of mental healthcare in general hospitals and in community health, services are often accessed only in tertiary hospitals located in city centers (WHO, 2021a). Initial contact with a psychiatrist is often delayed until the peak of a crisis. Subsequently, they may be referred to occupational therapy services.

Following the model of an acute care psychiatric ward in a major tertiary hospital in the Philippines, admitted service-users are situated together in a shared space called an "open ward" where they are free to interact with each other and are only isolated as needed. This is to counteract the alienation that they often experience prior to treatment. Milieu therapy is employed, wherein the environment is structured deliberately to facilitate recovery (Guimón, 2004). This includes a system where occupational therapy is integrated to facilitate a routine of self-care and social and leisure activities, bound within house rules and a system of therapeutic interaction. Participation and empowerment are promoted through establishing service-user organizations, sometimes called "patient government." Distinctly Filipino, a family member is asked to accompany the service-user in the ward as a *bantay* (24-hour watcher) to provide a sense of security and connectedness. This also equips the family to be therapeutic agents upon discharge. Regular ward meetings are held to coordinate care between the various professionals, including occupational therapists who play an important role in evaluation, treatment, and discharge planning, especially regarding occupational function.

Box 7.6 The case of Juan (*continuation*)

The occupational therapy staff in charge asked Juan what his goals are, to which Juan replied that he wanted to go home. Both agreed to reach this goal collaboratively. The therapist reminded Juan that he must be able to get back to caring for himself first. She guided him through a routine that incorporated personal hygiene and grooming, dressing, toileting, and feeding as part of his daily activities, as well as in managing his medications to prepare him for life outside the hospital. Juan was engaged in games, arts and crafts, cooking, and movie watching, both in individual and group sessions. These experiences helped shape Juan's daily repertoire of ADLs while undergoing psychiatric treatment.

Given that persons admitted to acute psychiatric care are those with identified mental disorders that impair daily function, occupational therapists can provide intensive interventions that address a person's ADLs, focusing on self-management (AOTA, 2016). Ecological models such as the Person-Environment-Occupation model are often used to frame the occupational therapy process. Notably, from our own experience and the interviews we had with mental health occupational therapists, neither psychoanalytic approaches such as the use of projective battery testing nor bottom-up approaches where specific client factors are targeted are commonly utilized nowadays.

Box 7.7 The case of Juan (*continuation*)

After two weeks of treatment consisting of both medication and occupational therapy, Juan was deemed ready for discharge by the psychiatrist. However, it was around this time that his family members suddenly went missing. He had to be transferred to an institution equipped for long-term, custodial care.

Here, he was once again referred to occupational therapy. As Juan's symptoms are already controlled and he is highly functional, maintaining his well-being and developing skills were the thrust of intervention. Upon conducting a dynamic performance analysis (Polatajko et al., 2000) and administering an interest checklist, balanced with what the facility can provide, they decided to focus on woodworking as a primary livelihood skill to work on. He was also included in a basketball team with other service-users, akin to how he would play the game with his friends during weekends.

Occupational therapy in long-term psychiatric care

Service-users in long-term residential psychiatric rehabilitation are often provided with targeted interventions that provide support for functioning in daily life, prevent relapse, and promote the development of skills for community living (AOTA, 2016). Treatment outcomes include community integration and quality of life and are achieved through the establishment and maintenance of functional skills. The Recovery Model orients mental healthcare towards allowing individuals to experience purpose and meaning in life activities, beyond simple remission of symptoms or even despite their continuation (Commonwealth of Australia, 2013). For occupational therapists, this emphasizes the value of outcomes related to quality of life, reintegration into society, establishment and maintenance of functional skills, and engagement in health-promoting occupations (Abenes et al., 2018). One common occupational therapy program in the Philippines with this thrust is called the "Grand Socialization." It brings together service-users from different wards to interact through different leisure and output-based activities. Vocational training is also conducted to promote productivity in the present and provide a source of livelihood in the future.

Box 7.8 The case of Juan (*continuation*)

After two months of institutionalization, Juan's mother unexpectedly came back for him. Tearfully, she admitted they had to leave him behind because they were afraid that they might not be able to handle him, but at the same time could not bear to be apart from him.

As an outpatient, Juan is on a monthly injectable antipsychotic medication. Despite being well, neighbors would still gossip about him and call him *baliw* [crazy]. This has made him wary to go outside. His family is just happy that he is "normal" again but is hesitant to let him work and go out, even with his occupational therapist's suggestion to attend the day center, lest he suffer another *sumpong* [breakdown]. Juan feels his recovery is not yet complete since he is always stuck at home.

The recovery-oriented approach discourages institutionalization and promotes community reintegration, as encouraged by national legislation (RA 11036) and the WFOT (Brintnell et al., 2019). However, clients who have been in long-term residential care may not be completely prepared for community integration. A day center is one such transitional program for former inpatients with chronic mental health concerns. Day centers organize regular group sessions led by occupational therapists during the week. Each day would focus on different priority areas, such as self-care, leisure, and work. Knowing that families are integral to recovery, a monthly family support group that focuses on psychoeducation and mutual support is facilitated. Occupational therapists can also liaise with other community-based efforts such as the annual mini-Olympics for Filipinos with mental health concerns (Lazo & Ignacio, 2019).

The majority of Filipino clients, however, are no longer able to receive occupational therapy services once discharged from long-term psychiatric care. The treatment gap ensues due to limited community-based mental health occupational therapy resources and its concentration in tertiary institutions (WHO, 2018). Interprofessional collaboration in the outpatient setting is also not well established (Sy et al., 2019). Stigma contributes to pushing service-users toward isolation and limits participation in community activities (WHO, 2018). At times, an overprotective and interdependent Filipino family culture may contribute to restriction in engaging in occupations. Most of all, there is a lack of pathways for supported employment for service-users due to the limited human resource and advocacy (WHO, 2018, 2021b). Together, these factors impede recovery beyond the institutional setting.

Mental health occupational therapy in the Philippines

The case of Juan is only one representation of mental health occupational therapy in the Philippines. Besides hospital-based settings, other settings exist in the Philippines, including community-based (see Chapter 8) and forensic mental health, as exemplified by the "Life Skills Program" for children in conflict with the law (CICL) (see Chapter 11). Another is on substance use rehabilitation, where occupational therapists work in the context of a therapeutic community. Mental health occupational therapists also frequently fulfill non-clinical roles like liaising with agencies, managing resources, advocating for service-users, and establishing clinical protocols. For instance, vocational programs entail not only teaching job skills but also forming linkages with the various government agencies for diploma completion and training, and establishing vocational avenues such as workshops or even farms.

Mental health settings are severely understaffed, with very few occupational therapists working in this practice area (Carandang & Delos Reyes, 2018; WFOT, 2022). From our interviews with mental health occupational therapists, some motivations to enter this field include an interest in human interactions and personal experiences with mental health. While Filipino occupational therapy students learn the foundational knowledge and skills for mental health practice, there is a consensus among those we interviewed that current occupational therapy education in the country tends to underplay mental health occupational therapy, especially its application in community settings. Self-driven learning and peer support are thus essential to provide not only cognitive but also emotional preparedness for future and current mental health practitioners. This is further supported by the initiation of a PAOT mental health special interest group in 2021.

Among occupational therapists, parallel to the situations of other mental health professionals, one of the biggest challenges is the lack of human resources (WHO, 2021b). To illustrate, in many settings, service-users may only be seen for a limited number of sessions to allow for ample turnover time. Licensed practitioners may have to take on a supervisory role and delegate intervention implementation to non-occupational therapists (Abenes et al., 2018). Factors that tend to dissuade practitioners from mental health practice include inflexible time schedules, concerns with remuneration, and limited exposure to mental health practice as students. Limited recognition of the profession and its roles in mental health among stakeholders lead to lack of prioritization in funding. For example, PhilHealth, the state-owned health insurance system, only stipulates occupational therapy services as an *optional* component for the accreditation of mental health service providers. Furthermore, it is not part of the recently approved mental health package for patients, which solely includes assessment, diagnostics, medical follow-ups, and psychotherapy (PhilHealth, 2023). Additionally, there is a lot of "heartache" from stories of human suffering. Nonetheless, the diversification and expansion of mental health occupational therapy allows many opportunities to be novel and creative (Sy et al., 2021). It reconnects the practitioner to the roots of occupational therapy—that of moral treatment and the restorative properties of occupation. There is a collective sentiment among practitioners that it is a highly fulfilling and stimulating field of practice, which allows one to impact other people's lives at a personal level while having one's own life touched as well.

> **Box 7.9 The case Juan (*continuation*)**
>
> Given how productive he was before, having little engagement in meaningful activities made Juan feel like a burden to his family. This state of emptiness led him to disengage from treatment. He was lost to follow-up, stopped his medications, and began to relapse. He was then re-admitted to the hospital only six months after his discharge due to the recurrence of psychosis. It is hoped that improved availability and continuity of community-based services for psychiatric rehabilitation will prevent this state of "unsustained recovery" from happening again.

Pediatric occupational therapy: Dominating practice to develop school-ready children

PhilHealth estimates that one in seven (5.1 million) Filipino children have disabilities (UNICEF Philippines, 2018). There is, however, no available data on the incidence and referral rates of developmental disabilities in the country (Valenzuela et al., 2022). Autism, considered the fastest-growing developmental disability globally, is estimated to affect 1.2 million Filipinos. Of these, only 10% are diagnosed and 5% receive intervention

(Autism Society Philippines, 2018). Meanwhile, cerebral palsy, the most common motor disability in childhood, is consistently among the top five cases referred to the pediatric rehabilitation service of the Philippine General Hospital (Hebreo et al., 2017).

Box 7.10 The case of Carlo

Carlo, a two-and-a-half-year-old boy, is the only child of a couple, both working as employees in private companies in Manila. As early as 18 months, his parents, Anna and Mike, noticed that he do not respond when his name was called and did not seem to engage with them, despite their attempts to play with him. However, they attributed this to his personality, describing him as *suplado* (snobbish), taking after his father. Carlo is also very active, always running around the house, climbing furniture, and jumping off them. Still suspecting that something might be wrong with their child, Anna began reading about autism on the Internet and in online "mommy groups." When her son turned two, she finally convinced her husband to bring Carlo to a developmental pediatrician, but they had to wait for three months for an appointment. They were concerned about his speech delay, as he usually communicated by grunting, crying, and leading their hand toward his wants and needs.

Upon Carlo's diagnosis of autism and subsequent referral to speech-language and occupational therapy, Anna decided to quit her job to focus more on their child. This also seemed to be the practical choice as they had difficulty finding a household helper and a caregiver for Carlo. Her mother, who lives with them, also provides childcare support. While waiting for an occupational therapy evaluation, which took four months, she searched the Internet for resources on teaching children with autism.

Due to their complex and multifaceted needs, children with disabilities will benefit from the services of an interprofessional team. In the Philippines, however, "systemic discrimination based on differences in culture and ethnicity, socio-economic factors such as affordability and accessibility, and predisposed health beliefs and lack of trust in health professionals" (Chiu et al., 2023, p. 5) were identified by Filipino parents and family members as barriers to receiving adequate and timely rehabilitation services for these children.

The experience of Carlo and his family is shared by many Filipino families who have children with disabilities. Services for children with autism in the country are delivered mostly by private entities, and parents must take the initiative in accessing needed services, which are often fragmented and uncoordinated (Gattud & Piduca, 2020). The same can be said for services for children with other developmental disabilities such as cerebral palsy and Down syndrome. Healthcare services are primarily an individual, out-of-pocket expense. Once a diagnosis and referral to professionals are obtained, parents must proactively take steps in seeking healthcare and support services due to the lack of social and healthcare policies and guidelines on the continuum of care for children with disabilities in the country (Chiu et al., 2023). Among families of children with autism, education, therapy services, and medications account for the highest expenses of families (Quilendrino et al., 2022). Households with children with disabilities incur costs that are 40–80% higher than households with typically developing children (Carraro et al., 2023).

Box 7.11 The case of Carlo (*continuation*)

After months of waiting, Carlo's family is introduced to Thea, an occupational therapist in a pediatric therapy center. Thea is in her second year of practice.

During the evaluation, Thea performed informal interviewing to learn about his daily routine and performance in self-care, and to screen for sensory processing difficulties. Anna's primary concerns were Carlo's lack of interaction with them, his delayed speech, and their worry about his safety. She describes him as always *on the go*—running, jumping, and spinning in his favorite corner of the house. His refusal to sit still makes it hard for her to teach him anything. She admits that she allows Carlo to use gadgets to keep him entertained while she does household chores. He usually watches videos on YouTube and plays educational apps. While Carlo's grandmother also helps to take care of him, she cannot keep up with him so she also allows him to use her mobile phone. He stays up until 1 a.m. and sleeps in until 11 a.m. the following day, disrupting the household's routines. They are planning to enroll Carlo in a preschool program in the coming school year, but are worried that no school will accept him because of his behavior and activity level.

Pediatrics is the most dominant occupational therapy practice area in the country (Carandang & Delos Reyes, 2018; Sy et al., 2021). Since the late 1990s, standalone, private pediatric therapy centers offering occupational physical and speech therapy services have increased rapidly. Some of the reasons why Filipino occupational therapists choose pediatrics are the flexibility in schedule that it offers, higher professional fees, and the constant, growing demand for services for children with disabilities, which ensures a viable client base. Pediatric practitioners also enjoy more autonomy in clinical decision-making, as they are not under the supervision of physiatrists, unlike practitioners in hospital settings. Instead, they usually obtain referrals from developmental pediatricians. Administrative duties are minimal compared with those required of practitioners working in public or private hospital settings. Over the years, Filipino occupational therapists developed a niche in pediatric practice because services provided were advertised as supporting occupational performance in the school setting, participation in which is highly valued in Philippine society (Lasco et al., 2022). Occupational therapy was sought after, as it opened the possibility for children with special needs to be included in mainstream or inclusive schools.

Box 7.12 The case of Carlo (*continuation*)

Thea observed Carlo during free and semi-structured play to learn more about behaviors and level of engagement during tasks, cognitive-language, and gross and fine motor skills. She administered the Sensory Profile, which showed that he scored "much more than others" in the sensory seeking and sensory sensitivity quadrants of the assessment. Thea recommended twice-a-week sessions, with intervention focused on addressing sensory processing challenges, promoting joint attention and engagement, and re-establishing daily routines in order to promote better sleeping patterns.

Thea educated Carlo's family about his hyperactive behavior being attributed to his sensory processing pattern of sensory seeking and sensory sensitivity. They worked together in modifying his daily routine to incorporate more movement and heavy work activities that will regulate his arousal and activity level. Instead of being given a tablet, his mother allowed him to help in household chores such as pushing heavy furniture and putting his toys away whenever she cleans the house. He was allowed to use the tablet in the afternoon for an hour, while his mother rested or napped. On days when they do not have therapy sessions, Carlo's mother would take him to the small neighborhood playground where he pedals his tricycle around and plays on the swing and slide.

Because preparing him for preschool is one of the family's priorities, they would then spend 20–30 minutes at home doing more structured tasks such as sorting Carlo's toys according to color or counting them, matching grocery items, and doing simple arts and crafts, which he enjoyed. Carlo initially refused to engage in these structured tasks, so Thea trained Anna on behavior management strategies. Providing a visual schedule of his daily routine reduced challenging behaviors. The family also designated a "study" corner in their home with a small table, chairs, and a shelf with books and toys. They provided a child-sized trampoline where Carlo can go whenever he needs a break during "study" time. In the late afternoon, he helped his grandmother water plants and pick up dried leaves in the garden. In the evening, it was agreed that his father would play with him to give his mother time to do more household chores. As Thea was certified in DIR-Floortime®, some therapy sessions were spent coaching the couple on how to engage Carlo in play. Gradually, they were able to adjust his sleep schedule so that he was asleep by 9 p.m. and awake by 7 a.m.

Filipino occupational therapists working with children with autism are guided mainly by behavioral, neurodevelopmental, acquisitional, and sensory integration frames of reference. However, as the Philippine occupational therapy undergraduate curriculum transitioned to a more "occupation" focus (Commission on Higher Education [CHED], 2017), in keeping with the WFOT's (2016) Minimum Standards for Occupational Therapy Education, using Person-Environment-Occupation models (Law et al., 1996) for assessment and intervention has also become more common. Moreover, the increase in seminars and workshops being offered online has enabled practitioners to access continuing education activities based on contemporary models, including relational and attachment theories and strengths-based approaches. Filipino occupational therapists are now gradually incorporating these novel perspectives into their practice.

Informal interviewing and clinical observation during play-based activities are the common assessment methods. This is partly due to the limited availability of standardized assessment tools developed and validated for Filipino children. In addition, the cost of purchasing the standardized tests and the training required for administering them could drive up the price of an evaluation session, making it less affordable for a middle-class family. This presents a dilemma that Filipino occupational therapists face: implementing evidence-based practice, promoting culturally relevant assessments and interventions, and balancing these with pragmatic considerations such as health financing.

Among Filipino families, educational participation—equipping the child with skills necessary for school—is usually prioritized. This is because Filipino parents consider education as an essential foundation for a successful future (Lasco et al., 2022). Independence in self-care and other activities of daily living and instrumental activities of daily living are prioritized less because of the Filipino collectivist culture (Meyer, 2010), especially at the family level, where immediate and even extended family members would provide care for a child with a disability. Consequently, Filipino children with disabilities do not have much opportunity to be independent at home.

Occupational therapists working in private pediatric centers are compensated based on the number of clients seen. Rates may vary, depending on whether they are a junior or senior therapist, which is based on the therapist's qualifications and number of years of practice. Moreover, more senior practitioners may be assigned other roles such as mentor, if the clinic has a mentoring system, or clinical educator, if the clinic is an affiliation site, or administrator/head of the occupational therapy department. Beyond these roles, practitioners in private clinics may have limited career mobility and opportunities for financial advancement.

While occupational therapy practice is concentrated in Metro Manila, a growing number of practitioners are now choosing to return to and establish a private practice in their hometowns in other regions of the country, thus expanding access to quality occupational therapy services in the Visayas (central Philippines) and Mindanao (southern Philippines) islands. Other practitioners choose to travel regularly to these regions where there are still few occupational therapists available to provide services to children with disabilities and their families (Gomez et al., 2012). The establishment of more occupational therapy schools in these regions has somewhat mitigated the lack of practitioners serving in the provinces (Sy et al., 2021); the training of Filipino occupational therapists for the purpose of migration and their resulting exodus abroad create a need for new ones (Dayrit et al., 2018; Pineda et al., 2023).

Physical rehabilitation occupational therapy: Navigating the environment towards meaningful participation

According to the latest available national census report, 12% of Filipinos older than 14 years' experience severe disability (Philippine Statistics Authority, 2019). While this report provided no information on the type of disability, a separate study of Filipinos with a disability in Metro Manila by Yap and colleagues (2009) showed that 34% have a physical mobility impairment. These Filipinos with disabilities have severely limited access to rehabilitation. Rehabilitation services are concentrated in regional and tertiary hospitals and in urban areas in the Philippines. The absence of universal healthcare in the Philippines also makes it difficult for persons in need of rehabilitation to cover the costs associated with it (Boyle et al., 2017; Dayrit et al., 2018). Thus, only 2% of persons with disabilities receive needed rehabilitation services (Olavides-Soriano et al., 2011). With 60% of people with disabilities being of working age (National Statistics Office, 2013), poor access to rehabilitation services, including occupational therapy, can have significant implications on work participation, particularly paid work, which emphasizes the contribution of disability in reinforcing poverty (Banks et al., 2017).

Box 7.13 The case of Anton

One day, a client named Anton was referred to Vangie, an occupational therapy staff in a rehabilitation unit of a tertiary hospital. He is a 25-year-old breadwinner living in the slum area of an urban city together with his wife and two children. He is a high school graduate and works as a lineman for an electrical company. Three weeks ago, he fell from an electrical pole while servicing an electrical line and sustained a level T6 incomplete spinal cord injury and head concussion.

Hospital-based physical rehabilitation

Typically, an occupational therapy section in the Philippines is overseen by the physical rehabilitation medicine department, which is headed by a physiatrist. Physiatrists thus function as the primary gatekeepers of rehabilitation services (Boyle et al., 2017).

Some clients may be referred for occupational therapy services as early as the acute phase, but others are only seen after secondary complications like bed sores, contractures, and deformities have become problematic. A referral for occupational therapy commonly contains the client's diagnosis and the doctor's orders for rehabilitation. Timing of such referral is crucial for ensuring successful outcomes for the client. However, wait times can be long for most government hospitals, delaying the service provision to the indigent clients.

Billing for occupational therapy services differs between inpatient and outpatient settings. Billing of therapy services for inpatient clients are integrated with other hospital expenses, which they pay on or just before discharge. PhilHealth members receive deductions in their hospital bill and others have additional private insurance (although most indigent people do not have one). Work-related disabilities of workers with an employer also receive financial assistance from the Employees' Compensation Commission. Any remaining cost must then be paid out of pocket. Informal ways to solicit money to pay this cost include appealing to organizations and politicians, sometimes with the assistance of a social worker, or borrowing from family and/or friends. As for outpatient settings, clients are billed per session. These are often paid out of pocket because PhilHealth does not cover outpatient occupational therapy services as of writing. Private health insurance coverage of occupational therapy is case-based.

Box 7.14 The case of Anton (continued)

That late afternoon, Vangie went to Anton's bed in the inpatient rehabilitation ward to perform an initial evaluation. Based on the physiatrist's note in the referral, Anton had to be evaluated while lying down and he was not allowed to sit until he received clearance from his orthopedist. Vangie observed that Anton wanes in and out of consciousness during their conversation and struggles with short-term recall. His wife reported that he struggles to sleep at night because of noise from other ward patients.

Vangie attempted to interview the couple about Anton's occupational profile and their goals for occupational therapy. Vangie learned that Anton's wife will work to support their children while he is in the hospital. The hospital bill, rent, utility bills, and their everyday expenses are major points of concern for the couple. In fact, Anton was left alone the whole day while his wife spent the day soliciting financial support from their mayor and other city officials. The wife joked that they have run out of family members to borrow money from. Anton then expressed his desire to return to work and be the breadwinner of his family or at least contribute to the household income upon discharge.

Occupational therapy process

An occupational therapy model commonly used in the Philippines is the PEO model (Law et al., 1996), which defines a person's performance based on the interaction between the person's innate skills and faculties, the environment they navigate in and the meaningful occupation they desire to engage in. Guiding the occupational therapy process in physical rehabilitation settings, two frames of reference often used in the Philippines are the biomechanical (McMillan, 2011) and rehabilitation (Dutton, 1993) frames of reference. The former is particularly relevant in the early acute phase of rehabilitation, where stabilizing the client's condition and preventing further complications are the priorities.

Prior to meeting the client for the first time, occupational therapists perform medical record review to obtain information about the client's medical history and any relevant information that will influence evaluation, such as current medications and contraindicated positions, movements, and activities.

During the initial evaluation and once the client's occupational therapy goals are identified, occupational therapists perform an assessment of occupations and person-factors (i.e., skills, body structures, and functions), and environment. Among occupations, ADLs are prioritized first while other occupations like leisure and work are delayed until a client can independently perform their ADLs. Person-factors such as the client's functional endurance, edema, range of motion, and muscle strength are also evaluated. Common tests used include dynamic performance analysis (Polatajko et al., 2000), as well several measurement devices (e.g., dynamometer and tactile monofilament) and rating scales (e.g., Functional Independence Measure and Barthel Index). In hospital-based settings in the Philippines, occupational therapists may not always have direct access to the client's natural environment where occupations are performed. Often it is due to distance and accessibility of the client's residence, especially for clients from remote places. Photographs, videos, or a verbal description of their house are used instead. Neighborhood and workplace environments are seldom evaluated.

> **Box 7.15 The case of Anton (continued)**
>
> Vangie establishes an intentional therapeutic relationship with Anton as they meet for their therapy session. This relationship facilitates Anton's openness to share his worries and fears with her. He divulges that they need to raise money for a spinal orthosis; otherwise he will not get clearance to sit. That is why he has decided to sell his motorcycle: "*Makagaan man lang sa pagiging pabigat ko*" ["To lighten the burden I am causing"], he says with a scoff. As he is still bed-ridden, they work to maintain mobility and strength of the upper extremity

through active range of motion exercises. Vangie also teaches Anton's wife compression bandaging to reduce edema in the lower extremity.

After much delay, Anton finally receives his spinal orthosis and the orthopedist clears Anton for upright sitting. Vangie re-evaluates Anton using the Barthel Index to assess his ADLs. Except for eating, where he scored 10 (independent), all other items were performed with complete or partial assistance. His daily sessions are geared towards improving his ADLs, particularly donning and doffing the spinal orthosis.

Two weeks later, Vangie noticed that Anton's wife never seems to be around of late and she is teaching what appears to be a different *bantay* [2] every day. When she probes Anton about it, he admits that his wife took a job at a wet market to help with finances and his other family members take turns being his *bantay*. Vangie then decides to leave written instructions, accompanied by a video recording taken from Anton's cell phone as needed, for exercises and activity adaptations. She then checks that his *bantay* of the day can follow the instructions left the day before correctly. This seems to help improve the consistency of Anton's exercise and ADL practice outside actual therapy sessions.

Because of delays in acquiring his spinal orthosis and more pressing needs for ADL training, his goal of return to work was postponed.

Guided by an expected prognosis of high spontaneous recovery in the early months post-injury, medical orders to occupational therapy are oriented towards a biomechanical frame of reference with the intention of recovering as much body function as possible to return to premorbid functioning. Many intervention techniques used by occupational therapists targeting range of motion, muscle strength, muscular and cardiovascular endurance, and edema fall under this frame of reference (McMillan, 2011). These include physical agent modalities, splinting, and exercise. Rehabilitation frame of reference is also often used to complement the recovery process to allow continued engagement in ADLs, work, and leisure despite the client's permanent disability (Dutton, 1993). Assistive devices, adapted techniques for doing occupations, and home modifications are possible strategies available to occupational therapists. The occupational therapist's professional reasoning balances the competing orientation of these two frames of reference. Depending on the extent of expected recovery, compensatory strategies should facilitate occupational performance but not to the extent that clients depend on them and neglect training body functions that have the potential to recover. As the client's status plateaus, however, compensating for body functions that are unlikely to return to premorbid state becomes the priority.

This time-based change in approach is motivated by: 1) the client being hopeful for a full recovery; 2) the confidence to invest all efforts towards recovery during the period when recovery is most likely; and 3) the occupational therapist working creatively with limited resources to assist the client in achieving optimal functioning (Yao et al., 2020). Occupational therapists working with indigent clients have to be creative and resourceful in fabricating needed assistive devices out of low-cost or readily available materials to achieve optimal functioning in their homes and in their communities. However, persons with mobility impairment are likely to encounter accessibility issues in the community (e.g., wheelchair ramps being too steep).

Box 7.16 The case of Anton (*continued*)

After four months of continuous therapy, the rehabilitation doctor expressed plans to discharge Anton in two days. Prior to that point, Vangie had interviewed him about his interests, previous work experience, and any work opportunities available to him in his community. While Anton had been recovering, he knew that he was far from being ready and able to return to work. Vangie wanted to continue providing intensive therapy for Anton but she could not influence discharge decisions. Vangie quickly wrote a discharge plan for Anton and advised him to see her for follow-up. Anton was never seen again after discharge.

The physiatrist holds the sole authority to discharge inpatient clients and occupational therapy goals may not always be the primary consideration. Due to long wait times, once the most urgent medical concern is resolved, clients may be discharged to make space for new client admissions. Discharge can be abrupt, with the therapist often learning about it when they find their client's bed empty. It is often impossible to adequately meet targeted occupational therapy outcomes within the existing timeline. Moreover, it can be challenging to design an ample discharge plan that matches the client's most recent level of performance and participation. This is the reason why it is advantageous to involve the caregiver early during therapy, so that instructions that will be useful at discharge can slowly be given during the duration of inpatient rehabilitation. Such an approach is possible in the Philippine context because, like Anton, clients admitted in the hospital often have a *bantay* with them.

Ideally, Anton's rehabilitation journey needs to continue through outpatient occupational therapy services in a community or local hospital. However, it is actually hampered by several obstacles, such as a limited number of such hospitals within one's residence, non-wheelchair-friendly public transportation system (Dabu et al., 2018), increased out-of-pocket costs for therapy services that are not covered by PhilHealth nor private insurance, and significant opportunity and income loss for the family member accompanying Anton. Obstacles like these trap people into a cycle of poverty and disability.

The case of Anton is the norm rather than an exception. Because of the relationship between disability and poverty, a large proportion of people with disabilities are also living in poverty (Banks et al., 2017). These people have very few options available for rehabilitation after discharge. As such, contact with occupational therapy also ends when they are discharged from the hospital. Anton (and many others like him) probably never returned to work and will have to live his life stuck inside the house due to the lack of support in receiving occupational therapy and other rehabilitation services, outdated Accessibility Law (see Chapter 13), lack of community resources, and the lack of opportunity to participate in society.

Conclusion

Many aspects of the local context, such as culture, socio-demographics, and the education and healthcare systems, influence a profession's practice landscape and its ability to serve the needs of society in both positive and negative directions. How these factors are configured in the Philippines has led to a significant majority of occupational therapists settling into pediatric practice. The irony is that there is a dominant pediatric practice yet it still does not meet the pediatric needs of society or is at the expense of increasing the gap of other disabilities not being addressed at all.

This foregrounds the point that many issues of the profession, such as a shortage and uneven distribution of professionals in the country (Carandang & Delos Reyes, 2018), economic migration and brain drain (Pineda et al., 2023), and poverty and lack of universal healthcare for all Filipinos (Boyle et al., 2017; Dayrit et al., 2018), affect the profession as a whole and not just certain practice areas. Nonetheless, it is important to acknowledge that certain practice areas are impacted more than others.

Recommendations for action

While these identified issues do not have easy fixes, the profession should leverage its creativity and resourcefulness to find solutions. PAOT, as the profession's national organization, has provided an important step in their workforce survey (Carandang & Delos Reyes, 2018), which provided some insights on the situation of the profession, in general, as well as individual practice areas, in particular. The survey should be run at regular intervals, similar to the WFOT workforce survey, to obtain current data about the profession and inform policies and programs that align with the realities and needs of professional practice. Furthermore, the workforce survey can be instrumental in developing a Filipino-contextualized model of practice and slowly weaning itself away from a mostly Westernized practice model, in observance with its own research agenda of advocating for more culturally relevant studies (PAOT, 2015)

Government and private healthcare facilities may never be able to compete with the higher salaries offered to occupational therapists abroad, making it unlikely that the migration of Filipino occupational therapists will stop (Pineda et al., 2023). However, public legislation and policies spearheaded or supported by PAOT should aim for expanding the access to occupational therapy services, as well as supporting retention policies to motivate occupational therapists to stay and serve Filipinos. For example, the implementation of the Philippine Inclusive Education Act (RA 11650) presents an opportunity to hire occupational therapists at local public schools. A similar opportunity can be created for mental health occupational therapy with the Philippine Mental Health Act (RA 11036).

Supporting non-traditional service models like telehealth (see Chapter 9), which was widely used and deemed helpful during the COVID-19 pandemic (Camden & Silva, 2021), can be promoted by government regulatory agencies (e.g., the Department of Health and Professional Regulation Commission) and occupational therapy program planners in private and public healthcare facilities as a mainstream intervention rather than simply an alternative (Chiu et al., 2023; Panotes et al., 2024). This can be a promising approach to expand occupational therapy reach to remote locations. However, it should be noted that telehealth as a service delivery model also amplifies inequity issues because of the technology needs, including Internet access, hardware requirements, and technology literacy.

Finally, we challenge Filipino occupational therapists to broaden their perspectives regarding the profession and create more opportunities for themselves, besides the typical clinician role. The profession has much more to offer to Filipino people than the traditional one-on-one, direct therapy services. It is vital to hone the skills and qualities necessary for clinicians to transition to other equally important roles, such as management and advocacy roles (Shams et al., 2019). Thus, occupational therapy curricula both at the undergraduate and graduate levels need to foster entrepreneurship and innovation (Anderson & Nelson, 2011). Aside from curricular alignment with local needs and advancing the profession through scholarly work, future occupational therapists are envisioned to be leaders and trailblazers involved with advocacy, program development, policy development, education, and research (Pitts, 2020) who influence change in the profession and are responsive to the ever-changing needs of Filipinos with disabilities.

Reflective and critical guide questions

1   Considering the current occupational therapy practice landscape, how can educational and employment policies be adapted to increase access to occupational therapy services and retention of occupational therapists?

2 Consider your preferred practice area and dissect the reasoning why you chose that specific practice area. Alternatively, interview an occupational therapy practitioner from any of the four traditional practice areas described in this chapter by asking about their practice and their motivations, i.e., why they chose that particular practice area.

3 The culture of migration among Filipinos is another driver of occupational therapy practice. Analyze the pros and cons of emigration of occupational therapists, both for the individual and the profession.

Notes

1 *Lola* translates to "grandmother" but is also typically used to address any older female adult.

2 *Bantay* refers to the person accompanying someone admitted in a hospital and often also functions as an informal caregiver.

References

Abenes, Z. J. D., Apigo, R. M., Elefante, G. A. D., Guevara, C. A. L., & Kang, J. J. C. (2018). *A qualitative study on the current occupational therapy mental health practice in two psychiatric care institutions in the Philippines* [Unpublished undergraduate thesis]. University of the Philippines Manila.

Anderson, K. M., & Nelson, D. L. (2011). Wanted: Entrepreneurs in occupational therapy. *American Journal of Occupational Therapy*, 65(2), 221–228. doi:10.5014/ajot.2011.001628.

Antonio, A. M. (2015). Challenges to the Filipino elderly as traditional caregivers: The changing landscape of long-term care management of the Filipino elderly. https://www.researchgate.net/publication/304019497.

AOTA. (2016). *Mental health promotion, prevention, and intervention: Across the lifespan.* https://www.aota.org/-/media/corporate/files/practice/mentalhealth/distinct-value-mental-health.pdf.

Autism Society Philippines. (2018). *Primer on autism in the Philippines.* Autism Society Philippines.

Banks, L. M., Kuper, H., & Polack, S. (2017). Poverty and disability in low- and middle-income countries: A systematic review. *PLoS One*, 12(12), e0189996.

Bhuyan, M. R., Lane, A. P., Moogoor, A., Močnik, Š., & Yuen, B. (2020). Meaning of age-friendly neighbourhood: An exploratory study with older adults and key informants in Singapore. *Cities*, 107, 102940. doi:10.1016/j.cities.2020.102940.

Boyle, P., Bhanbhro, S., & De Guzman, J. E. (2017). Universal healthcare in the Philippines and the scope of therapy and rehabilitation. *International Journal of Therapy and Rehabilitation*, 24(9), 403–408. doi:10.12968/ijtr.2017.24.9.403.

Brintnell E. S., Gunaranthne, P., Hitch, D., Ledgerd, R., Acevede, L. P., Pettican, A., Shafaroodi, N., & Stoffel, V. (2019). Occupational therapy and mental health [Position statement]. *WFOT.* https://wfot.org/resources/occupational-therapy-and-mental-health.

Cabatan, M. C., & Duque, R. L. (2020). Perspectives on occupational therapy education in Southeast Asia. In S. Taff, L. Grajo, & B. Hooper (Eds),

Perspectives on occupational therapy education: Past, present, and future (pp. 143–151). SLACK Incorporated.

Camden, C., & Silva, M. (2021). Pediatric telehealth: Opportunities created by the COVID-19 and suggestions to sustain its use to support families of children with disabilities. *Physical & Occupational Therapy in Pediatrics*, 41(1), 1–17. doi:10.1080/01942638.2020.1825032.

Carandang, K. A., & Delos Reyes, R. C. (2018). *Workforce survey 2017: Working conditions and salary structure of occupational therapists working in the Philippines survey*. PAOT.

Carraro, L., Robinson, A., Hakeem, B., Manlapaz, A., & Agcaoili, R. (2023). Disability-related costs of children with disabilities in the Philippines. *International Journal of Environmental Research and Public Health*, 20(13), 6304. doi:10.3390/ijerph20136304.

CHED. (2017). Policies, standards and guidelines for the Bachelor of Science in Occupational Therapy education (BSOT) program, Memorandum Order No. 52, s. 2017 (May 31) (Phil.). https://ched.gov.ph/wp-content/uploads/2018/04/CMO-No.-52-Series-of-2017-Policies-Standards-and-Guidelines-for-the-Bachelor-of-Science-in-Occupational-Therapy-Education-BSOT-Program.pdf.

Chiu, I., Sy, M., Oruga, M., & Bonito S. (2023). Children with special needs and their access to rehabilitation services in the Philippines: A Q-methodology study on perceived barriers by family members. *Public Health Challenges*, 2(2), e79. doi:10.1002/puh2.79.

Clark, F., Azen, S. P., Zemke, R., Jackson, J., Carlson, M., Mandel, D., Hay, J., Josephson, K., Cherry, B., Hessel, C., Palmer, J., & Lipson, L. (1997). Occupational therapy for independent-living older adults: A randomized controlled trial. *JAMA*, 278(16), 1321–1326. doi:10.1001/jama.1997.03550160041036.

Commonwealth of Australia. (2013). A national framework for recovery-oriented mental health services: Policy and theory. https://www.health.gov.au/resources/publications/a-national-framework-for-recovery-oriented-mental-health-services-policy-and-theory?language=en.

Cruz, C. J. P., & Cruz, G. T. (2019). Filipino older persons. In G. T. Cruz, C. J. P. Cruz, & Y. Saito (Eds.), *Ageing and health in the Philippines* (pp. 27–46). Economic Research Institute for ASEAN and East Asia.

Dabu, M. T. E., Galang, M. M. R. F., Galinato, A. B. S., Garcia, G. M., Igna, L. P., & Pineda, R. C. (2018). *Lived experiences of Filipino adults with mobility impairment in Pampanga towards receiving help* [Unpublished undergraduate thesis]. Angeles University Foundation, Philippines.

Dayrit, M. M., Lagrada, L. P., Picazo, O. F., Pons, M. C., & Villaverde, M. C. (2018). The Philippines health system review. *Health Systems in Transition*, 8(2). WHO Regional Office for South-East Asia. https://iris.who.int/handle/10665/274579.

Department of Budget and Management. (2024). *Staffing summary: Fiscal year 2024*. https://www.dbm.gov.ph/wp-content/uploads/Staffing/STAFFING2024/STAFFING-SUMMARY-2024.pdf.

Dominguez, J., Jiloca, L., Fowler, K. C., De Guzman, M. F., Dominguez-Awao, J. K., Natividad, B., … & Phung, T. (2021). Dementia incidence, burden and cost of care: A Filipino community-based study. *Frontiers in Public Health*, 9, 628700. doi:10.3389/fpubh.2021.628700.

Dominguez, J. C., Orquiza, M. G. S., Soriano, J. R., Magpantay, C. D., Esteban, R. C., Corrales, M. L., & Ampil, E. R. (2013). Adaptation of the Montreal Cognitive Assessment for elderly Filipino patients. *East Asian Archives of Psychiatry*, 23(3), 80–85.

Dutton R. (1993). Rehabilitation frame of reference. In H. L. Hopkins & H. D. Smith (Eds.), *Willard and Spackman's occupational therapy* (8th ed., pp. 79–81). Lippincott.

Gattud, V. I., & Piduca, M. J. C. (2020). Parent-initiated health and education services for children with autism in Baguio, Philippines. *Indonesian Journal of Disability Studies*, 7(1), 1–7. doi:10.21776/ub.ijds.2019.007.01.1.

Gomez, I. N. B., Paguyo, J. C., & Mamaril, A. R. (2012). The "travelling" team: Promoting health and wellness in the Northern Philippines. *Hong Kong Journal of Occupational Therapy*, 22(2), 97. doi:10.1016/j.hkjot.2012.12.005.

Guimón, J. (2004). *Relational mental health: Beyond evidence-based interventions.* Kluwer Academic.

Hebreo, A. R. P., Ang-Muñoz, C. D., Abiera, J. E. E., Dungca, M. L., & Mancao, B. D. (2017). Profile of pediatric patients with cerebral palsy at the department of rehabilitation medicine, Philippine General Hospital. *Acta Medica Philippina*, 51(4), 289–299. doi:10.47895/amp.v51i4.496.

Hocking, C., Clair, V. W. S., & Bunrayong, W. (2002). The meaning of cooking and recipe work for older Thai and New Zealand women. *Journal of Occupational Science*, 9(3), 117–127. doi:10.1080/14427591.2002.9686499.

Instituting a Policy of Inclusion and Services for Learners with Disabilities in Support of Inclusive Education Act, RA No. 11650. (2022, March 11). https://www.officialgazette.gov.ph/2022/03/11/republic-act-no-11650/.

Kadar, K. S., Francis, K., & Sellick, K. (2013). Ageing in Indonesia—health status and challenges for the future. *Ageing International*, 38, 261–270. doi:10.1007/s12126-012-9159-y.

Kondo, T. (2018). History and current practice of occupational therapy in Japan. *Annals of International Occupational Therapy*, 2(1), 43–52. doi:10.3928/24761222-20181116-01.

Ladrido-Ignacio, L. (2011). *Ginhawa: Well-being in the aftermath of disasters.* Flipside Publishing.

Lasco, G., Nuevo, C. E. L., Nolasco, M. L. P., Famaloan, F. R. A. N., Bundoc, J. R., Capili, D. I. S., & Bermejo, R. (2022). "It's as if I'm the one suffering": Narratives of parents of children with disability in the Philippines. *Acta Medica Philippina*, 56(7), 30–42. doi:10.47895/amp.vi0.658.

Law, M., Cooper, B. A., Strong, S., Stewart, D., Rigby, P., & Letts, L. (1996). The Person-Environment-Occupation Model: A transactive approach to occupational performance. *Canadian Journal of Occupational Therapy*, 63(1), 9–23. doi:10.1177/000841749606300103.

Lazo, L., & Ignacio, L. (2019). *National mental health research agenda in the Philippines 2019–2022.* World Association for Psychosocial Rehabilitation Philippines. https://www.pchrd.dost.gov.ph/wp-content/uploads/2022/03/Annex-4.-National-Mental-Health-Research-Agenda-2019-2022.pdf.

McMillan, I. R. (2011). The biomechanical frame of reference in occupational therapy. In E. A. S. Duncan (Ed.), *Foundations for practice in occupational therapy* (5th ed., pp. 179–193). Elsevier.

Mental Health Act, RA No. 11036. (2018, June 20). https://www.officialgazette. gov.ph/2018/06/20/republic-act-no-11036/.

Meyer, H.-D. (2010). Framing disability: Comparing individualist and collectivist societies. *Comparative Sociology*, 9(2), 165–181. doi:10.1163/156913210X125481460 54985.

Miao, J., Wu, X., & Zeng, D. (2022). Promoting ageing in place in Hong Kong: Neighbourhood social environment and depression among older adults. *Journal of Asian Public Policy*, 1–18. doi:10.1080/17516234.2022.2040087.

National Statistics Office. (2013). *2010 Census of population and housing—Report No. 2A: Demographic and housing characteristics (non-sample variables)*. http s://psa.gov.ph/system/files/main-publication/2010_PHIILIPPINES_FINAL% 2520PDF.pdf.

Olavides-Soriano, M. E., Ampo, E., & Escorpizo, R. (2011). Occupational rehabili- tation policy and practice in the Philippines: Initiatives and challenges. *Journal of Occupational Rehabilitation*, 21(Supp 11), S62–S68. doi:10.1007/s10926-010-9284-y.

Panotes, A., Jocson, J., Andigan, C. M., & Sy, M. P. (2024). Lived experiences of caregivers upon receiving occupational therapy through telehealth amidst the pandemic. *Cadernos Brasileiros de Terapia Ocupacional*, 32. doi:10.1590/2526- 8910.ctoao27853626.

PAOT. (2015, July). *The Philippine occupational therapy research agenda 2015*. http s://paot.org.ph/pdf/research/Philippine%20Occupational%20Therapy%20Resea rch%20Agenda%20(2015).pdf.

Park, S., & Ko, Y. (2020). The sociocultural meaning of "my place": Rural Korean elderly people's perspective of aging-in-place. *Asian Nursing Research*, 14(2), 97– 104. doi:10.1016/j.anr.2020.04.001.

Paterson, C. F. (2014). A short history of occupational therapy in mental health. In W. Bryant, J. Fieldhouse, & K. Bannigan (Eds), *Creek's occupational therapy and mental health* (5th ed., pp. 2–14). Elsevier.

Paz, C. J. (2008). Ginhawa: Well-being as expressed in Philippine languages. In C. J. Paz (Ed.), *Essays on well-being, opportunity/destiny, and anguish*. University of the Philippines Press.

PhilHealth. (2023, October 10). *PhilHealth circular 2023–0018*. https://www.phil health.gov.ph/circulars/2023/PC2023-0018.pdf.

Philippine Statistics Authority. (2019, May 3). Disability spares no one: A new perspective. https://psa.gov.ph/statistics/national-disability-prevalence-survey.

Philippine Statistics Authority. (2022, August 12). Age and sex distribution in the Philippine population 2020 census of population and housing. https://www.psa. gov.ph/content/age-and-sex-distribution-philippine-population-2020-census-pop ulation-and-housing.

Pineda, R. C., Abad-Pinlac, B., Yao, D. P. G., Toribio, F. N. R. B., Josephsson, S., & Sy, M. P. (2023). Unraveling the "greener pastures" concept: The phenomenology of internationally educated occupational therapists. *Occupational Therapy Journal of Research*. Advance online publication. doi:10.1177/15394492231205885.

Pitts, C. (2020). *Leadership roles in the field of occupational therapy* [Doctoral project, University of St. Augustine for Health Sciences]. SOAR @ USA: Stu- dent Capstone Papers Collection. doi:10.46409/sr.SNQM7186.

Polatajko, H. J., Mandich, A., & Martini, R. (2000). Dynamic performance analysis: A framework for understanding occupational performance. *American Journal of Occupational Therapy*, 54(1), 65–72. doi:10.5014/ajot.54.1.65.

Quiambao, A., Uy, S. J., & Guerrero, J. R. (2020). *Perspectives of selected Filipino occupational therapists on home assessment and modifications for the Filipino older adults* [Unpublished manuscript]. University of Santo Tomas Graduate School.

Quilendrino, M. I. O., Castor, M. A. R., Mendoza, N. R. N. P., Vea, J. R., & Castillo-Carandang, N. T. (2022). The direct cost of autism and its economic impact on the Filipino family. *Acta Medica Philippina*, 56(9), 24–30. doi:10.47895/amp.v56i9.5005.

Reyes, A. L., & Herrin, J. A. C. (2009). A five-year review of referrals to the developmental pediatrics section of a major tertiary hospital. *Acta Medica Philippina*, 43(3), 12–17. doi:10.47895/amp.v43i3.2683.

Shams, S. S., Batth, R., & Duncan, A. (2019). The lived experiences of occupational therapists in transitioning to leadership roles. *Open Journal of Occupational Therapy*, 7(1), 2. doi:10.15453/2168-6408.1513.

Strout, K. A., & Howard, E. P. (2012). The six dimensions of wellness and cognition in aging adults. *Journal of Holistic Nursing*, 30(3), 195–204. doi:10.1177/0898010112440883.

Struckmeyer, L. R., & Pickens, N. D. (2016). Home modifications for people with Alzheimer's disease. A scoping review. *American Journal of Occupational Therapy*, 70, 7001270020. doi:10.5014/ajot.2015.016089.

Sy, M. P., Martinez, P. G. V., Labung, F. F. T., Medina, M. A. K. G., Mesina, A. S., Vicencio, M. R. E., & Tulabut, H. D. P. (2019). Baseline assessment on the quality of interprofessional collaboration among Filipino mental health professionals. *Journal of Interprofessional Education & Practice*, 14, 58–66. doi:10.1016/j.xjep.2018.12.003.

Sy, M. P., Ohshima, N., & Roraldo, M. P. N. R. (2018). The role of Filipino occupational therapists in substance addiction and rehabilitation: A Q-Methodology. *Occupational Therapy in Mental Health*, 34(4), 367–388. doi:10.1080/0164212X.2018.1446206.

Sy, M. P., Yao, D. P., Panotes, A., Kaw, J., & Mendoza, T. (2021). Contemporary history: Progress and resilience of occupational therapy in the Philippines (2004–2020). *WFOT Bulletin*, 79(1), 80–93. doi:10.1080/14473828.2021.1995226.

Tiraphat, S., Peltzer, K., Thamma-Aphiphol, K., & Suthisukon, K. (2017). The role of age-friendly environments on quality of life among Thai older adults. *International Journal of Environmental Research and Public Health*, 14(3), 282. doi:10.3390/ijerph14030282.

UNFPA Asia-Pacific. (2017). *Perspectives on population ageing in the Asia-Pacific Region*. https://asiapacific.unfpa.org/sites/default/files/pub-pdf/Perspectives%20on%20%20Population%20Ageing%20Report_for%20Website.pdf.

UNICEF Philippines. (2018, July 24). No child left behind: Study calls for better care of children with disabilities. https://www.unicef.org/philippines/press-releases/no-child-left-behind-study-calls-better-care-children-disabilities.

Uy, S. J. (2011). *Perceived roles of occupational therapy in dementia care* [Unpublished manuscript]. Optimal Aging Center.

Uy, S. J. (2013). *Occupational therapy's therapeutic use of groups in dementia care* [Conference presentation]. Asian Society Against Dementia Congress, Cebu City, Philippines. http://www.asiandementia.org/pdf/7th-ASAD-Congress.pdf.

Valenzuela, R. L. G., Mendoza, J. E. D., Tantengco, O. A. G., & Ornos, E. D. B. (2022). Challenges in Philippine developmental paediatric care [Letter to the Editor]. *Journal of Paediatrics and Child Health*, 58(8), 1490. doi:10.1111/jpc.16055.

Vega, S. F. D., Cordero, C. P., Palapar, L. A., Garcia, A. P., & Agapito, J. D. (2018). Mixed-methods research revealed the need for dementia services and Human Resource Master Plan in an Aging Philippines. *Journal of Clinical Epidemiology*, 102, 115–122. doi:10.1016/j.jclinepi.2018.06.010.

WFOT. (2016, March). *Minimum standards for the education of occupational therapists*.   https://wfot.org/resources/new-minimum-standards-for-the-education-of-occupational-therapists-2016-e-copy.

WFOT. (2022). *Human resource project 2022: Global demographics of the occupational therapy profession* [PowerPoint slides]. https://wfot.org/checkout/29231/29230.

WHO. (2018). mhGAP Operations Manual: mental health Gap Action Programme (mhGAP). https://iris.who.int/bitstream/handle/10665/275386/9789241514811-eng.pdf?sequence=1.

WHO. (2021a). *Mental health ATLAS 2020: Member state profile [Philippines]* https://www.who.int/publications-detail-redirect/9789240036703.

WHO. (2021b, March 19). *Philippines—WHO Special Initiative for Mental Health: Situational assessment* [Full report]. https://www.who.int/publications/m/item/philippines—who-special-initiative-for-mental-health.

Yao, D. P., Inoue, K., Sy, M. P., Bontje, P., Suyama, N., Yatsu, C., Perez, D. A., & Ito, Y. (2020). Experience of Filipinos with spinal cord injury in the use of assistive technology: An occupational justice perspective. *Occupational Therapy International*, 6696296. doi:10.1155/2020/6696296.

Yap, J., Reyes, C., Albert, J. R., & Tabuga, A. (2009). *Preliminary results of the survey on persons with disabilities conducted in selected Metro Manila cities*. Philippine Institute of Development Studies. https://www.pids.gov.ph/publication/discussion-papers/preliminary-results-of-the-survey-on-persons-with-disabilities-conducted-in-selected-metro-manila-cities.

Chapter 8

Embracing *bayanihan*

Navigating occupational therapy practice in the community

Karen S. Sagun, Teresita C. Mendoza and Abelardo Apollo I. David Jr.

Chapter objectives

1   Understand the fundamental principles of community occupational therapy practice, which incorporate both local and international perspectives
2   Describe the evolution of community-based occupational therapy services in the Philippines, tracing its roots from traditional hospital settings to integration with community-based rehabilitation
3   Analyze the impact of legislative acts and policies on supporting occupational therapy in community-based healthcare
4   Discuss the process of developing community-centered occupational therapy programs, including key principles and best practices from pioneering Filipino community-based rehabilitation programs

Occupational therapy in the community serves a crucial role in developing not only individual members of the community but also the community as a whole. By recognizing the unique needs and challenges of a community, occupational therapists can develop tailored programs that address social, environmental, and cultural factors shaping occupational participation of the community. This chapter explores the evolution of occupational therapy in the Philippines, particularly its expansion from hospital settings into community-centered practice. It examines the profession's integration with community-based rehabilitation, delineating its characteristics, strategies, and growth. Furthermore, it offers practical guidelines for initiating community occupational therapy programs, reflecting the significant shift towards community reintegration for individuals with chronic disabilities as encouraged by the new Occupational Therapy Law (RA 11241).

Fundamentals of community practice in occupational therapy

The Filipino pamayanan *and its* bayanihan *spirit*

The interconnectedness of individuals within their communities holds a significant value in occupational therapy and is best captured by the concept of

DOI: 10.4324/9781003321217-8

pamayanan (Sy et al., 2021a, 2021b). It refers not only to the people of a community but also to the sense of belonging among its members, which fosters overall well-being, promotes active participation, and encourages collaborative efforts, shared resources, and collective problem-solving (Zialcita, 1996). Recognizing the cultural significance of *pamayanan* enriches the approach to community occupational therapy, ensuring interventions are culturally sensitive, effective, and empowering (Wittman & Velde, 2001). Occupational therapists tailor interventions to the specific needs of the community, considering cultural nuances and social dynamics, and collaborate with local leaders, traditional healers, and community members to ensure relevance and effectiveness (Bulan, 2023; Ramsey, 2011). This approach respects the inherent wisdom and strength within the *pamayanan* while introducing evidence-based practices that complement existing community resources to promote genuine development (Empuerto et al., 2022).

Bayanihan translates to being of a *bayan* (town or community; Ang, 1979). It reflects the Filipino value of communal unity and cooperation, where people work together to achieve common goals. The related term *bayani* refers to a hero or a person who has contributed significantly to society. A *bayani* embodies the spirit of *bayanihan* through their bravery, selflessness, and dedication to the common good. Their actions inspire others to come together and contribute to the betterment of the community. *Bayanihan* is a deeply ingrained cultural value that fosters a sense of unity and shared purpose and, in turn, encourages members to contribute their skills and resources to support their community. This concept plays a vital role in promoting health and well-being in occupational therapy (Eugenio, 1979; Roces & Roces, 2009). Embracing *bayanihan* involves recognizing the interconnectedness of individuals within their communities and actively involving not only the individual receiving therapy but also their family, caregivers, and the broader community in the therapeutic process (Duque, 2013).

Community-centered occupational therapy in the Philippines

Community-centered practice emphasizes health promotion, prevention, primary rehabilitation services, and community partnerships. In acknowledgment of widespread health inequity, these community services address not only medical but also social determinants of health such as socioeconomic status, education, employment, and healthcare access (Commission on Social Determinants of Health, 2008).

Its early roots came from community-based rehabilitation (CBR), which had a medical focus due to the influence of the WHO's (1980) International Classification of Impairments, Disabilities, and Handicaps. Early CBR programs' primary concerns were the prevention of impairment and restoring functional ability in persons with disabilities (PWD) to integrate them into their communities. The practice of CBR has evolved to include education, vocational training, social rehabilitation, and prevention, thus shifting the focus from restoring individual abilities to modifying community attitudes and contextual factors (WHO, 2010).

In the Philippines, the beginnings of community-centered occupational therapy can be traced back to 1976 when the University of the Philippines' School of Allied Medical Professions initiated a training program connected with the university's Comprehensive Community Health Program in Bay, Laguna (Mendoza, 1991). The aim was to train students in community primary healthcare, which encompasses promotive, preventive, rehabilitative, and supportive services that are person-centered, comprehensive, and participatory (WHO, 1978). At the conclusion of the Comprehensive Community Health Program in 1988, the training program was re-established in Rodriguez (formerly Montalban), Rizal, with a focus on bringing rehabilitation services to underdeveloped rural areas and empowering PWD (Magallona & Datangel, 2012). The Montalban model, a model of care that involved the client's family through a family care plan and delivered using a trans-professional approach, was an influential community rehabilitation model in the country (Magallona & Datangel, 2012).

National laws and policies have further reinforced community occupational therapy. The Magna Carta for Disabled Persons (Republic Act [RA] 7277, 1992) and Executive Order (EO) 437 (Office of the President, 2005) provided legal frameworks for CBR implementation and encouragement to local government units to adopt community-based programs for PWD. To ensure relevant competencies for community practice among entry-level occupational therapists, community-based health and rehabilitation is a mandatory course in undergraduate occupational therapy education (Commission on Higher Education [CHED], 2006). More recent national policies such as the Universal Health Care Act (RA 11223, 2018) and the Joint Administrative Order of the Department of Health, CHED, and PRC (2021) reflect the trend towards health inequity reduction by improving healthcare access in the country and reorienting the training of health professions towards primary healthcare. These developments collectively contributed to the recognition and integration of occupational therapy in community practice in the Philippines.

Community development approaches

PWD often face discrimination and barriers in various aspects of life. As a landmark international human rights treaty addressing these issues, the Convention on the Rights of Persons with Disabilities (CRPD) (United Nations, 2007) aims to uphold respect for the inherent dignity of PWD and promote, protect, and ensure their full and equal enjoyment of all human rights and fundamental freedoms (for further reading, see Chapter 13). It has since become a guiding framework for many approaches for community development, including CBR, community-based inclusive development, and disability-inclusive development, which we discuss below.

CBR is a strategy that brings rehabilitation services to the PWD's community rather than having them come to specialized institutions (WHO, 2010). Consistent with a multisectoral development approach, components of CBR programs target not only health issues of the community but also education, livelihood, social issues, and empowerment (see Figure 8.1). Moreover, CBR aims to create inclusive communities where PWD, their families, and the entire community are involved in the development process (Ayalew et al., 2020; Thomas, 2011).

Building upon CBR principles, community-based inclusive development's focus extends to broader development initiatives that promote genuine inclusion of every community member. The approach recognizes that sustainable development can be achieved only when all individuals are able to fully participate and contribute to their communities. Thus, the emphasis is on creating inclusive environments that address the diverse needs of all community members regardless of their abilities. The approach also values collaboration between various stakeholders, including government agencies, nongovernmental organizations, and community members, especially in the creation of inclusive policies, programs, and services.

Both models, however, have their shortcomings. Critics have argued that CBR places a heavy burden on already marginalized communities to provide care and resources for PWD. There is also a potential for tokenism within CBR initiatives, where the involvement of PWD in decision-making processes may be limited and not truly representative of their diverse needs and experiences. Moreover, neither CBR's provision of individual interventions nor

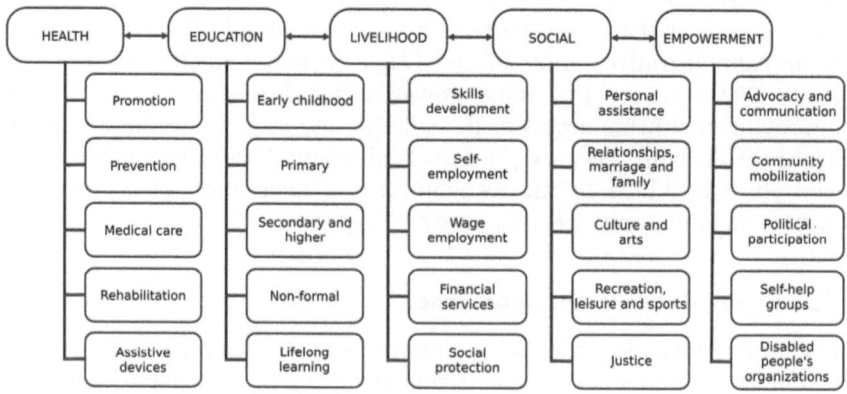

Figure 8.1 Community-based rehabilitation (CBR) matrix
Source: Reproduced from *Community-Based Rehabilitation Guidelines* [Introductory booklet], World Health Organization, © 2010.

community-based inclusive development's promotion of equal opportunities for participation and development reforms broader systemic issues (e.g., prejudice and non-inclusive practices) that cause social exclusion of PWD (Ayalew et al., 2020). Instead of empowering PWD, CBR and community-based inclusive development programs may inadvertently perpetuate paternalistic attitudes and marginalization within their communities.

Disability-inclusive development refers to the broader framework of development initiatives that explicitly consider and address PWD's needs and rights (United Nations, 2007). Central to the approach is the mainstreaming of disability issues across all sectors of development and the recognition of PWD's right to participate in and benefit from development efforts on an equal basis with others (WHO, 2010). Among the objectives of the approach is to identify and remove barriers, and create opportunities for PWD to fully engage in all aspects of community life. In effect, disability-inclusive development comprehensively combines the two aforementioned approaches, in recognition of the need to not only provide individual medical and social assistance but also address broader systemic barriers and discriminatory practices that limit the full participation of PWD in society (Thomas, 2011). The approach understands the needs for policy and structural changes to create an environment facilitative of inclusivity and equal opportunities for all.

These different approaches have implications for the role of occupational therapists in the community. In CBR, roles of occupational therapists may consist of assessing and managing the individual needs of PWD, as well as collaborating with community members and organizations to promote inclusion and accessibility. Occupational therapists working with a community-based inclusive development approach may collaborate with communities to identify and address barriers to participation and promote inclusive practices. For occupational therapists in disability-inclusive development settings, responsibilities may include not only individual rehabilitation and support of PWD but also advocacy for broader societal change and promotion of inclusive policies and practices at a macro level.

Essential to all community development approaches is the collaboration among involved individuals and agencies. Within health and social care professionals, Magallona and Datangel (2012) differentiated possible collaborative approaches (Figure 8.2). A multiprofessional approach to collaboration is when professionals work in parallel within their own specialized domains. An interprofessional approach demands greater collaboration between professionals but respective professional boundaries are maintained. These boundaries are transcended in a trans-professional approach, with professionals integrating and applying knowledge across professions to provide holistic care (Khalili et al., 2021). This spectrum of collaboration reflects the extent to which occupational therapists can contribute to individual and community health, as well as systemic change, depending on the context of their practice.

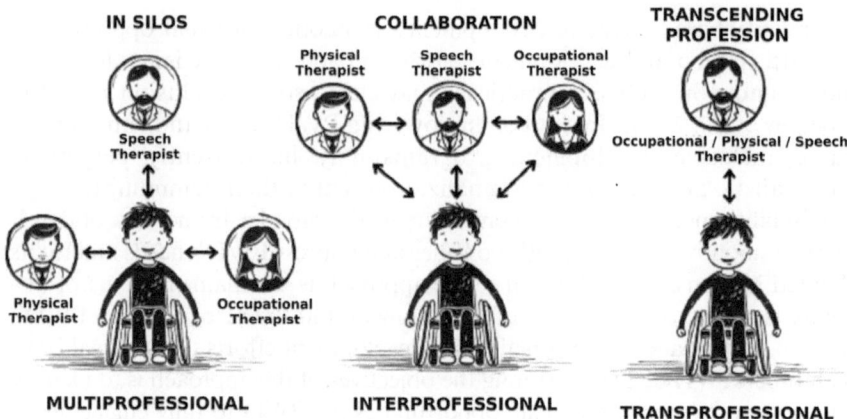

Figure 8.2 Collaboration approaches

Models of disability

Disability models provide a framework for understanding and addressing disability from different perspectives. Because these models have their use for specific purposes, it is crucial to critically examine these models to ensure that interventions and services are aligned with the needs and rights of PWD and their community.

The charity model views disability as a personal tragedy deserving of sympathy and assistance from the general population (Giampiero, 2014). The model perpetuates a paternalism, where PWD are passive recipients of others' charity rather than active participants in their own rehabilitation and empowerment. This model often leads to dependency and reinforces societal attitudes of pity and segregation, which are contrary to the principles of client-centered care and empowerment.

With an emphasis on fixing or curing an impairment, the medical model strives to diagnose, treat, and rehabilitate PWD. Although the model has facilitated scientific and technological advances in medical care, understanding disability as a purely biomedical issue (Green & Edwards, 2023) may result in a fragmented approach to rehabilitation. Non-medical factors contributing to the disability experience like physical and social barriers may be overlooked, thus allowing them to persist.

The social model of disability, in particular the *strong* social model, recognizes that disability is shaped by social, environmental, and attitudinal barriers (Shakespeare, 2013). In other words, individuals are disabled by society and its built environment, which ignores the spectrum of abilities among individuals. The model, however, fails to consider that impairments and illnesses can cause real pain and suffering regardless of the environment (Shakespeare, 2013). Nonetheless, the model cemented the significant role contexts play in shaping the lives of PWD, as well as the importance of creating enabling environments and promoting social inclusion.

Rather than reject the biomedical aspect of disabilities, the rights-based model accepts that disability is an integral facet of human diversity and does not diminish a person's inherent dignity (United Nations, 2007). As such, PWD have the same human rights as those without disabilities, which is consistent with CRPD principles. The model is particularly relevant to occupational therapy as it aligns with the profession's commitment to promoting human rights and social justice. Occupational therapists can play a vital role in advocating for the rights of PWD, ensuring their full participation in society and access to quality rehabilitation services.

Stories of Philippine community programs: Process of developing community occupational therapy programs from the ground up

Despite the Philippines' early adoption of community programs since the 1970s, many have struggled due to the absence of standardized guidelines for their establishment in developing countries. The succeeding section explores best practices from three pioneering Filipino CBR programs (Figure 8.3) noted for their innovative approaches and the authors' close involvement in their development and success. First, Project TEACH was initiated in 2007 by the REACH Foundation in partnership with the local government of Mandaluyong City. The project has garnered multiple awards, including the World Bank's Competition for Innovative Ideas Award and the United Nations Public Service Award. Second, the KABAHAGI Center offers comprehensive services for children with

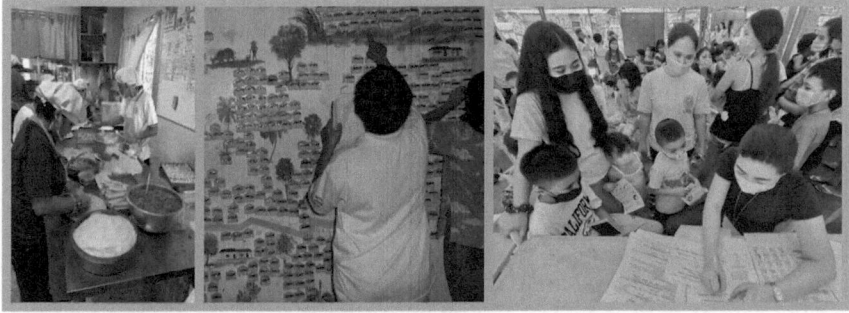

Figure 8.3 CBR programs in the Philippines. Photos from left to right: Project TEACH's cooking class for adolescents and young adults; UPM-CAMP CBR workers mapping disability in Rodriguez, Rizal; and disability screening in Quezon City by the KABAHAGI Center

disabilities and has been a Galing Pook Awards finalist. It was established in 2018 in Quezon City. Finally, the earliest community occupational therapy program in the country preceding WHO's promotion of CBR, is that of the UP-CAMP. Since its start in 1973, the program has been distinguished with several accolades, including the DOH-GTZ Bronze Award and the Pag-asa Award for outstanding public service from the Philippine Civil Service Commission.

Based on the authors' experience, a synthesis of the practical processes by which the aforementioned CBR programs have been established (David, 2021) is narrated. Moreover, snippets and examples of how the essential CRPD principles have been applied are highlighted to offer a better appreciation of how theories and models can reinforce community practice (Table 8.1).

Phase 1: Conceptualization and site selection

To plan any community program effectively, an understanding of the target community's specific needs is essential. This involves assessing the prevalence and types of disabilities through interviews, surveys, and records review. Additionally, identifying available local resources (e.g., facilities and professionals) and evaluating the socioeconomic status of the community are prerequisites for determining the affordability of planned services. High disability prevalence, a demonstrated need for services, and a lower economic profile are key factors indicating a community's suitability for a CBR program. Case in point: Mandaluyong City's dense urban poor settlements have a significant population of children with disabilities, which motivated the conception of Project TEACH. In Quezon City, the advocacy by parents led to the benchmarking with Project TEACH and subsequent creation of KABAHAGI Center for free therapy services. Meanwhile, Rodriguez, Rizal's high disability rate and supportive local leaders facilitated the implementation of the UP-CAMP CBR program.

Fostering partnerships among local disability champions and groups as well as with advocates and leaders from within the community can greatly determine the extent to which a community program is embraced, institutionalized, and sustained. Upon convening the stakeholders of a program, partnership among these entities should ideally be formalized through a memorandum of understanding. This step fosters equal opportunity and participation, and defines the terms of agreement, timelines, and the role of each member. For example, by engaging with heads of the local government to support CBR initiatives, UP-CAMP, KABAHAGI, and Project TEACH were able to more effectively elicit commitment and action from pertinent national and local government offices, such as the Department of Health, Department of Education, DSWD, Public

Table 8.1 Phases of development of the pioneer community-centered programs in the Philippines and the application of CRPD principles

Phases and relevant actions	*CRPD principles*
1. Conceptualization and site selection • Conduct a community and disability profile • Foster participation and commitment through formalized partnerships	*Participation and self-advocacy.* Taking ownership of the program, PWD and their family have the right to decide, plan, evaluate, manage, and implement programs in partnership with the community. They must organize themselves to ensure that they stay at the center of the rehabilitation process, advocate for change, and lobby for their rights and information to make the right decisions.
2. Laying down foundations • Develop programs and document service delivery protocols • Secure funding, prepare space and materials • Recruit, train, and empower human resources	*Empowerment and respect for autonomy.* PWD and their families must have opportunities to make their own informed decisions and control resources. This necessitates capacity building to acquire the necessary skills to act with authority, independent of the initiating agencies and the program managers. This principle ensures that the PWD are equipped to take on leadership roles within the program.
3. Program implementation • Conduct grassroots surveillance and eligibility screening • Assess, diagnose, and refer • Offer streamlined and holistic interventions	*Non-discrimination and inclusion of, and accessibility and respect for, children.* Inclusion encompasses respect of and acceptance of differences in culture, gender, and economic and religious realities, as a value and as a right. CBR must foster the convergence of PWD in other advocacies and campaigns as equal members of society. This can be achieved by breaking accessibility barriers, both physical and social.
4. Program evaluation and sustainability	*Sustainability.* A coordinated cooperation among stakeholders ensures that services remain effective and last beyond the support of the initiating agency.
5. Program expansion	*Growth.* Once a program becomes well established, it can be scaled up by expanding services or by replicating it in other similar communities. This is an addition to the CRPD principles as a potential direction for successful programs.

Information Office, Persons with Disabilities Affairs Division, Human Resources, Budget Office, and Public Employment Services Office. Inviting stakeholders from the private sector, such as academia, church-based organizations, and socio-civic and disability groups, can further augment the resources needed to set up a holistic community program.

Phase 2: Laying down foundations

The foundation of CBR initiatives are its programs, funding for its implementation, and dedicated manpower. In developing programs and protocols, it is ideal to conduct collaborative consultations and workshops with PWD, their families, and various stakeholders. The president of the *Kapisanan ng mga Magulang ng mga Batang may Kapansanan ng Mandaluyong* (Association of Parents of Children with Disabilities of Mandaluyong) plays a leadership role in Project TEACH, often serving as the program's main face and voice. The KABAHAGI and UP-CAMP have likewise helped empower the KABAHAGI Parent Advocates Organization and the *Kaibigang May Kapansanan* (Friends with Disabilities), respectively, to assume leadership roles in the program.

Several things must also be considered when crafting a CBR establishment and implementation plan. It should reflect the program objectives, consumer eligibility criteria, general methodology, timetable, management team, community participation mechanism, success indicators, sustainability mechanism, and budget. Stakeholders must craft a service-delivery framework that streamlines programs and services for PWD in accordance with their mandate. This deters redundancy and blurring of roles.

The resulting service delivery protocol should enable grassroots professionals, such as public school teachers, social workers, daycare center workers, government hospital workers, health workers, and civil society partners, to locate and identify individuals who have or who are at risk of having disabilities. Priority is given to the poorest among those identified who need the offered services.

Local government units and lead agencies have varying means and access to necessary resources and facilities. For instance, the city government was able to allocate a budget that fully subsidized KABAHAGI's payroll, construction of accessible facilities, and procurement equipment from the onset. Project TEACH was initially co-funded by the city government and REACH Foundation. The municipal government of Rodriguez created an official position for the municipal therapist and established the Occupational and Physical Therapy Rehabilitation Public Service Center. It also supported the local organization of PWD and the trained CBR workers managing the CBR clinics across ten barangays of the municipality.

One strategy to assist low-resourced communities is keeping abreast of pertinent disability laws and government programs, thereby allowing them to invoke their right to avail of appropriate support. In addition, applying for grants from big foundations and donor organizations can augment funds for community programs. Grants are typically awarded to proposals that clearly demonstrate mechanisms for community empowerment, efficient service delivery, and sustainability.

Establishing facilities and systematizing CBR program operations simplifies the process of recruiting and training personnel, whether by hiring new staff or reallocating existing local government or lead agency employees. Occupational, physical, and speech-language therapists employed in CBR initiatives provide not only direct therapy services but also consultations to other professionals and follow-ups of home carryover to assess effectiveness, correctness of application, and appropriateness for community setting.

With budget constraints, human resource needs can be achieved through volunteerism and opening the program for student trainees. Project TEACH trains parents of the project's service recipients as volunteer CBR workers who assist with various program implementations and support facility upkeep. Empowering PWD and their families to contribute their skills and resources to the program facilitates the *bayanihan* spirit without encouraging a culture of dependence on free services. As a training institution, UP-CAMP leveraged its need for community placement/internship places to supply community therapists to its CBR program. Meanwhile, both KABAHAGI and Project TEACH serve as accredited placement/internship sites for academic partners, with the latter also hosting international trainees. Such a strategy, however, also requires human resources in the form of clinical instructors.

Phase 3: Program implementation

CBR amalgamates a network of PWD and their families, advocates, agencies, and institutions from various backgrounds. This convergence widens the worldview of all parties involved, fosters a holistic appreciation of all the determinants of health, and offers opportunities to build on each other's work.

Through capacity-building efforts, grassroots community workers from partner agencies and organizations are oriented to the key characteristics and symptoms of various disability groups. With this knowledge, they can more easily identify individuals who have or appear to have a disability. Concerned individuals and their families are then advised to approach the CBR program's initial contact focal persons. These are usually the community centers' doctors and nurses.

Individuals referred to health centers are screened by medical personnel for impairments. Moreover, physiological and medical issues affecting their general health are addressed (e.g., medication provided to people with illness or vitamin and mineral deficiencies). Individuals in need of specialized diagnostic procedures are referred to specialists and/or laboratory facilities for appropriate tests. Upon diagnosis, doctors or social workers conduct family counseling to explain the implications of the diagnosis on the person's health, development, and well-being. The CBR program can then offer a comprehensive array of services and interventions which may include medical and dental services, therapy, education, counseling, character formation, assistive technology, vocational training, work placement, and sports and recreational programs (i.e., elements of CBR matrix). These CBR services are free for PWD, which helps them and their families attain a more positive and hopeful outlook.

For occupational therapy services, a staff member performs an initial evaluation in the first meeting with the client to identify the strengths, activity limitations, and context affecting occupational participation. Implementable and individually tailored home programs are then developed. The staff initially implements this program alongside a CBR worker and/or caregiver to demonstrate and explain its content. Eventually, the staff assumes a supervisory role as the CBR worker/caregiver begins to more actively implement the therapy sessions along with the client's family.

In case a person needs multiple services and there is a shortage of professionals, occupational therapists can employ a trans-professional approach to maximize resources, energy, and time. Here, therapists function as generalists wherein they safely implement interventions learned from within their profession as well as basic procedures endorsed by colleagues from other professions (Magallona & Datangel, 2012).

Phase 4: Program Evaluation and Sustainability

In KABAHAGI's *twin track approach* to CBR, the program's objectives are addressed and evaluated at both systemic and individual level wherein the program's effectiveness and relevance are appraised from an organizational and client-care level, respectively. Project TEACH regularly employs internal evaluation processes, which include objective assessments of the program's performance outcomes and surveys and interviews on client satisfaction. As an academic institution, UP-CAMP has conducted research studies to determine the impact of CBR on PWD, the community, and on student trainees.

Based on issues identified by the evaluation, practical strategies are crafted. When CBR programs demonstrate a significant impact in society and earn various recognitions, community leaders and policy makers are inspired to legislate policies institutionalizing CBR programs in their community. This guarantees an annual budget which is key to a program's sustainability.

Phase 5: Program expansion

When Project TEACH, KABAHAGI, and UP-CAMP CBR were institutionalized through a memorandum of agreement with their respective local government units and an approval of a city council ordinance, the stakeholders aspired to encourage other organizations and local government units to establish and/or strengthen CBR programs in their respective communities. Prompted by the COVID-19 pandemic, community programs have institutionalized remote CBR via online and digital service delivery modes. In February 2024, the REACH Foundation entered into a hallmark agreement with the Department of Interior and Local Government to open health centers that host telerehabilitation and family-mediated sessions nationwide.

UP-CAMP CBR, Project TEACH, KABAHAGI, and other CBR programs in the country collectively aspire to help the Philippines graduate from being a recipient to becoming an innovator that contributes new knowledge and systems for the global advocacy of barrier-free society for PWD.

Future of community-centered occupational therapy practice

The future of community-centered occupational therapy in the Philippines is poised for significant evolution, shaped by the establishment of regional chapters under PAOT. These regional chapters are instrumental in identifying unique local needs, resources, and cultural nuances that influence the nature of occupational therapy practice in various parts of the archipelago. By tailoring approaches to regional specificities, occupational therapy services in the community can become more relevant and effective. Moreover, strengthened public-private partnerships are expected to bolster the reach and quality of services in the community. Such collaborations can lead to more robust funding, innovative program development, and a broader scope of services available to communities, particularly in underserved areas.

The implementation of the Universal Health Care Act in the Philippines could be a game-changer for community occupational therapy. This legislation aims to provide all Filipinos with access to a comprehensive set of health services without causing financial hardship. As a result, services are likely to become more accessible, leading to an increased demand for occupational therapists in community settings. This expansion will necessitate a more substantial workforce and may also lead to the creation of new service models that prioritize cost-effectiveness and broad-based accessibility. The Act's emphasis on preventive healthcare will likely highlight the role of occupational therapists in community education, health promotion, and early intervention programs, further integrating occupational therapy into the fabric of community health services.

Conclusion

The establishment of community-centered occupational therapy programs is guided by fundamental concepts rooted in CRPD principles, which promote inclusive development. Drawing from the experience in the Philippines, there are five steps involved: conceptualization and site selection, establishing foundations, program implementation, program evaluation and sustainability, and program expansion. With *bayanihan* being innate to the Filipino *pamayanan*, the local landscape provides a fertile environment for occupational therapists to continue the legacy of serving Filipino communities.

Reflective actions and questions

1   Think back on your own personal experience of *bayanihan* (as an onlooker or as a receiver or provider of help). Appraise the advantages and disadvantages of *bayanihan*. If you are not from the Philippines, share an experience which echoes the *bayanihan* concept.
2   Consider your own community as a site for a community program. Justify the need for a community program and draft a proposal. You may use the five phases described in the chapter to organize the proposal.
3   Stories can serve as a valuable strategy to communicate the social significance of an advocacy and inspire people and organizations to commit their support to the advocacy. Identify personalities and/or organizations known to support a cause you hold close to your heart. Share a moving story (either real or imagined) that would convince them to support your advocacy.

References

Ang, G. R. (1979). The bayanihan spirit: Dead or alive? *Philippine Quarterly of Culture and Society*, 7(1/2), 91–93.

Ayalew, A. T., Adane, D. T., Obolla, S. S., Ludago, T. B., Sona, B. D., & Biewer, G. (2020). From community-based rehabilitation (CBR) services to inclusive development: A study on practice, challenges, and future prospects of CBR in Gedeo Zone (Southern Ethiopia). *Frontiers in Education*, 5, 506050. doi:10.3389/feduc.2020–.506050.

Bulan, P. M. (2023). Occupational therapy and the local context: Exploring opportunities for occupational therapy practice and education with stakeholders in Metropolitan Cebu. *World Federation of Occupational Therapists Bulletin*, 79 (2), 221–227. doi:10.1080/14473828.2020.1732680.

CHED. (2006). Policies, standards and guidelines for physical and occupational therapy education, *Memorandum Order No. 24, s. 2006* (May 26, 2006) (Phil.).

Commission on Social Determinants of Health. (2008). *Closing the gap in a generation: Health equity through action on the social determinants of health*. WHO. https://iris.who.int/bitstream/handle/10665/43943/9789241563703_eng.pdf.

David, A. A. (2021). Project Therapy, Education and Assimilation of Children with Handicap (TEACH): A community-based rehabilitation programme template for poor communities. In S. Kantartzis, N. Pollard, & H. V. Bruggen (Eds.), *And a seed was planted: Occupation based approaches for social inclusion. Volume 2: Inclusion projects and learning experiences* (pp. 127–137). Whiting & Birch.

Department of Health, CHED, & PRC. (2021). Guidelines for the reorientation of health professions education curricula and training programs to primary health care (PHC), *Joint Administrative Order No. 2021–0001* (June 3, 2021) (Phil.). https://law.upd.edu.ph/wp-content/uploads/2021/06/DOH-PRC-Joint-Memorandum-Order-No-2021-0001.pdf.

Duque, R. L. (2013). Thera-Free: Ten years of providing free and quality occupational therapy services to the underserved. *World Federation of Occupational Therapists Bulletin*, 67(1), 55–56. doi:10.1179/otb.2013.67.1.012.

Empuerto, C. C., Afable, A. M., Bardos, T. A., Oñes, G. K., Soriano, E. M., & Bulan, P. M. P. (2022). An occupational perspective on productive aging among older adults: Occupational therapy implications. *Occupational Therapy in Health Care*, 40(4), 405–418. doi:10.1080/02703181.2022.2053637.

Eugenio, D. L. (1979). *Philippine folk literature: The myths.* University of the Philippines.

Giampiero, G. (2014). Models of disability, ideas of justice, and the challenge of full participation. *Modern Italy*, 19(2), 147–159. doi:10.1080/13532944.2014.910502.

Green, H., & Edwards, B. (2023). *Models of disability: The great debate.* Routledge.

Khalili, H., Gilbert, J., Lising, D., MacMillan, K. M., & Xyrichis, A. (2021). Proposed lexicon for the interprofessional field. *InterprofessionalResearch. Global.* https://interprofessionalresearch.global/ipecp-lexicon/.

Magallona, M. L. M., & Datangel, J. P. (2012). The community-based rehabilitation programme of the University of the Philippines Manila, College of Allied Medical Professions. *Disability, CBR and Inclusive Development*, 22(3), 39–61. doi:10.5463/dcid.v22i3.110.

Magna Carta for Disabled Persons, RA No. 7277. (March 24, 1992) (Phil.). https://ncda.gov.ph/disability-laws/republic-acts/republic-act-7277/.

Mendoza, T. C. (1991). Training occupational therapy students in the primary health care setting. *World Federation of Occupational Therapists Bulletin*, 24(1), 12–15. doi:10.1080/14473828.1991.11785246.

Office of the President. (2005). Encouraging the Implementation of Community-Based Rehabilitation for Persons with Disabilities, *EO No. 437, s. 2005* (June 21, 2005) (Phil.).

Ramsey, R. (2011). Voices of community-practicing occupational therapists: An exploratory study. *Occupational Therapy in Health Care*, 25(2–3), 140–149. doi:10.3109/07380577.2011.569856.

Roces, A., & Roces, G. (2009). *CultureShock! Philippines: A survival guide to customs and etiquette.* Marshall Cavendish International Asia.

Shakespeare, T. (2013). *Disability rights and wrongs revisited* (2nd ed.). Routledge. doi:10.4324/9781315887456.

Sy, M. P., Roraldo, M. P. N. R., Reyes, R. C. D., Yao, D. P. G., & Pineda, R. C. (2021a). Occupational justice health questionnaire: Reflections on its application. *Cadernos Brasileiros de Terapia Ocupacional*, 29. doi:10.1590/2526-8910. ctoAO2244.

Sy, M. P., Yao, D. P. G., Panotes, A., Kaw, J., & Mendoza, T. C. (2021b). Contemporary history: Progress and resilience of occupational therapy in the Philippines (2004–2020). *WFOT Bulletin*, 79(1), 80–93. doi:10.1080/14473828.2021.1995226.

Thomas, M. (2011). Reflections on community-based rehabilitation. *Psychology and Developing Societies*, 23(2), 277–291. doi:10.1177/097133361102300206.

United Nations. (2007). *Convention on the rights of persons with disabilities.* https://www.ohchr.org/sites/default/files/Ch_IV_15.pdf.

Universal Health Care Act, RA No. 11223. (July 23, 2018) (Phil.). https://www.officialgazette.gov.ph/2019/02/20/republic-act-no-11223/.

WHO. (1978). *Report of the International Conference on Primary Health Care.* https://iris.who.int/bitstream/handle/10665/39228/9241800011.pdf?sequence=1.

WHO. (1980). *International classification of impairments, disabilities, and handicaps: A manual of classification relating to the consequences of disease.* https://iris.who.int/bitstream/10665/41003/1/9241541261_eng.pdf.

WHO. (2010). *Community-based rehabilitation: CBR guidelines* [Introductory booklet]. https://extranet.who.int/mindbank/item/2021.

Wittman, P. P., & Velde, B. (2001). Occupational therapy in the community: What, why, and how. *Occupational Therapy in Health Care*, 13(3–4), 1–5. doi:10.1080/J003v13n03_01.

Zialcita, F. N. (1996). The meanings of community. *Philippine Studies*, 44(1), 3–38.

Chapter 9

Telehealth and the use of technology in occupational therapy

Arden Panotes, Jomarx Jocson and Alexa Blas

Chapter objectives

1   Describe the use of technology in occupational therapy practice
2   Illustrate the contextual factors that shape the use of technology in occupational therapy practice in the Philippines
3   Discuss the process of acquiring assistive technology in the context of the Philippines
4   Discuss telehealth as a mode of service delivery in occupational therapy practice
5   Discuss the implications of using technology and telehealth in occupational therapy practice and its stakeholders

Technology plays an important role in occupational therapy, both in how occupational therapy services are delivered and during actual occupational therapy. Occupational therapists use technology to enable participation of individuals, groups, and communities to promote valued occupations. One example is the use of assistive technology in occupational therapy interventions. Before prescribing and acquiring assistive technology, a comprehensive evaluation is conducted. Evaluation tools, such as standardized assessments, are increasingly administered online in various settings. As occupational therapists analyze evaluation findings and plan service delivery, they engage in evidence-based practice, which also involves using different technologies to gather and identify the best available evidence. Technology is also used to support and deliver occupational therapy services through telehealth systems, in addition to the traditional communication and data management systems. Indeed, the use of technology in occupational practice is essential and growing. This chapter will discuss technology in occupational therapy practice in the Philippines with a focus on assistive technology and telehealth.

DOI: 10.4324/9781003321217-9

Assistive technology in occupational therapy in the Philippines

The World Federation of Occupational Therapists (WFOT) identifies assistive technology (AT) as encompassing mainstream and customized products, environmental modifications, services, and processes that enable participation in valued occupations. In occupational therapy, AT is intended to provide the best fit between the person, environment, and occupation (WFOT, 2019).

In the Philippines, AT can be tangible (e.g., enlarged spoon handles to support grip) or intangible (e.g., use of project management applications such as *Notion* to support executive function) supports towards occupational participation. Occupational therapists view the interaction between the client and the technology within the context of a meaningful activity situated in an environment. These technologies can range between low-cost and high-cost, with selection highly personalized and heavily influenced by cultural preferences, cost of acquisition, availability, and the environment or context in which they will be used (Yao et al., 2020, 2021; D. Yao, personal communication, January 28, 2024; T. Garcia, personal communication, January 29, 2024; J. Paulino, personal communication, January 30, 2024; J. R. Lucas, personal communication, January 31, 2024; P. Ching & F. Garcia, personal communication, February 9, 2024). Consequently, the acquisition and use of AT as part of occupational therapy interventions in the Philippines vary across contexts and health settings, with limited standardized, store-bought options. Occupational therapists and clients usually co-create their own devices using materials available in their immediate environment. Most AT acquisitions are out-of-pocket expenses or sponsored through grants, and health insurance only covers a limited type of AT such as prosthesis, orthosis, hearing aids, and optical devices (Philippine Health Insurance Corporation, 2014; Department of Social Welfare and Development, 2020; Cote, 2021; Ocampo, 2024). Repeated modifications of the AT to meet the client's changing needs and dynamic context are crucial in practice.

In some government hospitals in the Philippines, occupational therapists co-create assistive devices with their clients, utilizing available materials in the client's home or low-cost objects. For example, to create a long-handled sponge for bathing, occupational therapists may ask clients to bring a stick and a commercially available bath sponge. Occupational therapists take this approach considering that many clients in government hospitals have lowly salaries without personal insurance. On the other hand, financially capable clients often acquire assistive devices through friends and relatives living or traveling abroad, who have access to well-designed and commercially available AT products in other countries (D. Yao, personal communication, January 28, 2024; T. Garcia, personal communication, January 29, 2024).

Personal communication with occupational therapists in rehabilitation departments in hospitals in Metro Manila revealed that the most commonly prescribed assistive device is a universal handcuff (D. Yao, personal communication, January 28, 2024; T. Garcia, personal communication, January 29, 2024). Splints, when prescribed and used to enable participation in specific occupations, may be considered to be an assistive device and, thus, may be covered by the medical social service of the hospital but not the Philippine Health Insurance System (PhilHealth). In some cases, low-income clients request solicitation from charitable organizations of government officials for assistance to acquire AT. The need for assistive devices for clients is still often identified through referrals from medical doctors. This practice originated from the repealed Philippine Physical and Occupational Therapy Law of 1969 (Republic Act 5680), which mandated that occupational therapists require referrals from physicians to provide any service. Despite the passing of the Philippine Occupational Therapy Law of 2018 (Republic Act 11241), changing these processes will take time. Occupational therapists frequently work with people who use mobility aids such as wheelchairs, walkers, and canes, and closely coordinate treatment and discharge planning with clients' doctors and physical therapists. However, environmental accessibility issues sometimes obstruct clients from using their mobility aids effectively in their homes and communities (Yao et al., 2021; T. Garcia, personal communication, January 29, 2024; D. Yao, personal communication, January 28, 2024).

In community settings, the prescription and use of AT are adapted to users' needs within the constraints of the environment (J.R. Lucas, personal communication, January 31, 2024). Sometimes, the AT is repurposed and used differently from what was intended. For example, a community-based occupational therapist remarked how a wheelchair may function more as a positioning device at home because of physical barriers like high door thresholds, which limit its intended use for mobility. Families often adapt by carrying the wheelchair over the door threshold before using it for its intended purpose (P. Ching & F. Garcia, personal communication, February 9, 2024).

Another notable difference in the community setting is the long-term monitoring and actual use of the AT in context. Occupational therapists actively participate in fine-tuning the AT, considering improvements in client factors or overall participation in occupations. For instance, in providing a wheelchair to a child, the chair initially serves as a positioning device to facilitate postural control, which is a prerequisite for effective hand use while in an upright position. As the client gains more capacity to move the distal upper extremities, the occupational therapist may attach a tray to the wheelchair, so that a variety of activities can be done such as feeding, playing or writing while seated in the wheelchair. This increased occupational engagement allows for participation not only in the home but also in school settings. Wheelchair trays may provide a practical solution, instead of dealing with varying table heights and widths, which are common in the Philippines and can hinder access and use.

In the Philippine context, wheelchair service provision in the community setting is primarily funded out of pocket or through non-government or non-profit religious organizations that sponsor wheelchair acquisitions. These wheelchairs are often imported, with parts not readily available locally; hence, wheelchair adjustments are often limited, makeshift, or do-it-yourself (DIY). There is heavy reliance on a skilled technician who works under the guidance of trained occupational therapists. Occupational therapists frequently work in close collaboration with other health professionals (such as physical therapists, speech therapists, and wheelchair technicians) to ensure optimal adjustments. Although the occupational therapist's involvement in the wheelchair service provision model in the community setting is a growing practice, it is still in its early stages (P. Ching & F. Garcia, personal communication, February 9, 2024)

In contrast to ATs addressing mobility limitations and physical limitations, AT use in mental health settings is more subtle. One occupational therapist (J. Paulino, personal communication, January 30, 2024) reflected on using AT "without even knowing it." In mental health practice, AT often serves as an adjunct tool to support rehabilitation or as a compensatory strategy for specific client factors or process skills. Selection depends on what is available in the client's context and on the client's skills, beliefs, and financial capacity. For instance, holding a handkerchief may help ground a client during a panic attack, while social media messaging platforms (e.g., Facebook Messenger) may serve as a memory aid or a monitoring tool for a client undergoing executive functions training. Mobile applications that target specific mental health conditions, such as *Calm Harm* for clients with suicidal ideations, are used selectively when they are perceived to be helpful in enabling participation in the client's desired occupations.

Another common AT practice is the use of various learning support technologies and alternative and augmentative communication (AAC) devices to facilitate educational participation and social participation. Learning support ATs include both high-tech devices such as tablets and personal computers and conventional technologies such as peg boards, tripod pencil grips, and reading trackers (Campado et al., 2023). For AAC devices, occupational therapists collaborate closely with speech therapists to contextualize and customize the use of AAC devices. Speech therapists assess and identify a high-tech (e.g., tablet to communicate, speech-generating device) or low-tech (e.g., gestures, writing, pointing) AAC system best suited to the person and provide training for their use. Occupational therapists facilitate the use of AAC devices in occupations, such as in communicating food preferences during meals, greetings in a social situation, and participating in classroom activities.

Culture plays an important role in AT selection, acceptance, and use. For example, rosary beads, a religious tool, can be used for emotional regulation, reflecting cultural norms. Culture (family-centered culture) also influences the use of AT. Generally, AT is intended to promote independence in an activity or a task within the activity. However, the intended purpose of AT conflicts with the Filipino concept of *alaga*, which emphasizes the family members' active role in taking care or assisting relatives with disabilities, instead enabling participation in co-occupation (interdependence) and promoting independence. For example, a client may prefer to be assisted by a family member in bathing rather than using a long-handled sponge. The client appreciates this assistance as this makes him or her feel cared for, while the family member finds meaning or fulfillment in helping and considers this an act of service.

The benefits of ATs reported by the occupational therapists practicing in the Philippines are consistent with the studies on the effectiveness of ATs in various contexts over the years. The reported outcomes where ATs have significant impact include performance skills (Maor et al., 2011; Fteiha, 2016; Brims & Oliver, 2018) and engagement in occupations (Golding et al., 2019).

Locally, the selection and use of AT as an occupational therapy intervention is affected by the goals and needs of clients and their socio-economic status. AT serves as a means to achieve a goal—occupational performance, occupational participation, and occupational justice (Yao et al., 2020; Yamat et al., 2023). AT can be used to restore, maintain, or improve ability to perform occupations by enhancing underlying client factors and performance skills or compensating for impaired or loss of function. Its use can support occupational participation (Golding et al., 2019), enabling a person to live, work, and play in various socio-cultural contexts. Additionally, the use of AT can enable a person to uphold their right to choose, perform, and participate in meaningful occupations (Arthanat et al., 2012) as well as to achieve a balance in the amount of and variation between occupations (Wagman et al., 2012). With AT, a person develops what Amartya Sen's (Sen, 1999) *capability approach* describes as agency to make choices and the capability to lead a meaningful life and to contribute to the community.

Frames of reference and AT selection and prescription

Various frames of reference (FORs) can guide professional reasoning in the prescription and use of AT as an occupational intervention. In the Philippines, there are three common categories of FORs used to guide the reasoning process. These include FORs that describe the dynamic interaction of the person, environment, and occupation, influence occupational performance by augmenting or supporting performance skills, and improve underlying client factors that affect occupational performance (see Table 9.1).

Table 9.1 Examples of FORs used for AT selection and acquisition

Interaction between person, environment, and occupation

Frame of Reference	Description	Example of AT Utility
1. Person-Environment-Occupation Model (Law et al., 1996)	Posits that occupational performance results from the dynamic transaction between the person, environment, and occupation.	Occupational therapist considers a client's skill deficit, personal preferences, socioeconomic status, relevant skills and potential, learning capacity, access to tools, materials or equipment, and context and environment in selecting an AT.
2. Occupational Adaptation Model (Schkade & Schultz, 1992)	Highlights "press for mastery" where the person adapts to the environment by discovering new responses that work—or, simply put, an adaptive response.	Client is asked to hold a rosary or handkerchief to keep anxiety symptoms at tolerable levels.

Performance support or augmentation

1. Acquisitional FOR	Highlights the importance of teaching-learning in developing skills or appropriate behaviors within the context of an environment.	Occupational therapist teaches a client to use an application as a memory aid for a task.
2. Compensatory Approach	Prioritize the performance of the occupation despite underlying client factor concerns.	Client with a weak grip uses a spoon with a towel wrapped around the hand so they can scoop food.

Improvement of Underlying Client Factors

1. Biomechanical Model	Remediation specifically for range of motion (ROM), strength, and endurance.	Occupational therapist fabricates a functional hand splint and adjusts its fit to help maintain the ROM of a client who experienced a stroke.
2. Neurodevelopmental Model	Highlights the importance of kinesiology and biomechanics in addressing postural control and movement impairments.	Occupational therapist adjusts the positioning devices on a wheelchair to apply principles of mobility and stability.

The nexus of AT, ethics, and sustainability of care

We (the authors) reflected on the layers of complexity of OT practice and use of AT in the Philippine context. There is no one distinct Filipino-based AT except that it is an adaptation to limitations of the larger environment and the choice is culturally sensitive to the values of family even when guided by FORs that promote autonomy.

Despite having a similar client case and performance limitations, the resulting choice for AT is highly varied and often referred to as "DIY-ed." DIY or "Do it yourself" means that the AT was created or co-created by the therapist with a client using available materials within the context. The reason for this can be traced back to the difference in access and availability of ATs in a developing country such as the Philippines (Chakraborty, 2020). This raises the complex issue of poverty, availability, and access to healthcare, including occupational therapy services and even tools and equipment that support performance. At the practice level, an occupational therapist practicing in the Philippines faces the dilemma of where and how to acquire the needed tools and equipment to support the health and well-being of the person. It raises the question of sustainability of therapeutic care especially for AT practice and its supposed benefits. At present, these environmental factors create the limits to the selection and acquisition of AT for a client. Despite these limiting conditions, Filipino occupational therapists find creative ways to promote occupational performance using AT.

It is interesting to note that occupational therapy practice in the Philippines is guided by FORs developed in highly developed countries that highlight strong values of autonomy and independence. Pooremamali (2012) substantiated the need for culturally adjusted interventions because the "ambivalence between striving for empowerment and wanting support" as well as the difference between collectivistic versus individual worldviews influence how a client views empowerment, support and well-being. Hammell (2009) asserted that independence is "not universally prized." This is important because the FORs guide the occupational therapist's perspective on function and dysfunction, especially in the selection and acquisition of AT. From the interviews, it is evident that the family, especially the primary caregiver, shapes the selection and acquisition of AT. Considering the case of the caregiver making bathing a co-occupation and finding meaning in caring for the family member, this raises the question: is assistance in bathing considered a dysfunction?

Case vignettes: Local use of AT

We outline below two cases regarding the use of AT from the local context in order to give you the context of the function of AT for people with disabilities, how it is acquired, the importance of collaborative practice, and the influence of socioeconomic factors in sustaining its use.

Box 9.1 Case of Jose: A child receiving home care for training of self-care tasks and home mobility

Jose is a male, non-verbal adolescent with apraxia of speech who lives with his family and a helper. He is receiving occupational therapy in a private pediatric clinic. Additional services through home care were given to generalize learned skills in the home environment. Because of the restrictions brought about by the pandemic, frequency of home care services were increased. During these sessions, his occupational therapist focuses on developing skills needed for self-care, which involves the use of both high- and low-technology devices such as a tablet and a set of picture exchange cards. He uses these devices mainly for communication. His speech-language therapist prescribed and trained him in using these devices while his occupational therapist ensures the use of these in his daily living activities. For example, during feeding, Jose uses his tablet to communicate hunger and choice of food. He taps the picture on the application and he shows the screen to his family member. He also uses this to express his thoughts and feelings such as when he feels unready to engage in an activity. For his picture exchange cards, these are used as visual cues in his environment. His drawer at home has pictures of the objects that it contains. He also has a schedule board with pictures and words that represent his routine. Every morning, a family member discusses his schedule for the day on the board. Every time he finishes a task, he flips the picture. This helps him anticipate his tasks for the day and organize his time. There are also posters posted in different rooms of the house such as in the bathroom where he has pictures of the steps of bathing and brushing teeth. His family members were trained by the occupational therapist in facilitating the use of these devices for Jose. With the help of these devices, he became independent in most self-care activities at home as well as simple household tasks such as washing the dishes and mopping the floor.

Box 9.2 Case of Liam: A child needing an alternative augmentative communication device

Liam is a five-year-old child diagnosed with autism. He is non-verbal yet he shows good visual perceptual skills. His occupational therapist, in collaboration with his speech-language therapist, is considering the use of a high-technology augmentative and alternative communication (AAC) device. He has shown good progress with his low-technology AAC device—a board with pictures. However, his communication is currently being limited by it. With high-technology AAC, there will be more opportunities for him to practice learned concepts for communication in a way that can be easily understood by communication partners, such as in expressing thoughts and requesting wants. Shifting to a high-technology AAC device entails the need for a tablet and a software that costs more than PhP 10,000.00 (or approximately USD 200). Therapy to train him on the use of the device will also be shouldered out of pocket by his parents as therapy services are not covered by the government health insurance system.

Telehealth in occupational therapy

Telehealth in occupational therapy pertains to the use of information and communication technologies to deliver services including evaluation, intervention, monitoring/supervision, and consultation when there are differences in location between the therapist and the client (WFOT, 2014). WFOT asserts that services delivered via telehealth shall demonstrate the same standards as those delivered in person and comply with set policies from governing bodies. Ethical considerations are emphasized to ensure the welfare and best interest of clients. Occupational therapists must employ mechanisms to ensure confidentiality for both the synchronous and stored data of clients.

Telehealth can be synchronous, where the therapist and client are interacting at the same time through videoconferences, remote monitoring, and virtual applications, or asynchronous, where data such as videos, photos, and documents are transmitted using electronic means by the occupational therapist or the client. There are low-technology strategies such as phone calls, electronic mails, and text messages. Mid-tech strategies include videoconferencing and use of commercially available applications. High-tech strategies are those that can cater to personalized and specialized intervention (Camden & Silva, 2020).

As the COVID-19 pandemic brought physical restrictions, occupational therapists in the Philippines were prompted to shift to deliver services through online means. This is when the use of telehealth in practice gained relevance in the country. Prior to this, telehealth was rarely used, as the primary mode of service delivery was in-person. This is also in relation to the technological infrastructure available in the country. The occupational therapy community then worked collaboratively to establish guidelines, develop competencies for telehealth, and educate clients about the platform. The Philippine Academy of Occupational Therapists (PAOT) released guidelines on the utilization of telehealth together with a series of online webinars and forums to upskill occupational therapy practitioners on the use of technology. The guidelines specify the professional standards, ethical considerations, monitoring mechanisms, continuous quality improvement, cost of services, documentation, and resumption to direct service delivery, as telehealth is perceived as an alternative form of occupational therapy service provision (PAOT, 2020).

Telehealth in the form of a synchronous video conference then was mainly used for the continuity of provision of occupational therapy intervention for existing clients. Private and government facilities created their own protocols from the set guidelines. Most protocols involve a trial session where the therapist explains how occupational therapy will be delivered via telehealth and assesses if the technical requirements are met. Internet connection problems and power interruptions in rural areas posed a challenge for clients and therapists (Delos Reyes et al., 2021). Some clients also do not have a device that can run a videoconference application. In such instances, occupational therapists provide home programs that are sent via email. These home programs contain the activities that can be done at home to achieve therapy goals.

From providing direct intervention, occupational therapists shifted to using a family coaching approach in educating and training clients and their families in implementing therapy strategies at home. They maximize the materials and equipment available in the client's home and send printable information packets as needed. Families and carers acknowledge that they have a role as learners in learning therapy principles and strategies for their family members (Panotes et al., 2024)

Most occupational therapists conduct telehealth on a work-from-home set-up with those in private center–based practice using their own laptops and computers. Those working with children with developmental disabilities reported that delivering services via telehealth had increased demand for time and energy as they had to prepare online materials and resources and integrate them with structured activities (Eguia & Capio, 2022). After the online session or consultation, occupational therapists also prepare documentation in a computerized format to be given to the client.

Therapy managers and center owners also made efforts in establishing telehealth by developing delivery services protocols and providing training for their therapists. They also oriented parents on this relatively new service delivery model for the country. In the protocol, ethical principles and professional standards were considered and policies were applied consistently throughout the process of receiving telehealth. Therapists were initially uncomfortable with the new platform due to unfamiliarity and concerns with the transition from onsite to online services. This was mediated through a series of training sessions for the therapists. Similarly, clients had second thoughts on using technology for therapy due to unstable internet connections and worries of being able to carry over or follow the instructions of the therapist. To address these challenges, online consultations were provided by the therapy managers to discuss telehealth with them. Similarly, trial sessions for synchronous telehealth were offered to let the therapist and the client experience how a session would be conducted. Most therapists and clients had positive experiences with telehealth after the trial session, which led to their continuous use of the service. However, some did not proceed with availing telehealth services due to concerns about readiness for using technology to manage a child's behavioral problems. They were given other options through asynchronous means such as home program booklets and short consultations through phone calls.

Making telehealth more accessible to the Filipino public

Below we provide a case on how telehealth was used in a community-based rehabilitation program, sponsored by the local government. This case highlights how occupational therapists made services accessible to the clients through telehealth. It is also observed in this case that occupational therapists used technology as a new tool for providing training for families to continue receiving therapy at home.

Box 9.3 Utilization of telehealth in community-based programs

A community-based program initiated by a local government in Metro Manila was created to be a training center for parents and caregivers who belong to low-income families to help them access assistance and support for their children with additional needs. In the succeeding years, it evolved into a training center for allied health interns in, for example, occupational therapy, speech therapy, and physical therapy fields. When physical distancing was implemented during the COVID-19 pandemic, the center transitioned from in-person to telehealth. The center developed protocols and training modules based on the PAOT's (2020) guidelines. The telehealth program involved both asynchronous and synchronous approaches. Asynchronous sessions typically consist of giving materials ahead of time and having a phone call to give feedback on how the carers implemented it. Facebook Messenger was used during synchronous telehealth since it requires low bandwidth and the clients are familiar with it. The interns and clinical supervisors made an account specifically for telehealth while the clients used their personal accounts. The center provided 50 tablets to the families in need of therapy delivered via telehealth. Internet connectivity would be at the expense of the family receiving therapy. The center orients the interns regarding the process of conducting training to the families and community-based rehabilitation (CBR) workers at the start of the program. However, due to the limited number of CBR workers available during that time, the interns were instructed to perform the telehealth directly with the children and their carers. In a day, each intern would cater to four clients and the clinical supervisor would rotate in the ongoing therapy sessions to check the implementation of the program. The main goal of telehealth is to provide caregiver education and training of families on how to deliver therapy at home. Initially, the families showed apprehension about the new approach of receiving services. Based on the survey conducted by the center, most of the parents and carers still opt to get services in-person, as they are concerned about the effectiveness of using technology to access therapy. However, they were willing to still give it a try and eventually adapt and appreciate its potential benefits. They also showed their gratitude for receiving therapy even in the midst of the pandemic. Currently, the center still utilizes telehealth for group sessions, targeting social enterprise and managing business at home.

Telehealth provided continuity of services during the pandemic in the Philippines. It has made occupational therapy accessible for clients and their families without the need to travel to a hospital or clinic. Given that most facilities offering occupational therapy are in urban areas, clients in rural areas were able to access services through telehealth. However, access to technology was also a requirement for both the occupational therapist and the client. Occupational therapists and their clients need to have a computer or laptop that can support the platforms that will be used together with a stable internet connection to be able to engage in telehealth. Usability is also a consideration such that both occupational therapists and their clients can effectively use emails and videoconferencing for telehealth. The need for service shall be balanced with the need for data security and privacy. Occupational therapists shall consider the level of security offered by the platforms that will be used in telehealth and have strategies in place to ensure safety of information in the online space.

Emerging technologies in occupational therapy practice

At present, there are parallel efforts to improve the service delivery of occupational therapy in the Philippines. Included in these efforts are upgrades with the materials, tools, and equipment or a direct improvement in the occupational therapy processes (e.g., evaluation and monitoring). An occupational therapist and a speech therapist who are both wheelchair service providers are developing affordable and appropriate intermediate wheelchair models for the Philippines by collaborating with the University of the Philippines Discovery Hub (P. Ching & F. Garcia, personal communication, February 9, 2024). Another notable development led by an occupational therapist, who is also a data scientist, is the development of Scalable Intelligent Note-taking and Teaching-learning Assistant (SINTA), which is an AI-powered note-taking application that records a session in real time, translates recorded audio to text, and organizes the notes according to the practice format (K. Carandang, personal communication, June 10, 2024). These trailblazing initiatives demonstrate how occupational therapists in the Philippines continuously learn and identify efficient and effective ways to provide therapy services that consider the person, environment, and occupation.

Reflection questions

1   In a small group, discuss practical ways to enable occupational participation and justice using AT while promoting sustainability given scarce resources from both therapists and clients as well as environmental restrictions?

2 In relation to ethical use (specifically on data privacy and confidentiality), discuss among your peers in school or at work what ethical considerations must be taken into account when using AT for the delivery of occupational therapy services?

3 There is a scarcity of local research about occupational therapy using telehealth and assistive technologies. Looking through the local publications available in this chapter and the limitations they offered, what research questions and objectives can you come up with to further research these areas?

References

Addy, L. (2006). *Occupational therapy evidence in practice for physical rehabilitation*. Oxford: Blackwell.

Arthanat, S., Simmons, C., & Favreau, M. (2012). Exploring occupational justice in consumer perspectives on assistive technology. *Canadian Journal of Occupational Therapy. Revue canadienne d'ergothérapie*, 79, 309–319.

Barthel, K. A. (2010). A frame of reference for neuro-developmental treatment. In P. Kramer & J. Hinojosa (Eds.), *Frames of reference for pediatric occupational therapy* (3rd ed., pp. 187–233). Philadelphia: Lippincott Williams & Wilkins.

Brims, L., & Oliver, K. (2018). Effectiveness of assistive technology in improving the safety of people with dementia: A systematic review and meta-analysis. *Aging & Mental Health*, 23(8), 942–951. 10.1080/13607863.2018.1455805.

Camden, C., & Silva, M. (2020). Pediatric telehealth: Opportunities created by the COVID-19 and suggestions to sustain its use to support families of children with disabilities. *Physical and Occupational Therapy in Pediatrics*, 41(1), 1–17. 10.1080/01942638.2020.1825032.

Campado, R. J., Toquero, C. M. D., & Ulanday, D. M. (2023). Integration of assistive technology in teaching learners with special educational needs and disabilities in the Philippines. *International Journal of Professional Development Learners and Learning*, 5(1), ep2308. 10.30935/ijpdll/13062.

Chakraborty, S. (2020). Assistive technologies: Addressing the divide between the developed and developing world. *Journal of Science Policy & Governance*, 16. 10.38126/JSPG160204.

Cote, A. (2021). Social protection and access to assistive technology in low- and middle-income countries. *Assistive Technology*, 33(1), S102–S108. 10.1080/10400435.2021.1994052.

Delos Reyes, R., Aceremo, J. A., Acosta, A., Atienza, R. L., & De Castro, J. C. (2021). Beliefs of Filipino caregivers on occupational therapy through telehealth. *Annals of Physiotherapy & Occupational Therapy*, 4(1). 10.23880/aphot-16000187.

Department of Social Welfare and Development. (2020, June 30). DSWD provides assistive devices to persons with disability. https://www.dswd.gov.ph/dswd-provides-assistive-devices-to-persons-with-disability/#:~:text=These%20devices%20may%20include%20talking,wheelchair%2C%20tri%2Dwheelchair%20bike%2C.

Eguia, K. F., & Capio, C. M. (2022). Teletherapy for children with developmental disorders during the COVID-19 pandemic in the Philippines: A mixed-methods evaluation from the perspectives of parents and therapists. *Child: Care, Health and Development*, 48(6), 963–969. 10.1111/cch.12965.

Fteiha, M. A. (2016). Effectiveness of assistive technology in enhancing language skills for children with autism. *International Journal of Developmental Disabilities*, 63(1), 36–44. 10.1080/20473869.2015.1136129.

Golding, C., Bond, C., Fernandez, V., & Barrientos, E. (2019). Assistive technology and the impact of occupations [Capstone project]. 10.33015/dominican.edu/2019.ot.10.

Hammell, K. W. (2009). Sacred texts: A sceptical exploration of the assumptions underpinning theories of occupation. *Canadian Journal of Occupational Therapy*, 76(1), 6–13. 10.1177/000841740907600105.

Law, M., Cooper, B., Strong, S., Stewart, D., Rigby, P., & Letts, L. (1996). The Person-Environment-Occupation Model: A transactive approach to occupational performance. *Canadian Journal of Occupational Therapy*, 63(1), 9–23.

Maor, D., Currie, J., & Drewry, R. (2011). The effectiveness of assistive technologies for children with special needs: a review of research-based studies. *European Journal of Special Needs Education*, 26(3), 283–298. 10.1080/08856257.2011.593821.

McMillan, I. R. (2011). The biomechanical frame of reference in occupational therapy. In E. A. S. Duncan (Ed.), *Foundations for practice in occupational therapy* (5th ed., pp. 179–194). Edinburgh: Churchill Livingstone.

Ocampo, J. (2024, June 13). Bridging the gap: The state of assistive technology in the Philippines. *Ateneo Special Education Society*. https://www.ateneospeed.org/our-stories/bridging-gap-state-assistive-technology-philippines/.

Panotes, A., Jocson, J., Andigan, C. M., & Sy, M. P. (2024). Lived experiences of caregivers upon receiving occupational therapy through telehealth amidst the pandemic. *Cadernos Brasileiros de Terapia Ocupacional*, 32. 10.1590/2526-8910. ctoao27853626.

PAOT. (2020). *Guidelines on the use of telehealth as an alternative form of occupational therapy service provision*. World Federation of Occupational Therapists. https://wfot.org/assets/resources/PAOT-Guidelines-on-the-Utilization-of-Telehealth.pdf.

Philippine Health Insurance Corporation. (2014). Benefits. https://www.philhealth.gov.ph/benefits/.

The Philippine Occupational Therapy Law of 2018, Republic Act 1124. (2018). https://lawphil.net/statutes/repacts/ra2019/ra_11241_2019.html.

Philippine Physical and Occupational Therapy Law, Republic Act 5680. (1969). https://www.prc.gov.ph/uploaded/documents/PHYSICALTHERAPY-LAW.pdf.

Pooremamali, P. (2012). *Culture, occupation and occupational therapy in a mental health care context* [Doctoral Dissertation, Malmö University]. https://mau.diva-portal.org/smash/get/diva2:1404262/FULLTEXT01.pdf.

Schkade, J. K., & Schultz, S. (1992). Occupational adaptation: Toward a holistic approach for contemporary practice: I. *American Journal of Occupational Therapy*, 46(9), 829–837.

Sen, A. (1999). *Development as freedom*. Alfred A. Knopf.

Wagman, P., Håkansson, C., & Björklund, A. (2012). Occupational balance as used in occupational therapy: A concept analysis. *Scandinavian Journal of Occupational Therapy*, 19(4), 322–327. 10.3109/11038128.2011.596219.

WFOT. (2014). *Position statement on occupational therapy and telehealth*. World Federation of Occupational Therapists. https://wfot.org/checkout/25960/26409.

WFOT. (2019). *Position statement on occupational therapy and assistive technology*. https://wfot.org/resources/occupational-therapy-and-assistive-technology.

Yamat, K., Bondoc, J. A., Delasas, G. E., Lacson, M. A., Rodriguez, R. V., & David, A. A., Jr. (2023). SAKLAY: A guide to an assistive technology service delivery process in the Philippines. *Philippine Journal of Allied Health Sciences*, 6(2). 10.36413/pjahs.0602.010.

Yao, D. P. G., Bontje, P., Inoue, K., Tanaka, A., & Lacsamana-Manalaysay, J. (2021). Coping with bereavement: The experience of a Filipino who lives life using a wheelchair. *World Federation of Occupational Therapists Bulletin*, 77(1), 58–64. 10.1080/14473828.2020.1868164.

Yao, D. P. G., Inoue, K., Sy, M. P., Bontje, P., Suyama, N., Yatsu, C., Perez, D. A., & Ito, Y. (2020). Experience of Filipinos with spinal cord injury in the use of assistive technology: An Occupational Justice Perspective. *Occupational Therapy International*, 1–10. 10.1155/2020/6696296.

Chapter 10

Occupational therapy in disaster pre-crisis phase

Maria Menierva Lagria and Roi Charles Pineda

Chapter objectives

1 Describe disaster risk reduction (DRR) principles and their relationship with socioeconomic development
2 Identify international and national policies shaping DRR activities in the Philippines and within the occupational therapy profession in the Philippines
3 Describe occupational therapy roles in DRR, using the example of the MARCH Village community development project

In everyday parlance, a disaster describes an adverse event that affects us negatively. We may indiscriminately use the term to describe a broad range of personal crises. For example, a particularly nasty haircut may be called a *disaster*!

In the humanitarian system, however, a disaster has a more specific meaning. For example, the United Nations International Strategy for Disaster Reduction (UNISDR, 2009) defines a disaster as "a serious disruption of the functioning of a community or society involving widespread human, material, economic or environmental losses and impacts, which exceeds the ability of the affected community or society to cope using its resources" (p. 9). An event therefore qualifies as a disaster when its direct or indirect consequences (e.g., physical injuries and deaths, psychological trauma, human displacement, infrastructure destruction, and/or economic loss) are substantial and widespread, and where external help, in the form of assistance from national or international actors, is necessary to overcome its impact.

The topic is particularly relevant to the Philippine context, considering that the country has had one of the highest number of disasters in the world over the last 20 years, according to the United Nations Office for Disaster Risk Reduction (UNDRR, 2020). Due to its geographic location, the country is visited, on average, by 19 typhoons yearly (Cinco et al., 2016), often causing destruction of properties and crops. Moreover, seismic

DOI: 10.4324/9781003321217-10

and volcanic activities frequently occur in the country. Consequent disasters from these natural hazards can disable individuals, groups, and populations from engaging in daily occupations, performing established routines, and fulfilling valued life roles (American Occupational Therapy Association [AOTA], 2011). In this regard, occupational therapists are in a prime position to not only provide direct interventions to help individuals and groups resume their occupations but also contribute to local, national, and international DRR actions.

In this chapter, we discuss the principles of DRR, related international and national policies, and practices adopted in the community. Because the impact of a disaster extends well beyond the disaster event itself, DRR is often broken down into pre-, in-, and post-crisis phases. DRR activities are organized around the needs, risks, and priorities of each phase (UNISDR, 2015). The cyclical configuration of these phases and activities (see Figure 10.1) represents the recurring nature of many disasters. While we acknowledge the early call of the World Federation of Occupational Therapist (WFOT, 2014) for occupational therapists' involvement in all phases of DRR, this chapter focuses on the pre-crisis phase because it was found to be the phase where Filipino occupational therapists are least involved (Ching & Lazaro, 2021). This aligns with the global and national paradigm shift to managing disaster risks rather than merely responding to disasters.

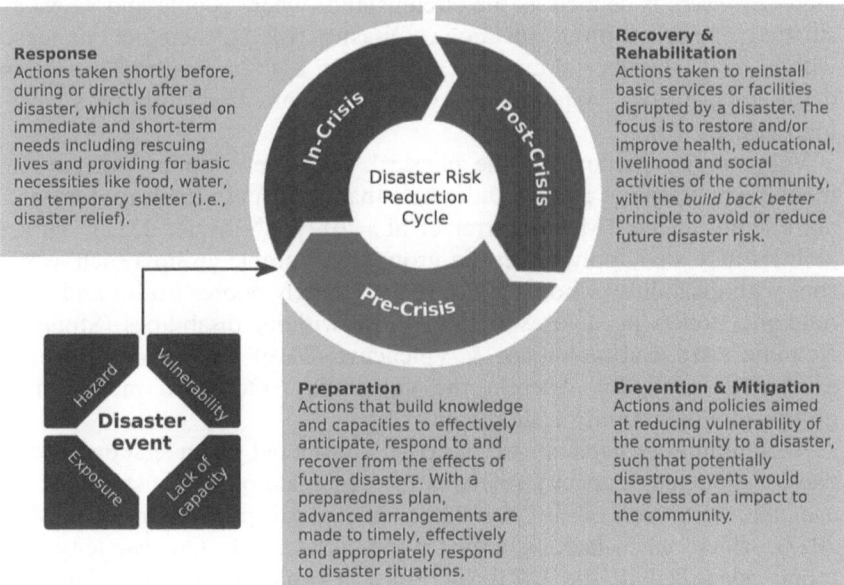

Figure 10.1 Disaster risk reduction cycle, the actions associated per phase of the cycle (United Nations General Assembly, 2016; UNISDR, 2017), and the disaster risk elements

DRR principles

A wide range of events or processes can result in a disaster. It is now widely recognized that most disasters are not random unavoidable events but occur because of a combination of social and natural processes. Based on current disaster risk models (Marin-Ferrer et al., 2017; UNISDR, 2017), the occurrence of disasters and intensification of their impact are shaped by four elements: presence of hazards, exposure to hazards, vulnerability of the population affected, and low capacity to overcome the impact of a hazard event. No disaster occurs if any one of these elements is absent (Marin-Ferrer et al., 2017).

A hazard is a natural phenomenon, substance, or human activity that has the potential to cause injury or death, damage infrastructure, disrupt social and economic activities, or deteriorate the environment (UNISDR, 2017). Hazards are often categorized as natural or human-induced. However, it has become clear that many hazards are socio-natural because they arise from interacting natural and anthropogenic processes (UNISDR, 2017). For example, deforestation by humans increases the risk of typhoon-related hazards such as flooding and landslides. Deforestation also contributes to global warming, resulting in more adverse weather conditions.

Disasters cannot happen if people and infrastructure are not exposed to the hazard, regardless of the hazard's severity (Marin-Ferrer et al., 2017). Here, *exposure* is defined as the circumstance where people and assets are situated in hazard-prone locations. Disaster risk is, therefore, increased with a greater number of exposed elements in a given locality. Population-dense low-elevation coastal zones where typhoons frequently pass have a high disaster risk.

Vulnerability pertains to the physical, social, economic, and environmental conditions of people and assets that predispose them to a hazard's detrimental effects (Marin-Ferrer et al., 2017; UNISDR, 2017). Vulnerabilities may also apply to certain groups (vulnerable groups) such as persons with disabilities who have disproportionately poorer health and social outcomes following a disaster than those without disabilities (Stough & Kelman, 2018; Subramaniam & Villeneuve, 2019). This underscores disaster risk inequality, wherein the vulnerable, often also marginalized, groups in a community bear the most risk.

A community's capacity needs to be considered in understanding why disasters happen. Capacity refers to the aggregate of all the strengths and available resources of an individual, group, or population (UNISDR, 2017), which, when lacking, elevates the disaster risk. One capacity commonly identified in the DRR literature is *resilience* or the ability of a community to restore its basic structures and functions following exposure to hazards (UNISDR, 2009). It has become a buzzword in the Philippines, particularly as it relates to post-disaster imagery of Filipinos smiling or practicing *bayanihan* [1] instead of despairing. This is supported by Filipinos' strong self-perception of resilience against disasters, which is grounded in several positive characteristics such as *malasakit* (empathy), *tiwala* (trust), *pagtitiis* (fortitude), *pagkamasayahin at palabiro* (cheerfulness and sense of humor), and *pananalig sa Diyos* (faith in God) (Adviento & de Guzman, 2010; Usamah et al., 2014). Although positive attitude and communal unity undoubtedly contribute to recovery, they are usually insufficient to rely upon for DRR planning (Alcayna et al., 2016). Moreover, overreliance on a community's resilience pushes all the responsibilities for DRR onto the community itself rather than demanding better governmental policies that holistically address all elements of disaster risk (for further critique of resilience, see Walch, 2017).

Risk reduction

DRR is the anticipation and reduction of the individual and interactive risk associated with these four aforementioned elements (UNISDR, 2017). Managing disaster risk is best considered with a context-specific, human-centric, and multi-sectoral approach that targets multiple elements of disaster risk. This involves planned actions to avoid new and existing disaster risk (prevention), curb the effects of hazards and consequent disasters (mitigation), shift a specific risk's financial impact from one entity to another (transfer), and build resources and capacities for effective disaster anticipation, response, and recovery (preparedness; UNDRR, n.d.). Risk management often focuses on preventing, mitigating, transferring, or developing preparedness for issues related to exposure, vulnerability, and lack of capacity of a given community or population (UNISDR, 2015), with the assumption that natural hazards are typically outside our control. However, the rise in frequency and intensity of hydro-meteorological hazards like typhoons attributed to anthropogenic climate change (UNDRR, 2020) has shown that hazards can also be managed to an extent. This is the reason why DRR and climate change activities are intimately connected.

Success in DRR activities is best achieved when structural changes to governance (top-down) and local community-led initiatives (bottom-up) work in concert (UNDRR, n.d.; UNISDR, 2015). Moreover, disaster risk is strongly tied to socioeconomic development and strength of governmental institutions (Marin-Ferrer et al., 2017; UNISDR, 2015). It has long been recognized that the primary drivers of poverty and people's vulnerability to hazards are interrelated (UNDRR, 2020). People in poverty are likely to live in poorly constructed dwellings that lie in hazard-prone locations, have fewer resources and capacities to avoid and recover from hazards, and succumb to deeper poverty from the cumulative impact of successive hazard exposure. Weak governance and political will prevents effective DRR planning and implementation, especially when DRR and climate policies conflict with the objective of short-term economic growth (UNISDR, 2015). This highlights the importance of integrating DRR strategies with not only climate policies but also poverty reduction and sustainable development programs. After all, environmentally degrading practices and poor economic and urban development undermine the success of any DRR strategies.

Occupational perspective on disaster and development

What has been clear thus far in the chapter is that many of the drivers of disasters are strongly linked to issues of development such as sustainability and social justice (for further reading, see Chapter 11). Rushford and Thomas's (2015) disaster and development occupational perspective framework reflects this link. At its core is occupation and its various functions in a disaster and development context. We suggest that disaster and development is defined by occupation (*occupation in context*). We can comprehend the impact of disaster and development from the disruption of occupations and speed of recovery of occupational patterns and activities post-disaster. Occupation also serves as a tool to achieve our goals related to DRR activities (*occupation as medium*). With these two functions, occupational therapists can be occupational stewards and leverage the transformative use of occupation to build resilient, equitable, and sustainable societies that are able to avoid or recover from disasters. The use of occupation in DRR work is embedded in layers of contexts, including the DRR cycle, and the ecological, sociocultural, political, and economic aspects that shape societies (Figure 10.2).

Box 10.1 Caught unprepared by a typhoon like no other before it

Liza is from a 50-household islet whose primary livelihood is fishing. The islet is part of a *barangay* off the main island of Bantayan, one of the smaller Visayan islands in Cebu province. The area is frequented by typhoons. Thus, the islet residents are no stranger to heavy rains or strong winds.

The day prior to super-typhoon Yolanda's (Haiyan) landfall, community officials informed the islet residents to stock up on essential supplies and be ready to evacuate, in case the need arose. However, to Liza and her neighbors, it was just another passing typhoon, not to mention it was sweltering hot that day. They proceeded to have a small birthday celebration that night. The following morning, no typhoon came, not even a drizzle. Everybody continued their routines—preparing fishing implements and selling fish. Suddenly, around ten in the morning, the clouds darkened, shortly followed by deafening rainfall and gushing winds. Seawater surged inside homes, taking lives, houses, and livelihoods. After several hours, the sun shone again like nothing had happened. In Yolanda's wake was unimaginable devastation, along with grief and hopelessness enveloping the community.

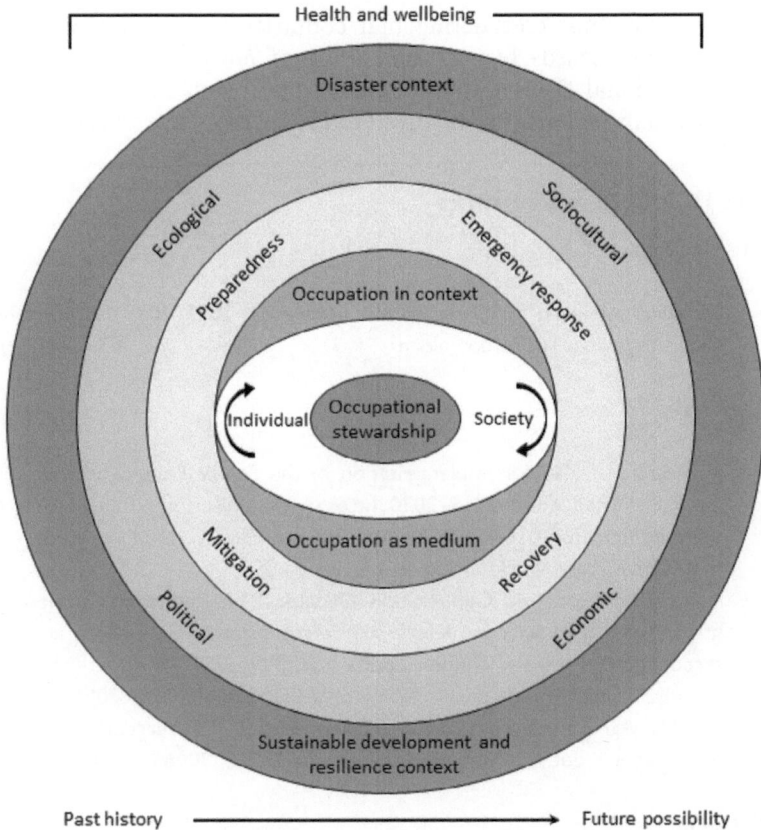

Figure 10.2 The disaster and development occupational perspective (DDOP) framework
Source: Reproduced with permission of Elsevier Science & Technology Journals, from
Disaster and development: An occupational perspective, Rushford, N. & Thomas, K.,
©2015; permission conveyed through Copyright Clearance Center, Inc.

DRR policies

Given the country's long history of experiencing disasters, the Philippines
recognizes the importance of DRR and has strong DRR frameworks,
policies, and plans in place (Alcayna et al., 2016; UNISDR, 2015). It is a
signatory of the Sendai Framework for Disaster Risk Reduction (and its
predecessor, Hyogo Framework for Action), which provides guidance for
preventing and decreasing disaster risk for resilient and sustainable development (UNISDR, 2017). One of the landmark advances of the Sendai
Framework was the inclusion of the needs of persons with disabilities in
DRR policies and plans (Bennett, 2020). Furthermore, the framework
emphasizes the need for mechanisms that would allow regional

collaborative actions, considering that countries in a region often share similar natural hazards (e.g., *Pacific Ring of Fire*). This gave rise to a number of regional DRR frameworks and agreements in Asia-Pacific and Southeast Asian regions that involve the Philippines (Box 10.2).

Box 10.2 DRR frameworks

International

- Sendai Framework for Disaster Risk Reduction 2015–2030 https://www.undrr.org/media/16176/download

Regional

- Asia Regional Plan for Implementation of the Sendai Framework for Disaster Risk Reduction 2015–2030 https://www.unisdr.org/2016/amcdrr/wp-content/uploads/2016/11/FINAL-Asia-Regional-Plan-for-implementation-of-Sendai-Framework-05-November-2016.pdf
- Asia-Pacific Economic Cooperation Disaster Risk Reduction Framework https://www.apec.org/docs/default-source/groups/epwg/2024/apecdisasterriskreductionframework_endorsed.pdf?sfvrsn=8d9ce067_2#:~:text=The%20APEC%20DRRF%20consists%20of,for%20all%20(ANNEX%20B).
- ASEAN Agreement on Disaster Management and Emergency Response https://agreement.asean.org/media/download/20220330063139.pdf

National

- NDRRMC Disaster Risk Reduction Management Framework and Plan 2020–2030 https://ndrrmc.gov.ph/attachments/article/4147/NDRRMP-Pre-Publication-Copy-v2.pdf

---

While the Philippines' early policies centered primarily in response and aid during disaster events, more recent laws have increased focus on risk management (Table 10.1). The key DRR legislation in the country is the Philippine Disaster Risk Reduction and Management Act of 2010, which formed the National Disaster Risk Reduction and Management Council (NDRRMC), the highest decision-making body composed of heads of agencies (e.g., Department of Health, Department of Social Welfare and Development, Philippine National Red Cross, and PhilHealth) and headed by the Secretary of National Defense. One of the most important functions of the NDRRMC is to develop a holistic, all-hazards, inter-agency, and community-based plan to guide DRR efforts in the country.

Table 10.1 Evolution of national policies affecting DRR actions in the Philippines

Policy	Year enacted	Objective(s)
EO 159	1968	• Direct the establishment of disaster control units in government, health, and educational institutions
PD 1566	1978	• Strengthen the national disaster response capability • Establish the National Disaster Coordinating Council • Lay out a national disaster preparedness plan
Local Government Code	1991	• Decentralize governance, including that of disaster response activities
Climate Change Act	2009	• Incorporate climate change issues into government policy • Establish the framework strategy and program on climate change • Establish the Climate Change Commission
Philippine Disaster Risk Reduction and Management Act	2010	• Strengthen national DRR system • Constitute the NDRRMC, which took over and expanded the scope of the National Disaster Coordinating Council • Institutionalize a national DRR plan and allocate funds for it
Disaster Risk Reduction Management Plan 2011–2028	2011	• Identify the expected outcomes, outputs, activities, and actors of the national DRR plan
Disaster Risk Reduction Management Plan 2020–2030	2020	• Update the previous DRR plan

Despite strong policies underscoring the Philippines' well-developed DRR framework, the country regularly reports high casualties from natural hazards (Walch, 2017). Alcayna et al. (2016) identified several reasons for this. First, there is poor policy implementation stemming from a shortage of financial resources and qualified personnel. Second, the private sector, which contributes significantly to DRR efforts, has grown distrustful of collaborating with the government due to real or perceived corruption. As a consequence, DRR initiatives from the private sector are not always well coordinated with local and national DRR activities. Walch

(2017) has also argued that DRR policies of the Philippines appear good on paper but actually neglect the underlying vulnerabilities of the population (e.g., high social and income inequality, and increasing number of *squatters* or informal settlers) that ultimately lead to disasters.

Framework for occupational therapy in DRR

Occupational therapists are traditionally seen as healthcare professionals working in clinical settings. It was not until the 2004 Indian Ocean tsunami that occupational therapists' role in DRR became more widely recognized through the effort of the WFOT (Sinclair et al., 2005). The Federation has since released two position statements affirming the significant role occupational therapy plays across all phases of DRR. Furthermore, their recent publication (2022) concretized seven principles underlying occupational therapy in DRR, which are as follows:

1   Identification of community's needs related to DRR
2   Initiation of services for individuals and communities affected by disasters to facilitate their occupational participation and performance
3   Implementation of DRR policies at all levels of governance
4   Inclusion of people with disabilities and at-risk populations in DRR
5   Implementation of the *build back better* philosophy in all DRR activities
6   Development of educational and professional competence for implementing occupational therapy in DRR
7   Engagement in research for occupational therapy in DRR

These principles can be applied to occupational therapy in DRR initiatives focused at the level of the individual (micro), community (meso), and national/international stakeholders and policy makers (macro) (WFOT, 2022).

In light of the globally recognized role of occupational therapists in DRR, the Philippine Academy of Occupational Therapists (PAOT) formulated a DRR plan for the profession in 2013 (Duque et al., 2013). The plan has seven objectives, which address the most essential needs at the time: integrating DRR into occupational therapy education, establishing interagency collaboration to ensure involvement of occupational therapy in local and national disaster-related activities, and institutionalizing a DRR program within PAOT. Since the plan's formulation, no formal evaluation of its achievements has been implemented. Progress has been made, such as the establishment of a subcommittee on DRR within PAOT and relatively recent publications reporting the involvement of occupational therapists in community and national disaster-related activities, notably in the in- and post-crisis phases (Bulan & Eturma, 2018; Ching & Lazaro, 2021).

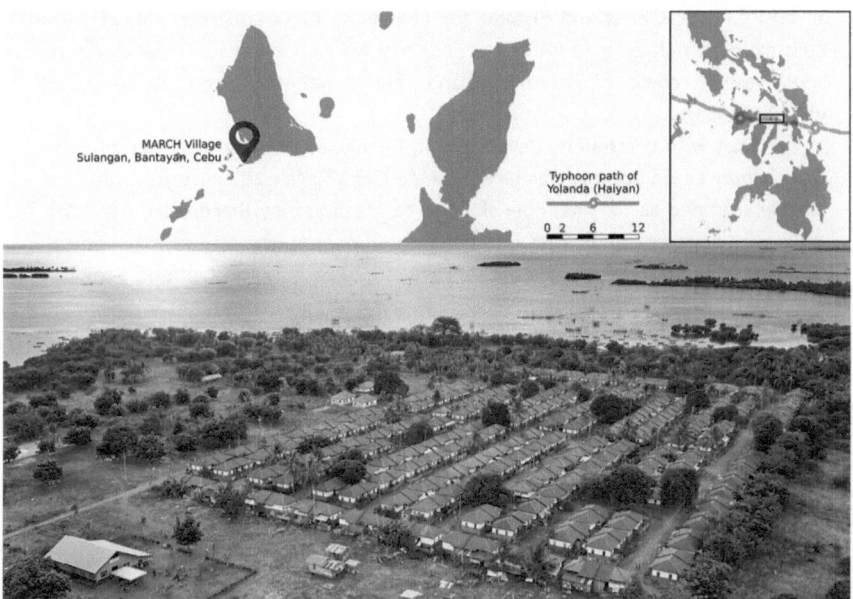

Figure 10.3 Geographic location of MARCH Village in Sulangan, Bantayan island (top) and aerial shot of the constructed cement houses for the relocated residents (bottom)
Source: ©2019 Tommy Chia, "MARCH Village aerial shot." Reproduced with permission.

Meanwhile, there is still a general lack of awareness of occupational therapy roles in DRR, even among healthcare professionals, which hinders interagency collaboration for disaster-related activities (Bulan & Eturma, 2018). DRR has not yet been successfully incorporated into undergraduate occupational therapy curricula (Commission of Higher Education [CHED], 2017) and continues to be a specialized practice area requiring additional training. The PAOT organizes these training workshops sporadically. Besides an evaluation, an update of the professional organization's 2013 DRR plan is necessary to harmonize it with the WFOT's (2022) principles on occupational therapy DRR roles and actions, as well as with more recent national and international frameworks (Box 10.2).

Box 10.3 Rebuilding after devastation: What can occupational therapists do?

After the typhoon's devastation, several islets near Bantayan island were declared red high-hazard zones and the local government mandated the permanent relocation of its residents. The relocation was supported by the joint venture of the local government and several non-governmental organizations, such as MARCH for Christ and Habitat for Humanity. New concrete houses were built from scratch on a 15.9-hectare property with a 1.2-km shoreline along the southwestern coast of Bantayan island. The community came to be called MARCH Village.

To assist with community development, Minnie, an occupational therapist and this chapter's lead author, was hired as MARCH Village's administrator. She was initially stumped as to what role she had to play because there were no individuals with apparent disabilities in the relocated community. She quickly noticed, however, the occupational disruption caused by not only the typhoon itself but also the consequent relocation. She knew she had a job to do.

DRR practice: Facilitating disaster resilience and community development

With the sudden and permanent resettlement, MARCH villagers needed assistance to develop and reorganize a disaster-resilient community. This community development project called for a sustainable development strategy combining DRR principles with the WHO's (2010) CBR matrix (see Chapter 8). Fundamental to DRR is managing risk elements. The post-Yolanda relocation's objective was to reduce the exposure of residents to hazards associated with living in isolated, low-lying, typhoon-prone islets. The CBR matrix provided a framework for capacity building, taking into consideration the community's needs, priorities, and available resources.

Disaster-displaced MARCH villagers were relocated to an unfamiliar environment, which disrupted their usual roles, habits, and routines. To address occupational disruption at the micro and meso levels, Minnie facilitated the acquisition of new skills relevant to changes in occupations and the adoption of new roles, habits, and routines. Identifying priority occupations was facilitated by the involvement of the villagers who are self-aware of their own needs. Perhaps one of the silver linings of the villagers' situation is that a restructuring of their occupations afforded more freedom to adopt new ways and patterns of "doing" that are aligned to DRR strategies. This exemplifies the disaster and development occupational perspective framework's *occupation as medium*.

Based on identified DRR and community development needs of the community, Minnie coordinated several programs corresponding to components of the CBR matrix during her stay in MARCH Village in 2015–2023 (Table 10.2). Among the most notable are in livelihood, education, and empowerment programs. A significant vulnerability of the community identified was the heavy reliance on fishing and selling fresh fish as a livelihood. Although several boats were distributed to replace those wrecked by Yolanda, to *build back better*, the need for a diversified livelihood was clear. Several viable options were identified by the community and through

Table 10.2 Occupational therapy activities in MARCH Village across the components of the CBR matrix (WHO, 2010)

Component	*Element*	*Activity*
Health	Health promotion and prevention	Collaborating with other health professionals to conduct mental health psychosocial support, and vision and hearing screening
	Rehabilitation	Providing occupational therapy services to people with disabilities
	Assistive devices	Assessing need for and providing mobility aids (e.g., wheelchair and crutches)
Education	Early childhood	Facilitating opening of daycare center
	Non-formal	Collaborating with nearby secondary school for alternative learning system, and with the technical education and skills development authority for skills training
	Lifelong learning	Raising preparedness through hazard drills, *e-balde* for essential supplies, etc.
Livelihood	Skills development	Facilitating capacity building to diversify livelihood (e.g., baking, welding, cell phone repairing, etc.)
Social	Personal assistance	Liaising with social services for family interventions and social grants
	Culture and arts	Organizing international cultural experiences with foreign volunteers and guests
	Recreation, leisure, and sports	Organizing recreational events
Empowerment	Community mobilization	Facilitating and collaborating with stakeholders in community meetings
	Political participation	Training leadership skills and supporting the election of youth and community leaders
	Disabled people's organizations	Integration of villagers with disabilities in *barangay* and municipal disability organizations

skills training, as well as networking and advocacy to obtain funds for necessary equipment, these options were realized. Two of these (i.e., fish drying and market gardening) are detailed in WFOT's (2022) DRR manual.

Education to increase awareness of DRR was another priority area. From the villagers' recent experience of Yolanda, everyone understood the consequences of failing to be prepared. The MARCH administrative team developed several disaster preparedness plans that are cognizant of existing DRR initiatives in the area. This was to avoid giving conflicting instructions that may have confused rather than educated. One such existing program is *emergency balde* (bucket), *e-balde* for short, which utilizes a ubiquitous household item in the Philippines as a storage space for emergency supplies of essential items (e.g., food, water, medicine, and documents) that can easily be brought along in case of evacuation. Additionally, the bucket can be used to collect and store water as needed. Hazard response drills were also implemented, including tying down boats and other objects that can be moved by the wind or storm surge, understanding the meaning of typhoon warnings, and learning assembly points in the village. Due to the regularity of typhoons, effectiveness of these drills was tested and adjusted regularly.

Finally, the empowerment component of the CBR matrix ensured the community's active involvement in all aspects of development, through the Village Community Association, with the intention of fostering leadership and self-sufficiency within the community. This is apparent from the villagers undertaking income-generating initiatives that enabled them to meet their own needs and reduce reliance on donations and organizational support from the MARCH administrative team. Moreover, empowered community members have taken leadership roles in many programs of the community.

Box 10.4 Empty classrooms on a rainy day: Occupations in transition

It is impossible to foresee every aspect of MARCH villagers' transition to their new environment, especially for the MARCH administrative team who have no experience of the villagers' life pre-Yolanda. On one of the first rainy days since the relocation, Minnie was approached by a concerned school teacher. The teacher was puzzled why she walked into an empty classroom that morning.

Talking with the students and parents, Minnie and the teacher learned that students had to take boats to reach the schools on Bantayan island because there were no schools in the surrounding islets. This meant that, with unfavorable tides and inclement weather, no one went to school because it was not safe to travel by boat. Although the schools are now within walking distance from the students' new homes in MARCH Village, the carried-over knowledge of the weather and tides' immense influence still directed their school attendance.

Conclusion

Occupational therapy has created its role in DRR with its unique perspective in seeing disasters from its subsequent occupational disruption (occupation in context) and the use of occupations to foster disaster-resilient communities. Due to the potential magnitude of the tasks-at-hand in DRR practice, occupational therapists may have to *doff* their clinical smocks and *don* their multi-role jackets that would allow better navigation of the demands (e.g., organizational, administrative, clinical, advocative, consultative, etc.) of community development. Unshackling from its clinical boundary, occupational therapy could learn to address occupational disruptions not only for persons with disabilities but also in seemingly well individuals coming from life crises such as disasters. Fortunately, prospective occupational therapists now have several frameworks and manuals that can help them guide their practice. The case of MARCH Village demonstrates the application of the amalgamation of several framework principles and manual guidelines, including those from the UNDRR disaster risk reduction, WHO CBR matrix, WFOT DRR manual, and the disaster and development occupational perspective framework.

Questions for reflection and suggestions for action

1 A discourse on disaster and development is incomplete without discussing justice-related issues (see Chapter 11). Think of your own local community and identify injustices that are likely to elevate disaster risk of individuals or groups experiencing these injustices. What roles do occupational therapists play in alleviating them?

2 Do you have a disaster response plan for your own household, community, or workplace? If so, evaluate how well it incorporates the various elements of disaster risk (hazard, exposure, vulnerability, and lack of capacity). Alternatively, devise a plan that matches the needs of the household, community, or workplace with disaster risk in mind.

3 Occupational therapists use many words, such as occupations, in very specific ways in discussions of theory and practice with each other. How does the use of occupational therapy jargon impact communication with leaders, laypeople, and other professions, particularly in interagency DRR work? Discuss ways occupational therapists can better communicate what the profession can offer in relation to DRR objectives.

Note

1 *Bayanihan* is the collective action of a community to help others in need (Adviento & de Guzman, 2010). For further discussion, see Chapter 8.

References

Adviento, M.L., & de Guzman, J.M. (2010). Community resilience during Typhoon Ondoy: The case of Ateneoville. *Philippine Journal of Psychology*, 43(1). 101–113.

Alcayna, T., Bollettino, V., Dy, P., & Vinck, P. (2016). Resilience and disaster trends in the Philippines: Opportunities for national and local capacity building. *PLoS Currents Disasters*, 8. doi:10.1371/currents.dis.4a0bc960866e53bd6357ac135d740846.

AOTA. (2011). The role of occupational therapy in disaster preparedness, response, and recovery. *American Journal of Occupational Therapy*, 65(*Suppl.*), S11–S25. doi:10.5014/ajot.2011.65S11.

Bennett, D. (2020). Implementation of the four priorities of the Sendai Framework for inclusion of people with disabilities. *International Journal of Disaster Risk Science*, 11, 155–166. doi:10.1007/s13753-020-00267-w.

Bulan, P.M.P., & Eturma, C.M. (2018). Practising occupational therapists' attitudes towards disaster management. *WFOT Bulletin*, 74(2), 99–105. doi:10.1080/14473828.2018.1533154.

CHED, Policies, standards and guidelines for the Bachelor of Science in Occupational Therapy education (BSOT) program, Memorandum Order No. 52, s. 2017. (2017, March 28). https://ched.gov.ph/wp-content/uploads/2018/04/CMO-No.-52-Series-of-2017-Policies-Standards-and-Guidelines-for-the-Bachelor-of-Science-in-Occupational-Therapy-Education-BSOT-Program.pdf.

Ching, P.E., & Lazaro, R.T. (2021). Preparation, roles, and responsibilities of Filipino occupational therapists in disaster preparedness, response, and recovery. *Disability and Rehabilitation*, 43(9), 1333–1340. doi:10.1080/09638288.2019.1663945.

Cinco, T.A., de Guzman, R.G., Ortiz, A.M.D., Delfino, R.J.P., Lasco, R.D., Hilario, F.D., Juanillo, E.L., Barba, R., & Ares, E.D. (2016). Observed trends and impacts of tropical cyclones in the Philippines. *International Journal of Climatology*, 36(14), 4638–4650. doi:10.1002/joc.4659.

Duque, R.L., Grecia, A., & Ching, P.E. (2013). Development of a national occupational therapy disaster preparedness and response plan: The Philippine experience. *WFOT Bulletin*, 68(1), 26–31. doi:10.1179/otb.2013.68.1.008.

Local Government Code of 1991, RA No. 7160. (1991, October 10). https://www.officialgazette.gov.ph/1991/10/10/republic-act-no-7160/.

Marin-Ferrer, M., Vernaccini, L., & Poljansek, K. (2017). *Index for risk management INFORM: Concept and Methodology Report Version 2017*. European Union. doi:10.2760/094023.

Max-Neef, M.A., Elizalde, A., & Hopenhayn, M. (1991). Development and human needs. In M.A. Max-Neef (Ed.), *Human scale development: Conception, application and further reflections* (pp. 13–54). Apex.

Parente, M., Tofani, M., De Santis, R., Esposito, G., Santilli, V., & Galeoto, G. (2017). The role of the occupational therapist in disaster areas: Systematic review. *Occupational Therapy International*. doi:10.1155/2017/6474761.

Philippine Disaster Risk Reduction and Management Act of 2010. RA No. 10121. (2010, May 27). https://www.officialgazette.gov.ph/2010/05/27/republic-act-no-10121/.

Rushford, N., & Thomas, K. (2015). An occupational perspective on disaster and development and a conceptual framework. In N. Rushford & K. Thomas (Eds.), *Disaster and development: An occupational perspective* (pp. 235–241). Elsevier.

Sinclair, K., Pattison, M., & Thomas, K. (2005). The World Federation's response to the Indian Ocean tsunami disaster: Situational assessment and recommendations for future action. *WFOT Bulletin*, 52(1), 5–8. doi:10.1179/otb.2005.52.1.002.

Stough, L.M., & Kelman, I. (2018). People with disabilities and disasters. In H. Rodriguez, J. Trainor, & W. Donner (Eds.), *Handbook of disaster research* (2nd ed. pp. 225–242). Springer.

Subramaniam, P., & Villeneuve, M. (2019). Advancing emergency preparedness for people with disabilities and chronic health conditions in the community: A scoping review. *Disability and Rehabilitation*, 42(22), 3256–3264. doi:10.1080/09638288.2019.1583781.

UNISDR. (2009). *2009 UNISDR terminology on disaster risk reduction.* https://www.preventionweb.net/files/7817_UNISDRTerminologyEnglish.pdf.

UNISDR. (2015). *Making development sustainable: The future of disaster risk management. Global assessment report on disaster.* https://www.undrr.org/media/14914/download.

UNISDR. (2017). *Words into action guidelines: National disaster risk assessment.* https://www.undrr.org/media/20847/download.

United Nations General Assembly. (2016). *Report of the open-ended intergovernmental expert working group on indicators and terminology relating to disaster risk reduction.* https://www.preventionweb.net/files/50683_oiewgreportenglish.pdf?_gl=1*r5coi8*_ga*MjA0NzkzMDc5MS4xNjkyMzQwODkx*_ga_D8G5WXP6YM*M TY5MjM0MTA2NC4zLjEuMTY5MjM0MTM0OS4wLjAuMA.

UNDRR. (n.d.). Disaster risk reduction and disaster risk management. https://www.preventionweb.net/understanding-disaster-risk/key-concepts/disaster-risk-reduction-disaster-risk-management.

UNDRR. (2020). *The human cost of disasters: An overview of the last 20 years 2000–2019.* https://www.preventionweb.net/files/74124_humancostofdisasters2002019reportu.pdf.

Usamah, M., Handmer, J., Mitchell, D., & Ahmed, I. (2014). Can the vulnerable be resilient? Co-existence of vulnerability and disaster resilience: Informal settlements in the Philippines. *International Journal of Disaster Risk Reduction*, 10 (A), 178–189. doi:10.1016/j.ijdrr.2014.08.007.

Walch, C. (2017). Typhoon Haiyan: Pushing the limits of resilience? The effect of land inequality on resilience and disaster risk reduction policies in the Philippines. *Critical Asian Studies*, 50(1), 122–135. doi:10.1080/14672715.2017.1401936.

WFOT. (2014). *Occupational therapy in disaster preparedness and response (DP&R).* https://wfot.org/resources/occupational-therapy-in-disaster-preparedness-and-response-dp-r.

WFOT. (2022). *Disaster preparedness and risk reduction manual.* https://wfot.org/resources/wfot-disaster-preparedness-and-risk-reduction-manual.

WHO. (2010). *Community-based rehabilitation: CBR guidelines* [Introductory booklet]. https://extranet.who.int/mindbank/it.

Chapter 11

Justice work and social care practice in occupational therapy

Michael Sy, Anna-Liza Yap Tan Pascual, Daryl Patrick Yao and Roi Charles Pineda

Chapter objectives

1   Discuss occupational justice as a concept within the contexts of health and social care systems
2   Cite examples of occupational injustices as an experience for people and groups
3   Describe how occupational justice principles can be applied into practices that promote occupational participation within and outside occupational therapy
4   Narrate how occupational justice concepts and applications are contextualized in a sample practice within the social care setting in the Philippines

Unpacking occupational justice and related concepts

Occupational justice is the recognition and provision of the occupational needs of individuals and communities as part of a fair and empowering society (Wilcock & Townsend, 2000). Given that occupational justice is a relatively emerging concept in occupational therapy, especially in the Philippines, much of its conceptual underpinning may appear too abstract and detached from traditional occupational therapy practice (Hocking et al., 2019). A good place to begin understanding occupational justice and its application in practice is by looking at the construct of *justice.*

As an ethical principle, justice refers to the promotion of fairness and equitable treatment of individuals within populations (Feinsod & Wagner, 2008). Fairness usually is associated with *equality*, i.e., every individual possesses exactly the same human rights, while *equity* starts with the assumption that individuals' social standing, as determined by their race, gender, class, and other factors, differ. Therefore, society's resources must be allocated with these social inequalities in mind. Justice that guarantees full participation of people in society and equitable

DOI: 10.4324/9781003321217-11

distribution of benefits and burdens to its members demands the acknowledgment of two propositions: (1) inequities are created by societies beyond the forces of nature or god's will, and (2) societies are responsible for altering policies and programs to make situations for humans more equitable (Hocking, 2017). In modern societies, the goal for its members is to achieve health and social outcomes that are equitable rather than equal. This entails the distribution of health and social care based on need (*need* principle) to bring about the best possible outcomes (*maximizing* principle), including the allocation of resources to reduce, if not to eradicate, health and social inequities (*egalitarian* principle; Cookson & Dolan, 2000).

Occupational justice is taken to be an aspect, subset, or derivative of, or complementary to, social justice (Hocking, 2017). Whereas social justice means having equitable access to resources, occupational justice entails being able to participate and engage in occupations given equitable opportunities. To guide the application of occupational justice concepts, the *Framework for Occupational Justice* was developed by occupational justice theorists led by Stadnyk, Townsend, and Wilcock in 2010. The framework describes how structural and contextual factors largely influence a person or community's occupational engagement and occupational justice outcomes. Structural factors include underlying occupational determinants such as international or national policies, as well as occupational instruments or programs (e.g., employment, housing, education, transportation, and technology use). Contextual factors include personal information and demographics of person and groups. Structural and contextual factors are interrelated to determine outcomes of justice, which can either be upholding occupational rights or reinforcing occupational injustice. Chichaya et al. (2018) indicate that because occupation is socially constructed, international and local policies form part of the structural factors that shape contextual factors where justice and injustices in occupational participation are formed.

An example of structural factors that shape occupational justice in daily living is the *Ottawa Charter for Health Promotion*, a set of written legislations developed by the WHO (1986) to promote public health globally. The charter identified key prerequisites of health, including peace, shelter, education, food, income, a stable ecosystem, sustainable resources, social justice, and equity. These prerequisites, also known as social and/or justice determinants of health, underpin what we consider as *occupational rights*. Occupational rights are defined as "the right of all people to engage in meaningful occupations that contribute positively to their own well-being and the well-being of their communities" (Walley-Hammell, 2008, p. 62). In a position statement for the WFOT, Hocking et al. (2019) broadly defined occupational justice as the universal rights for all people to engage in occupations that will let them survive, find meaning, and promote their own and community's well-being. Specifically, these rights include:

• Participating in a range of occupations that support survival, health and well-being so that populations, communities, families, and individuals can flourish and realize their potential, consistent with the Ottawa Charter
• Choosing occupations without pressure, force, coercion, or threats but with acknowledgment that with choice comes responsibility for other people, lifeforms, and the planet
• Freely engaging in necessary and chosen occupations without risk to safety, human dignity or equity

Ideally, occupational rights are meant to be possessed by all people. Occupational justice may be achieved when people can participate in occupations based on their needs and are given equitable opportunities to do so. With this in mind, occupational therapists are expected to promote the occupational rights of their clients. Walley-Hammell (2015) challenged occupational therapists to cultivate their competency in identifying socially structured inequalities that diminish an individual or group's occupational opportunities. Occupational therapists pursuing structural competency should first and foremost "identify and understand their own inequitable access to power, opportunities and resources, and to identify, understand and seek to engage with those structural conditions that unfairly reduce the opportunities available to disabled and other marginalized and disempowered people" (p. 450). The lack or absence of justice in everyday life prevents people and groups from engaging in daily activities. This is occupational injustice, which is a violation of human and occupational rights. Table 11.1 illustrates the relationship between justice, social justice, occupation, occupational justice/rights, and occupational injustice.

Table 11.1 Viewing source of income as a social determinant and how it is translated within the concept of occupation, social justice, occupational justice/rights, and occupation injustice

Social/justice determinant	*Occupation (doing)*	*Social justice*	*Occupational justice/rights*	*Occupational justice*
Source of income	Finding work; work engagement; sustaining a livelihood	Establishing social policies that will support a level of income sufficient for healthy living for all	The right to seek equitable employment with reasonable working conditions and appropriate remuneration	Engaging in work with unfavorable work conditions, unreasonable working hours, without just compensation

Occupational injustices

Occupational justice can be achieved when occupational rights are exercised by people and communities. When these occupational rights are abused or violated, there is occupational injustice. In no particular order or hierarchy, we outline below the examples of occupational injustices described in occupational therapy and science literature (Kronenberg et al., 2005; Nizzero et al., 2017; Stadnyk et al., 2010):

- **Occupational alienation**: denying people from engaging in meaningful occupations
- **Occupational deprivation**: restricting people from health-promoting occupations while residing in diverse contexts
- **Occupational disruption**: disturbing a person's normal pattern of occupational engagement brought about by a significant life event, personal event, or environmental change (typically a temporary or transient state)
- **Occupational imbalance**: having too little to do or excessively burdened to do things on a daily basis
- **Occupational marginalization**: lacking the opportunity to engage in occupations due to invisible expectations on who, when, where, and how one participates in occupations
- **Occupational apartheid**: denying access to meaningful occupations on the basis of socio-political, sexual, and religious characteristics

These occupational injustices are context-specific, can occur simultaneously, and can be described from varying degrees of intensity. With a Philippine context in mind, specifically from the perspectives of Filipinos with physical disabilities, Yao et al. (2020) identified varying and complex occupational injustices related to limited opportunities, physical and social barriers, and unfavorable employment conditions (e.g., job insecurity and lower wages). Furthermore, a critical piece by Sy et al. (2021) noted that a neat categorization of occupational injustices must be avoided because injustices can be experienced and interpreted differently between individuals and contexts, its form can mutate across contexts, and discriminatory mechanisms may interact to intensify the injustice experience in a phenomenon called *double marginalization*.

Occupational justice work in occupational therapy

Occupational therapists have a professional duty to facilitate how occupations can be achieved equitably through participation, engagement, and experience. Despite occupational therapy's root in justice work (Bailliard et al., 2020), many occupational therapy practitioners still see the dissonance rather than the consonance between occupational justice and occupational therapy (Gupta, 2016). It is indeed an unrealistic goal for the profession to totally eradicate injustices or inequities with occupations. We can nevertheless help identify and reduce their occurrence and consequently advocate for equitable occupational opportunities for all.

There is increasing awareness among occupational therapists of their role in promoting occupational justice. Serrata-Malfitano and colleagues' (2019) systematic review ascertained that occupational justice and its related concepts are already informing contemporary occupational therapy practice using varying approaches. These include individual approaches, collective/social approaches that address justice issues at a macro-structural level, and a combination of both (individual-integrated-with-collective/social approaches), with most studies focused on individual and combined approaches. They further stressed that occupational therapists and justice practitioners must be cognizant that occupational injustices stem from systemic factors and thus require collective/social approaches. Integral to such approaches is structural competency, which would allow *social transformation through occupation* (Benjamin-Thomas & Laliberte-Rudman, 2018). Social transformation through occupation is an emerging concept referring to collaborative approaches where occupation is perceived as means and ends in restructuring practices, systems, and structures in order to develop a just society (Farias et al., 2019).

To facilitate the application of occupational justice in practice, we will discuss the Participatory Occupational Justice Framework (POJF) and provide some possibilities on how occupational therapists and justice workers can actuate the processes drawn from the framework. While this chapter highlights POJF because it has been used the most in occupational justice studies in the Philippines, we invite you to read further and learn more on other occupational justice frameworks and models, such as the Framework of Occupational Justice (Stadnyk et al., 2010), Social Transformation Model of Occupational Therapy (Frank & Zemke, 2008), Occupational Enablement to Facilitate Social Change in Community Practice Framework (Janse van Rensburg, 2018), and Occupation, Capability and Wellbeing Framework for Occupational Therapy (Walley-Hammell, 2023).

Participatory Occupational Justice Framework

The POJF was designed as a tool to guide rather than prescribe practice (Townsend & Whiteford, 2005). It is a non-linear framework (see Figure 11.1) that intends to prompt practitioners (occupational therapists, justice workers, and anyone producing justice-related practices) to engage in collaborative processes. These processes are carried out with people; together, they identify the occupational injustices being experienced

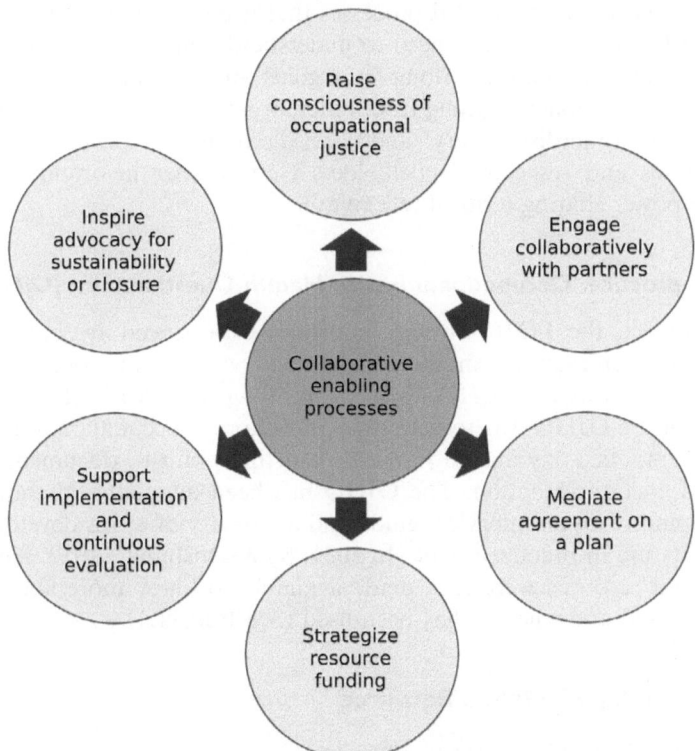

Figure 11.1 Participatory Occupational Justice Framework. From Whiteford, G., Jones, K., Rahal, C., & Suleman, A. The Participatory Occupational Justice Framework as a tool for change: Three contrasting case narratives. *Journal of Occupational Science.* ©2018 The Journal of Occupational Science Inc.
Source: Reproduced by permission of Informa UK Ltd., trading as Taylor & Francis Group, www.tandfonline.com on behalf of 2018 The Journal of Occupational Science Inc.

within a specific context and develop a plan to actively tackle it. Whiteford and Townsend (2011) devised six enabling processes to guide the non-linear practice processes.

Being non-linear (i.e., no starting or ending point), the POJF can commence at any enabling process. It is, however, suggested to start with *raising consciousness of occupational injustice* and conclude with *inspiring advocacy for sustainability or closure* (Whiteford & Townsend, 2011). While designed with occupational therapists in mind, the POJF does not require an occupational therapist to be present across all the enabling processes. The role of the occupational therapist is to facilitate these enabling processes directly or indirectly. Specific competencies and guiding questions per enabling process were outlined by Whiteford and Townsend (2011) to help practitioners apply the conceptual bases of the POJF.

Knowing that there are several processes that need to be undertaken when using the POJF, practitioners need to understand that the POJF entails the following: time commitment (long-term goals and sustainability), commitment from practitioners coming from different professional and disciplinary backgrounds (interdisciplinary and transdisciplinary), partnership with communities and respective stakeholders (service user involvement), and enacting power sharing (critical reflexivity).

Tool for practice: Occupational Justice Health Questionnaire (OJHQ)

To commence the POJF, current injustices experienced by individuals, groups, and communities should be identified. Among the tools available for this purpose is the OJHQ (Wilcock & Townsend 2014). The original purpose of the OJHQ was to help draw attention to occupational injustice in a busy practice day and to provide a starting point to document injustices and encourage action. The OJHQ has been adapted and translated into Filipino, with an interview guide and a glossary of terms developed to support its use in practice (Sy et al., 2021; Sy & Ohshima, 2019). An open educational resource website is made available to know more about how OJHQ is used and where it has been used (See Box 11.1).

Box 11.1 OJHQ Online Resource

Website: https://www.drmikesyot.com/ojhq
   Purpose of the resource site:

1   To disseminate OJHQ materials and resources easily and freely
2   To document inquiries from occupational therapists and justice workers who would like to know more about occupational justice and the OJHQ

Contents:

- OJHQ in English and Filipino versions
- Interview guide
- Glossary of terms
- Video demonstration
- Sample studies using the OJHQ as a tool in practice

Like any occupational therapy tool, the OJHQ requires contextualization and some level of training before use and application. Practitioners who intend to use the OJHQ in the future must be aware of its benefits and considerations. Benefits of using the OJHQ include the enhancement of clinical and professional reasoning competencies and provision of non-clinical data to add the layer of social determinants of health (Sy et al., 2021). Furthermore, utility considerations include user competency in interviewing and interpersonal skills; literacy in occupational justice concepts, the OJHQ tool, and situational contexts; and awareness and openness to critical occupational therapy principles.

A story of hope: Occupational therapy and justice for Filipino children in conflict with the law (CICL)

CICL are individuals aged 15 to 18 who committed an offense or those currently in detention facilities who are under 18 years. Although their legal cases are handled under the Department of Justice, it is the Department of Social Welfare and Development (DSWD) that provides social support for these minors. The Philippines' Comprehensive National Juvenile Intervention Program for 2018–2022 aimed to reduce new CICL cases, as well as rehabilitate and reintegrate CICL into their families and communities by 2022. To achieve this, one of the intended outcomes included breaking the recidivism cycle, which entails strategies for training for positive behavior, self-management and life skills, promoting positive parenting, and strengthening organizational structures of the national and local juvenile justice and welfare systems.

The United Nations Standard Minimum Rules for the Administration of Juvenile Justice (The Beijing Rules) and the Philippine Juvenile Justice Law (RA 9344 as amended) advise against that committing of CICL in a closed facility. In cases where this is the most appropriate option, the shortest possible period should be considered. However, due to the lack of effective and comprehensive community-based interventions in the country, many CICL are detained for periods lasting years, with some eventually intermingling with adult offenders (Paule et al., 2020). Moreover, juvenile justice's main goals of rehabilitation and reintegration are hindered due to the dearth of individualized, multidisciplinary, and comprehensive programs for children's rehabilitation and effective reintegration into their families and communities.

Based on a situational analysis study (Paule et al., 2020), in 2018 there were a total of 6,049 children in detention, including jails, but this number has decreased over the years. There has been a similar decrease in the number of CICL living in *Bahay Pag-asa* (translated as "House of Hope"; these residential youth care facilities are located nationwide) from 1,333 in 2019 to 668 in 2022 (Juvenile Justice and Welfare Council [JJWC], 2022). Although these figures provide some optimism for the state of CICL in the Philippines, Paule and colleagues' (2020) report explicitly highlights the absence of a consistent definition and categorization of detention for CICL. Moreover, Save the Children Philippines and Convention of the Rights of the Children Asia (2021) estimated the ideal number of *Bahay*

Pag-asa to be 118, but only 63 had been built as of 2021. A mere 13% of these facilities comply with DSWD (2005) standards for CICL detention centers, which require the following: at least one social worker for every 25 young people; a multidisciplinary team with rehabilitation programs; and one bed per resident; as well as nutritious meals, clothing, and toiletries. From what we have personally seen, juvenile correction centers are essentially prisons where CICL are locked inside *dorms* (see Figure 11.2), which is contrary to the home-like environments advised by the law.

Under-investment in children is a recognized problem in low-income, developing countries (UNICEF Innocenti—Global Office of Research and Foresight, 2023). Public investments in relevant policies, services, facilities, and programs for Filipino CICL remain very low (JJWC, 2017). The identified human resources needed for rehabilitation include social workers, psychologists/psychiatrists, medical doctors, vocational trainers, security personnel, house parents, and teachers. While there is a position for occupational therapists in the revised implementing rules and regulations of the Bureau of Corrections Act of 2013, there are no known occupational therapists employed in any of the correctional facilities. Historically speaking, occupational therapists have had roles in correctional prisons in the Philippines. However, at present, occupational therapy services are not in the policy recommendations when it comes to servicing CICL.

The lack of quality and adequate health and social care services in most youth detention homes and jails is clear. Thus, instead of rehabilitation integration, detained CICL are faced with "hopelessness and trauma, fostered aggressiveness, assimilation to the culture of crimes, longingness for

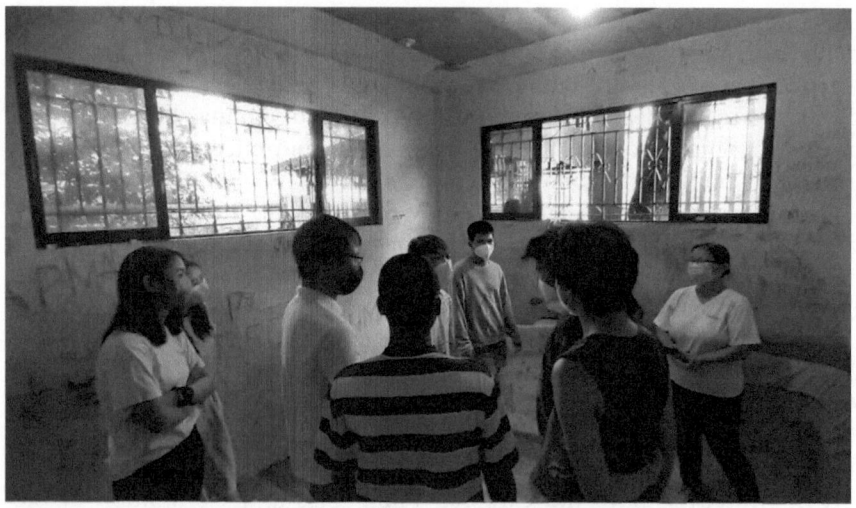

Figure 11.2 A typical correctional facility dorm in the Philippines

family, stigmatization, and creation of dependency among caregivers" (Paule et al., 2020, p. 21). While the policies and resources are still underdeveloped, a group of occupational therapists has been making sustainable efforts to support and partner with CICL towards their rehabilitation, reintegration, and participation. In the succeeding section, we tell the story of the Restart HOPE project, described through the lens of Anna (chapter co-author) and underpinned by the POJF.

Engage collaboratively with partners

In 2018, a group of volunteer occupational therapists began Restart Hope in CICL (Restart). Our group's aim is to uphold the principles of occupational justice among CICL. Restart envisions a Philippines where youth in correctional settings are recognized by their inherent worth, are valued by others, hopeful for the future, and equipped to become productive members of society. To this end, we see that our mission is to empower and instill hope in the Filipino youth who are in correctional settings. Soon after we established Restart, we received permission from the city division of the DSWD to implement the *Life Skills Program* in one of their corrections facilities that housed almost 200 CICL. Through a close collaboration with the officer in charge of the facility, we agreed to develop the program containing specific topics beneficial to CICL.

Mediate agreement on a plan

Although we have observed that the facilities have some structure for the children, in reality little time was used to engage in valued occupations. Paule et al. (2020) determined that the ratio of human resources to CICL is less than ideal and physical facilities to provide mental health interventions were inadequate or substandard. At the moment of writing this chapter, there has been no local data about the efforts in supporting CICL to engage in meaningful activities that develop skills for successful community reintegration.

Our goal was to teach life skills, including self-awareness, social skills, life planning, job finding, money management, and healthy living. Based on our first-hand experience, we saw the eagerness of CICL to learn in groups, do project-based and hands-on activities, and play games. There were several instances when they expressed their appreciation to the occupational therapists, since they recounted that these life skills were never introduced to them before. It was also relieving for them to have a safe space where someone would listen to their own stories— about their families, the events that led to their arrest, their dreams and aspirations, and their frustrations. Figure 11.3 illustrates a timeline output from one of the CICLs in a *Bahay Pag-asa* dorm.

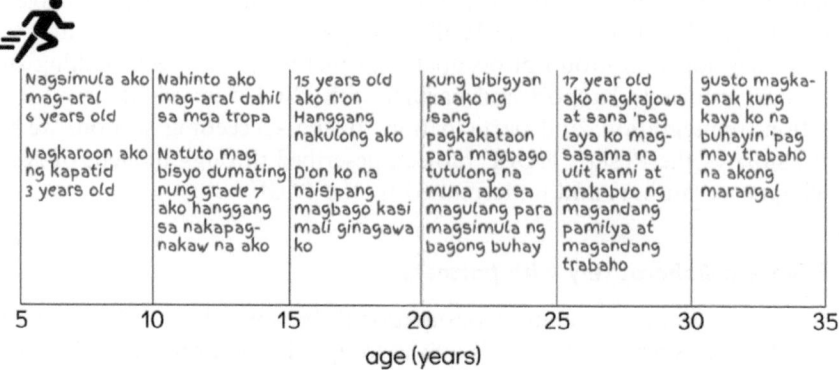

Figure 11.3 Timeline of a CICL showing their life history and dreams for the future. Translation: [5–10 years] I started school at 6 years old. I had a sibling at 3 years old. [10–15 years] I stopped going to school because of my gang. I learned vices until I committed theft when I was in grade 7. [15–20 years] I was 15 years old when I got detained. That was when I thought of reforming because I have been doing the wrong things. [20–25 years] If I were given a chance to change, I would first help my parents to start a new life. [25–30 years] I was 17 years old when I had a girlfriend. I hope to reunite with her when I get released and start a good family and a good job. [30–35 years] I would like to have a child once I am able to have a stable job to provide for them

Strategize resource finding

The *Life Skills Program* has since been implemented in other CICL facilities through both in-house and online arrangements, especially during the COVID-19 pandemic. Our group realized that core occupational therapy competencies are an adequate and sustainable resource to support this marginalized group, which are as valuable as the support given by our partners in the government and community through direct resource provisions. These competencies include maintaining therapeutic relationships, active listening, basic counseling skills, facilitating groups, interpersonal and intrapersonal communication, clinical reasoning, sound decision-making and judgment, teamwork and collaboration, and therapeutic use of self, activities, and groups. Through constant continuing professional education and consultation with experts and partners, we are able to gain more confidence in optimizing our occupational therapy skills to support individuals and groups towards occupational justice in a sustainable way.

Support implementation and continuous evaluation

Focus group discussions and interviews are done with CICL and staff members at the end of each program. Doing so has reinforced the value and relevance of the *Life Skills Program* in the shelter homes for CICL. For instance, *Money Game*, one of the favorite activities of CICL, uses real-life situations to challenge their thinking about financial decisions. Qualitative data gathered from focus group discussions and interviews are used to help Restart identify areas of improvement for the program and best practices that can be re-used for the future.

Raise consciousness of occupational injustice

In addition to direct services, Restart has been raising awareness of the need for occupational therapy services in this population through social media campaigns, conference presentations, and research. As of the writing of this chapter, our group has on-going research that explores the roles and potentialities of occupational therapy in correctional facilities and juvenile justice practice in the Philippines. Through this research, we intend to use occupational justice frameworks and tools to guide the effective identification of social and occupational injustices faced by CICL and, from there, propose justice-oriented solutions for policy development and practice.

Inspire advocacy for sustainability or closure

Occupational justice work will not prosper without sustainability. Since we began, we have been pursuing partnerships with universities who can host occupational therapy students for fieldwork training. The aim of this strategy is to immerse students in this less-frequented area of practice. Our plan is to initially set up services in a CICL facility, bring in occupational therapy students as part of the human resource, and then turn over the program to the university for continuity. When this happens, our group will have other opportunities to initiate the same plan in another facility.

It has been gratifying to see more occupational therapists interested in this area of practice underpinned by occupational justice principles. The *Life Skills Program* is still evolving to make it more relevant and suited to the dynamic needs of Filipino CICL. However, since all our services are being provided for free, it has been challenging to mobilize occupational therapists and volunteers to get involved in this population. In the future, we hope to see paid positions in both public and private facilities where occupational therapists can be employed while championing occupational justice.

Critical reflection on occupational justice as applied in the Filipino context

Because justice issues are context-specific, we must consider the (non-) applicability or (re)contextualization of some occupational justice-related concepts in our own practice contexts. This is to encapsulate the authenticity of the injustice experiences under investigation. To do so, it is important to acknowledge some realities when applying occupational justice concepts in practice in the Philippines.

First, we need to realize that the injustices being described in this chapter may not be perceived as an actual injustice by the individual or groups experiencing them. The apathy or *blindness* of many Filipinos to these issues may stem from having these injustices heavily threaded into the tapestry of their daily life, making them the norm of life. Hence, the occupational therapist's role to educate about human and occupational rights and how these rights could be violated directly and indirectly by people and systemic structures is pivotal, especially for the marginalized and subjugated.

Second, *colonial mentality* or the tendency to view Western ideas as superior to indigenous Filipino ideas is deeply ingrained in the Filipino psyche (David & Okazaki, 2010). Consequently, Filipino occupational therapy practitioners and researchers may favor Western over indigenous ideas and practices without regard to its applicability in practical contexts. Filipinos may uncritically prioritize occupational justice–related issues (e.g., promoting individual agency or emphasizing leisure participation) in the occupational therapy process, which can sometimes conflict with Filipino values and culture.

Third, in a country such as the Philippines, where religion can influence laws and policies, it is important to consider that some people's understanding of justice comes from a religious rather than a sociopolitical perspective. In other words, justice is served when one does something in accordance with God's laws. People who see justice from a religious perspective may perceive social and occupational justice as a political instrument. When left unexplained, the principles of occupational justice can be seen as a set of agendas with the intention of blaming a dominant group (oppressors) reinforcing injustices and inequities in Philippine society.

Conclusion

This book chapter intends to help our readers understand that the nature of injustices is grounded in socially constructed contexts and are formed, in part, by structural and contextual factors beyond the individual or group. To the future users of the POJF and the OJHQ, it is important to contextualize their application. This should not be limited to translation and adaptation, but rather through collaborative and participatory efforts by the client, practitioners, and institutions towards a transformed way of life. We urge the consideration of indigenous knowledge, participant voices, cultural values, and spiritual beliefs in applying occupational justice concepts into practice.

Reflective actions and questions

1 Form a small group (students and/or practitioners) and choose one of the three realities above for your discussion. The discussion could be guided by these broad questions: What is your understanding of "occupational justice"? Do you resonate with this reality; why or why not? What roles do social privilege, colonization, and/or religion play in upholding justice and perpetuating injustice in our society today?

2 Visit the OJHQ resource site to learn more about OJHQ. As a tool intended for practice, do you think the OJHQ can be utilized in your workplace; why or why not? Can you list the benefits of using this tool for your clients as well as the challenges that this might cause you and your team?

References

Bailliard, A. L., Dallman, A. R., Carroll, A., Lee, B. D., & Szendrey, S. (2020). Doing occupational justice: A central dimension of everyday occupational therapy practice. *Canadian Journal of Occupational Therapy*, 87(2), 144–152. doi:10.1177/0008417419898930.

Benjamin-Thomas, T. E., & Laliberte-Rudman, D. (2018). A critical interpretive synthesis: Use of the occupational justice framework in research. *Australian Occupational Therapy Journal*, 65(1), 3–14. doi:10.1111/1440-1630.12428.

Chichaya, T., Joubert, R., & McColl, M. (2018). Analysing disability policy in Namibia: An occupational justice perspective. *African Journal of Disability*, 7, a401. doi:10.4102/ajod.v7i0.401.

Cookson, R., & Dolan, P. (2000). Principles of justice in health care rationing. *Journal of Medical Ethics*, 26(5), 323–329. doi:10.1136/jme.26.5.323.

David, E. J. R., & Okazaki, S. (2010). Activation and automaticity of colonial mentality. *Journal of Applied Social Psychology*, 40, 850–887. doi:10.1111/j.1559-1816.2010.00601.x.

DSWD. (2005). Standards for youth detention homes. *Administrative Order 15, Series of 2005*. https://www.dswd.gov.ph/issuances/AOs/AO_2005-015.pdf.

Farias, L., Laliberte-Rudman, D., Pollard, N., Schiller, S., Serrata-Malfitano, A. P., Thomas, K., & van Bruggen, H. (2019). Critical dialogical approach: A methodological direction for occupation-based social transformative work. *Scandinavian Journal of Occupational Therapy*, 26(4), 235–245. doi:10.1080/11038128.2018.1469666.

Feinsod, F. M., & Wagner, C. (2008). The ethical principle of justice: The purveyor of equality. https://www.hmpgloballearningnetwork.com/site/altc/article/8210.

Frank, G., & Zemke, R. (2008). Occupational therapy foundations for political engagement and social transformation. In N. Pollard, D. Sakellariou, & F. Kronenberg (Eds.), *A political practice of occupational therapy* (pp. 111–136). Churchill Livingstone.

Gupta, J. (2016). Mapping the evolving ideas of occupational justice: A critical analysis. *Occupational Therapy Journal of Research*, 36(4), 179–194. doi:10.1177/1539449216672171.

Hocking, C. (2017). Occupational justice as social justice: The moral claim for inclusion. *Journal of Occupational Science*, 24(1), 29–42. doi:10.1080/14427591.2017.1294016.

Hocking, C., Townsend, E., & Mace, J. (2019). Position statement: Occupational therapy and human rights. WFOT. https://wfot.org/resources/occupational-therapy-and-human-rights.

Janse van Rensburg, E. (2018). A framework for occupational enablement to facilitate social change in community practice. *Canadian Journal of Occupational Therapy*, 85(4), 318–329. doi:10.1177/0008417418805784.

JJWC. (2017). *Philippines' Comprehensive National Juvenile Intervention Program 2018–2022*. https://jjwc.gov.ph/wp-content/uploads/2020/06/Comprehensive-National-Juvenile-Intervention-Program-CNJIP.pdf.

JJWC. (2022). Updated 2022 situational analysis: Children in conflict with the law and children at risk in the Philippines. https://storage.googleapis.com/request-attachments/o57tbPgVeP3SZlZb7rncAr2eTSy2XERBTJmErM9HP5NFxGRSlvj8vWsl28H1HokUuCoYRe2xOmbQmDZL3xsmB60qZ5QlsG6r3hTt/2022%20Situational%20Analysis%20on%20CICL_Final.pdf.

Kronenberg, F., Algado, S. S., & Pollard, N. (2005). *Occupational therapy without borders: Learning through the spirit of survivors*. Elsevier/Churchill Livingstone.

Nizzero, A., Cote, P., & Cramm, H. (2017) Occupational disruption: A scoping review. *Journal of Occupational Science*, 24(2), 114–127. doi:10.1080/14427591.2017.1306791.

Paule, M., Bagadiong, J., Favila, A., Cuerdo, A., & Fortich, S. (2020). Situational analysis on children in detention facilities in the Philippines. *JJWC*. https://www.jjwc.gov.ph/wp-content/uploads/2021/07/SitAn-on-Children-in-Detention-JJWC.pdf.

Save the Children Philippines and Convention of the Rights of the Children Asia. (2021). *The challenging plight of Filipino children: Children's rights in the Philippines in the new normal*. https://www.csc-crc.org/wp-content/uploads/2022/02/FINAL-Child-Situationer-2021.pdf.

Serrata-Malfitano, A. P., da Mota-de Souza, R. G. M., Townsend, E. A., & Lopes, R. E. (2019). Do occupational justice concepts inform occupational therapists' practice? A scoping review. *Canadian Journal of Occupational Therapy*, 86(4), 299–312. doi:10.1177/0008417419833409.

Stadnyk, R., Townsend, E., & Wilcock, A. (2010). Occupational justice. In C. H. Christiansen & E. Townsend (Eds.), *Introduction to occupation: The art and science of living* (pp. 329–358). Pearson.

Sy, M. P., & Ohshima, N. (2019). Utilizing the Occupational Justice Health Questionnaire (OJHQ) with a Filipino drug surrenderee in occupational therapy practice: A case report. *WFOT Bulletin*, 75(1), 59–62. doi:10.1080/14473828.2018.1505682.

Sy, M. P., Roraldo, M. P. N. R., Delos Reyes, R. C. R., Yao, D. P. G., & Pineda, R. C. S. (2021). Occupational Justice Health Questionnaire: Reflections on its application. *Cadernos Brasileiros de Terapia Ocupacional*, 29, e2961. doi:10.1590/2526-8910.ctoAO2244.

Townsend, E., & Whiteford, G. (2005). A participatory occupational justice framework: Population-based processes of practice. In F. Kronenberg, S. Simó Algado, & N. Pollard (Eds.), *Occupational therapy without borders: Learning from the spirit of survivors* (pp. 110–126). Elsevier.

UNICEF Innocenti—Global Office of Research and Foresight. (2023). *Too little, too late: An assessment of public spending on children by age in 84 countries.* https://www.unicef.org/innocenti/media/2851/file/UNICEF-Too-Little-Too-La te-Report-2023.pdf.

Walley-Hammell, K. (2008). Reflections on … well-being and occupational rights. *Canadian Journal of Occupational Therapy*, 75(1), 61–64. doi:10.2182/ cjot.07.007.

Walley-Hammell, K. (2015). Occupational rights and critical occupational therapy: Rising to the challenge. *Australian Occupational Therapy Journal*, 62(6), 449– 451. doi:10.1111/1440-1630.12195.

Walley-Hammell, K. (2023). Focusing on "what matters": The Occupation, Capability and Wellbeing Framework for Occupational Therapy. *Cadernos Brasileiros de Terapia Ocupacional*, 31, e3509. doi:10.1590/2526-8910.ctoAO269035092.

Whiteford, G., & Townsend, E. (2011). Participatory Occupational Justice Framework (POJF 2010): Enabling occupational participation and inclusion. In F. Kronenberg, N. Pollard, & D. Sakellariou (Eds.), *Occupational therapies without borders: Towards an ecology of occupation-based practices* (pp. 65–84). Elsevier.

Wilcock, A., & Townsend, E. (2000). Occupational terminology interactive dialogue. *Journal of Occupational Science*, 7(2), 84–86. doi:10.1080/ 14427591.2000.9686470.

Wilcock, A. A., & Townsend, E. A. (2014). Occupational Justice Health Questionnaire. In B. A. Boyt Schell, G. Gillen, & M. E. Scaffa (Eds.), *Willard & Spackman's occupational therapy* (20th ed., pp. 548–549). Lippincott Williams & Wilkins.

WHO. (1986). *Ottawa Charter for Health Promotion.* https://apps.who.int/iris/ha ndle/10665/349652.

Yao, D. P., Inoue, K., Sy, M. P., Bontje, P., Suyama, N., Yatsu, C., Perez, D. A., & Ito, Y. (2020). Experience of Filipinos with spinal cord injury in the use of assistive technology: An occupational justice perspective. *Occupational Therapy International.* doi:10.1155/2020/6696296.

Chapter 12

Strengthening research in occupational therapy

Ivan Neil B. Gomez, Caroline Fischl and Michael Sy

Chapter objectives

1 Map current occupational therapy research in the Philippines
2 Describe challenges and explore strategies on how to strengthen research and evidence-based practice in the Philippines
3 Through stories on knowledge development, translation, and implementation in the local context, reflect on your own needs and contribution to support occupational therapy research in the Philippines

Tanya, a newly licensed occupational therapist at a tertiary hospital, manages adults with neurological disorders at the outpatient stroke unit. She observed varying referral times from the onset of stroke, with some clients referred immediately and others after days or weeks. Early referrals seemed to result in better occupational outcomes. She consulted her colleagues, who encouraged her to investigate research evidence on the correlation between referral time and outcomes.

Introduction

Research ensures the continuous development of occupational therapy (OT) and its effectiveness (Taylor, 2017). Besides advancing practice, the Philippine Academy of Occupational Therapists (PAOT) advocates for a research agenda to describe practice areas and develop education and the profession locally (PAOT, 2015). Yet, there is a dearth of OT publications in the Philippines (Sy et al., 2021). This chapter examines the current state of OT research in the Philippines. As part of this examination, we mapped studies within OT conducted from 2000 to early 2023, using information collected through educational programs, professional networks, and searches in databases. Subsequent sections detail findings from this mapping.

Research in OT and occupational science in the Philippines is primarily embedded in education at undergraduate and graduate levels. The World Federation of Occupational Therapists' (WFOT) minimum standards for

DOI: 10.4324/9781003321217-12

education require active and up-to-date research in programs to address local needs (WFOT, 2016). These standards are further translated into the requirements for undergraduate OT programs in the country (Commission on Higher Education [CHED], 2017). Education on research at the undergraduate level includes an introduction to research methods, basic biostatistics, and their application in evidence-based practice. At the graduate level, students learn advanced methodologies. Students at both levels apply this knowledge in a thesis. Research projects are often driven by both OT students and educators. Situated within occupation-based curricula, topics on the relevance of occupations to support health and well-being are encouraged. Additionally, in professional courses, students learn to search for and appraise research evidence to support clinical reasoning. Although research enhances evidence-based practice, participation in research diminishes after entry-level education due to various factors.

This chapter illustrates the process of evidence-based OT through a case study, structured around the five steps of evidence-based practice: *Ask, Access, Appraise, Apply,* and *Evaluate* (Sackett et al., 1996; Straus et al., 2019). It concludes with a reflection on how to support research and evidence-based practice in OT in the Philippines beyond undergraduate programs.

Ask

Research involves systematically examining a complex issue or phenomenon that affects people and societies. It starts by asking clear, specific, and relevant questions. To formulate questions, it is important to understand what is real in the world and can be known (ontology), how knowledge is generated and applied (epistemology), and the values guiding the inquiry (axiology).

> *Tanya's observation prompted her to reflect on how to search for evidence. She recalled learning to frame research questions during her undergraduate studies and used her internship experience to transform her research question into a clinical query.*

Ontology

Ontology deals with the nature of reality (Varpio & MacLeod, 2020) and helps researchers determine what is real about the issue or phenomenon they are examining. Our mapping exercise showed that research in the Philippines is dominated by inquiries into pediatric practice, followed by adult/geriatric physical dysfunction, psychosocial/mental health, and community-based OT. Education, professional development, and work rehabilitation have received less attention in research. This finding mirrors OT practice trends in the country (Carandang & Delos Reyes, 2018).

Aligning research with practice fosters a mutually beneficial relationship. To strengthen research in both traditional and emerging practices, occupational therapists need to practice and enhance the visibility of the profession in these areas. Simultaneously, empirical research in specific domains is essential to inform and improve professional practice. Capitalizing on this parallelism can enhance the understanding of reality, fostering research-practice alignment that positively impacts OT in the Philippines.

Epistemology

Epistemology is concerned with the nature and scope of knowledge (Varpio & MacLeod, 2020). Understanding how knowledge is generated, validated, and applied helps researchers design studies to ensure that the generated knowledge is robust and contextually relevant. Quantitative research traditions dominate Philippine OT research (Figure 12.1). However, there is a recent shift towards qualitative methods, reflecting a worldwide recognition of occupation as a phenomenon beyond mere numbers and statistics (Taylor, 2017).

Review methodologies have gained prominence in recent years due to COVID-19 pandemic restrictions on community mobility and in-person social contact, which prompted the need for online methods. Prior to the pandemic, courses on review methodologies were only offered at the graduate level. This adjustment challenged the expected outcomes for undergraduate research, which has primarily focused on empirical research. The emergence of review, mixed, and multi-methods in Filipino OT research necessitates changes in undergraduate curricula.

Axiology

Axiology delves into the nature of values and their impact on research (Varpio & MacLeod, 2020). When formulating research questions, it is

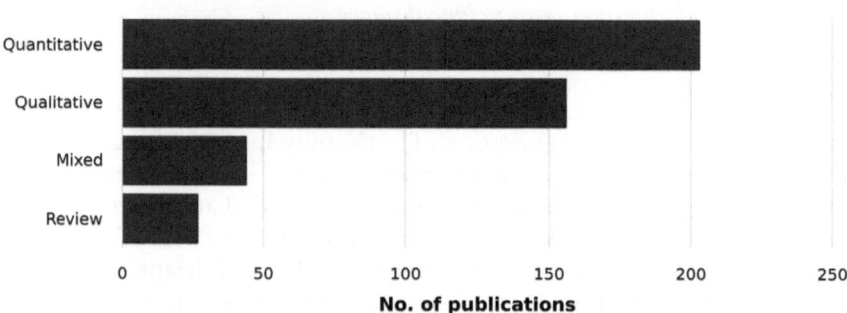

Figure 12.1 Distribution of methodologies in Filipino occupational therapy research (n=430)

essential to clarify the underlying values and motivations driving the inquiry. Are the research questions aimed at validating a predetermined understanding or comprehending a specific situation? Researchers, whether students or educators, must critically assess their positionality as it shapes the research process. Positionality includes one's identity and social position in relation to the research and its participants (Bukamal, 2022).

Student- and faculty-led occupational therapy research

In the Philippines, student-driven research projects dominate OT research, outnumbering published journal articles. Students often choose topics aligned with their interests or those of preferred academic staff. Typically, undergraduate students work in groups to develop a thesis proposal and conduct their study within two to three academic terms.

A recent shift toward research discipleship has been noted, where educators lead research projects and mentor students who contribute at various stages. With more graduate and postgraduate degrees in OT and allied health programs, and more Filipino occupational therapists pursuing higher degrees, an increase in published OT articles in peer-reviewed journals is expected (Sy et al., 2021).

Acquire

Access to credible information sources is essential for addressing questions. This subsection focuses on the availability of these platforms and databases in the Philippines.

Tanya began a fact-finding mission to answer her clinical question. Finding limited and outdated print journals in the hospital's library and scarce online resources, she used her alumni status to access her former university's library. The librarian suggested exploring local government publications, university resources, and relevant medical and professional association websites.

Information sources and access

Students receive practical support within their programs for accessing information sources. However, OT practitioners not affiliated with hospitals or higher education institutions (HEIs) often face challenges to access up-to-date research (Carandang & Delos Reyes, 2018). Most Filipino occupational therapists work outside these settings, limiting access to databases and journals due to paywalls. Google Scholar, while a free alternative, lacks advanced search capabilities compared to established search platforms like EBSCO and OVID (https://ovidsp.ovid.com/).

PubMed (https://pubmed.ncbi.nlm.nih.gov/) is another option but may not provide full-text access to all relevant journals. Filipino occupational therapists can explore open access sources like Directory of Open Access Journals (https://doaj.org/) and the Western Pacific Region Index Medicus (https://www.globalindexmedicus.net/biblioteca/wprim/) for free scientific articles. Textbooks offer foundational information but may lag behind current developments.

Another challenge is the limited availability of culturally relevant and locally applicable knowledge. Many OT theses do not progress to publication in journals and remain archived within HEIs, inaccessible to non-students, staff, or alumni. Some educational programs have taken steps to address this issue by publishing undergraduate thesis titles and abstracts on their HEI library websites or through government-hosted research information management systems, such as the Health Research and Development Information Network (HERDIN) (https://www.herdin.ph/) and the Philippine Health Research Registry (PHRR) (https://registry.hea lthresearch.ph/index.php/registry).

Clinical Practice Guidelines (CPGs) can inform practice and are based on research that has been filtered, critically appraised, and synthesized. Since creating CPGs is resource-intensive, this endeavor has yet to be fully implemented in OT in the Philippines. Nevertheless, existing CPGs approved by the Philippines' Department of Health (DOH) can provide related information to occupational therapists. CPGs will be discussed later in this chapter.

Philippine occupational therapy–related journals

The *Philippine Journal of Occupational Therapy* (*PJOT*) was launched in 2005 and published articles until 2010, focusing on locally relevant peer-reviewed content. Its subsequent inactivity has limited the availability of local OT knowledge sources. While OT journals are available, adapting and contextualizing this knowledge for local use is necessary. Filipino researchers have published in international journals, but funding constraints for journal subscriptions and open access publishing charges limit accessibility. In recent years, local peer-reviewed journals have emerged as viable alternatives, addressing the absence of a dedicated Filipino OT journal. Examples include:

- *Acta Medica Philippina*
  (https://actamedicaphilippina.upm.edu.ph/index.php/acta/)
- *Education Quarterly* (https://journals.upd.edu.ph/index.php/edq/index)
- *Journal of Management and Development Studies*
  (https://jmds.upou.edu.ph/index.php/journal)
- *Journal of Social Health* (https://socialhealthjournal.ust.edu.ph/)

- *Philippine Journal of Allied Health Sciences* (https://pjahs.ust.edu.ph/)
- *Philippine Journal of Health Research and Development* (https://pjhrd.upm.edu.ph/index.php/main)

Open access and the democratization of knowledge

The lack of access to valuable research evidence in the Philippines needs urgent and potentially radical solutions. Initiatives like *Plan S* (https://www.coalition-s.org/), which aims to make research fully and immediately accessible, can benefit Filipino occupational therapists. Research should be democratized and not hidden behind paywalls, especially for those who need it the most (Gomez, 2019). HEIs should transition from isolated research efforts to collaborative coalitions to collectively address problems and avoid redundancy. Publishing research titles and abstracts should become standard practice to inform occupational therapists on the current scope of Philippine OT knowledge. Government programs like HERDIN and PHRR can facilitate knowledge dissemination.

OT researchers worldwide acknowledge the importance of open access to their research. However, challenges such as high article processing charges for open access imposed by publishers often burden research groups and institutions. Some state research grants require publishing research findings open access without an embargo period. Additionally, there are efforts within professional associations to transform their scientific journals into fully open-access publications; the *Scandinavian Journal of Occupational Therapy* (*SJOT*) serves as a notable example. Benchmarking against journals like the *SJOT* could help revitalize local journals like the *PJOT*.

Appraise

Appraising the evidence entails thoroughly examining the credibility of the evidence. This includes ensuring that ethical and valid methods were used as well as assessing the validity, relevance, and recency of the results.

> *Tanya reviewed several CPGs and recommendations concerning stroke. She discovered that the American Heart Association recommends early referral to and the start of rehabilitation within the first 24 hours of stroke onset, with evidence suggesting that more than three hours of daily therapy lead to better functional improvements. The American Occupational Therapy Association specifies OT interventions tailored to various outcomes. In the Philippines, the Stroke CPG of the Philippine Academy of Rehabilitation Medicine (PARM) advises ensuring medical stability before rehabilitation and integrating outpatient rehabilitation into discharge planning.*

Ethical approval in research

This section discusses ethical approval in research. More information on ethics is discussed in Chapter 14.

Obtaining ethical approval is essential before conducting research, whether for a student thesis or independent research. Despite limited information on this practice in OT research programs in the Philippines, it should be the standard (Enriquez, 2019). Ethical approval ensures that participants are fully informed of the study aims, procedures, risks, benefits, and their rights before, during, and after the study. The process of acquiring ethical approval takes time, so this must be considered when planning research projects.

The Philippine Health Research Ethics Board (PHREB) ensures adherence to universal ethical principles in health research by providing Good Clinical Practice (GCP) training and accrediting institutional review boards (IRB) (https://ethics.healthresearch.ph/). The PHREB requires researchers conducting health research in the Philippines to undergo GCP training, or its equivalent. GCP training can be expensive, but several organizations offer free GCP training and certification. Examples are provided below. Contact your local IRB for clarification.

- Global Health Training Centre:
  https://globalhealthtrainingcentre.tghn.org/ich-good-clinical-practice/
- National Drug Abuse Treatment Clinical Trials Network:
  https://gcp.nidatraining.org/
- PharmaLessons: https://www.pharmalessons.com/free-courses/gcptraining/

The PHREB includes professionals and representatives from the Department of Science and Technology (DOST), DOH, and CHED. OT professionals should engage in IRBs to ensure occupation-based outcomes are considered in health research. Additionally, the feasibility of creating a national OT-specific IRB to ensure scientific, ethical, and occupation-based soundness of OT research protocols should be explored.

Critical appraisal and risk of bias

Not all published research possesses good methodological quality. While there is a common belief in the superiority of published, randomized controlled trials, or filtered and synthesized evidence, this is not always applicable. Each research study should be approached critically, by assessing its trustworthiness or validity and reliability, as well as recency, relevance, impact, and applicability. Examining biases before accepting authors' conclusions is also important.

Critical appraisal and risk of bias are similar constructs but use different terminologies (Barker et al., 2023). Critical appraisal has been criticized for its score-based quantification of methodological quality, leading to the emergence of risk of bias assessment. However, risk of bias assessments have limitations due to their focus on quantitative measures. In contrast, critical appraisal tools facilitate appraising the evidence across various research designs, providing occupational therapists options beyond intervention and diagnostic accuracy. Both approaches help occupational therapists understand research before applying it. OTSeeker (https://www.otseeker.com/default.aspx) provides valuable resources for learning about critical appraisal. Examples of critical appraisal checklists and risk of bias assessments are available through:

- Critical Appraisal Skills Programme:
  https://casp-uk.net/casp-tools-checklists/
- JBI: https://jbi.global/critical-appraisal-tools
- McMaster University: https://merst.healthsci.mcmaster.ca/
- Risk of Bias Info: https://www.riskofbias.info/welcome
- University of Oxford Centre for Evidence-Based Medicine:
  https://www.cebm.ox.ac.uk/resources/ebm-tools/critical-appraisal-tools

Filipino occupational therapists should discern the difference between critical appraisal checklists and reporting checklists. The former investigates biases affecting evidence quality, while the latter addresses the minimum information that should be reported in a research article. Similar criteria may exist, but critical appraisal assesses believability. The EQUATOR Network (https://www.equator-network.org/) provides reporting guidelines across research methodologies, useful for occupational therapists intending to publish their articles.

Journal clubs

One strategy to enhance critical appraisal skills is engaging in journal clubs, which regularly review research and reflect on the relevance of research findings. This practice is common in clinical placements for OT interns in the Philippines. It should be expanded to include more clinicians, structured evaluations of research bias, and reflections on translating evidence into practice. Several resources and platforms are available to guide occupational therapists starting a journal club or engaging in research discussions, like the ones listed below:

- American Occupational Therapy Association:
  https://www.aota.org/practice/practice-essentials/evidencebased-practiceknowledge-translation/kt-toolkit-journal-club-guide

- Occupational Therapy Australia:
  https://www.otaus.com.au/cpd-and-events/teapot-talks
- Occupational Therapy International Online Network by the WFOT:
  https://otion.wfot.org/
- Royal College of Occupational Therapists (RCOT): https://www.rcot.co.uk/
  sites/default/files/Developing-Specialist-Section-ejournal-club-Dec2019.pdf
- The Occupational Therapy Hub:
  https://www.theothub.com/forum/the-ot-journal-club

Apply

Once evidence is found, occupational therapists must decide its applicability and develop strategies to apply the findings. This involves reflection on the quality of the evidence, client's values and circumstances, staff expertise, and practice context. This section discusses the current state of evidence-based practice (EBP) in the Philippines and ways to support evidence-based OT practice.

> *Having limited and indirect evidence, Tanya encountered opposition from her senior colleagues who prioritized experience and expertise over evidence and questioned the relevance of international guidelines. Proactively, Tanya engaged her colleagues in reflecting on the evidence and contextualizing it for their practice. Together, they consulted hospital stakeholders to develop strategies for integrating evidence-based recommendations, bridging the gap between evidence and experience.*

Evidence-based practice in the Philippines

Evidence-based OT practice in the Philippines is relatively new, with the first known article on EBP-related capacity published just over 20 years ago (Cabatan et al., 2010). While EBP concepts are integrated in educational programs (Rotor & Gorgon, 2011; Sy et al., 2021), training for clinicians should also be available (Dizon et al., 2014a, 2014b).

In a country with limited research generation, health professionals often apply practice-based evidence, centering clinical decision-making on their expertise and clinical experience. This challenges EBP and highlights practice gaps.

Recent personal communications with OT students in clinical placements revealed the concept of "book-based evidence," where students base their clinical decisions on textbook knowledge. Despite having access to HEI library resources, it is concerning that students do not use more up-to-date knowledge. Continuing book-based practice as professionals may diminish the quality of care due to the lack of current knowledge.

Translating evidence to practice

Addressing the limitations of the conventional EBP model from the 1990s, JBI proposed a model of evidence-based healthcare (see https://jbi.global/jbi-model-of-EBHC). This JBI model incorporates practice contexts as an important variable when applying evidence, considering the varied clinical questions healthcare professionals encounter. It goes beyond intervention and diagnostics, making it more relevant to OT practice, as it provides a framework that transcends culture, capacity, communication, and collaboration.

Previous attempts at capacity-building in evidence-based healthcare in the Philippines include a tailored training program described by Dizon et al. (2012, 2014a, 2014b). While participation of occupational therapists was limited, the program has effectively improved their EBP knowledge and skills. Unfortunately, such programs are currently unavailable for Filipino occupational therapists. Investment in similar EBP training for Filipino occupational therapists is needed. Besides knowledge and skills, translating evidence into practice involves reflective practice (described in Chapter 5). Table 12.1 is a recommended guide for applying evidence to practice.

Table 12.1 Evidence translation checklist (adapted from Dizon et al., 2012)

Component	Guide prompts
Clinical relevance or applicability	• Similarities of the participants' characteristics and values described in the evidence and with those that you serve • Description of the intervention or approaches to be replicated • Necessary skills, facilities, equipment, and resources available to the occupational therapist to replicate the intervention or approach
Validity of the evidence	• Validity of the findings based on critical appraisal of the evidence • Validity of the outcome measures used • Consideration of other factors that may have affected the results
Magnitude of effects or clinical impact	• Findings go beyond statistical significance but present clinical significance • Expected effects address the intended outcomes
Applicability	• Occupational therapist's confidence in applying the findings based on clinical relevance, validity, and magnitude of effects
Barriers to applying the evidence	• Barriers to applying the evidence • Identification of potential barriers to the application of the evidence
Strategies to address barriers	• Identification of realistic strategies to address the barriers

Clinical practice guidelines

CPGs are documents with recommendations to standardize practice and ensure optimal client care. Unfortunately, CPGs are not available for the OT profession in the Philippines. While the PAOT provides position statements and practice recommendations, these are not CPGs. Examples of OT CPGs from other countries are provided below:

- American Occupational Therapy Association: https://research.aota.org/collection/7219/AOTA-Practice-Guidelines
- Canadian Association of Occupational Therapists: https://caot.ca/site/prac-res/pr/hub?nav=sidebar&banner=4
- RCOT: https://www.rcot.co.uk/practice-resources/rcot-practice-guidelines
- WFOT: https://wfot.org/resources

Terminologies related to clinical practice recommendations can be confusing. Definitions are presented in Table 12.2.

Adopt, Contextualize, Adapt

While CPGs are useful, their applicability to the local context can be problematic. Most CPGs are from developed countries, where OT practice may differ from the Philippines. Even if evidence is valid and clinically significant, client values, occupational therapists' expertise, resources, and practice contexts will vary, raising questions about the recommended interventions' effects.

Developing new CPGs requires extensive resources, which may not be feasible in the Philippines. Instead, contextualizing CPGs from other countries is recommended. The South African Guideline Evaluation Clinical Practice Guideline Development Framework (SAGE Framework) (Dizon et al., 2016) provides a good starting point and has been used by PARM. Replicating similar methods to support Philippine OT practice should be considered. The SAGE Framework suggests utilizing available CPGs and developing a contextualized version through expert and stakeholder consultations. This multi-tier process ensures evidence uptake and compliance. The evidence is evaluated using the *Adopt, Contextualize, Adapt* analogy. The goal is to involve local experts to complement existing evidence and develop locally relevant practice recommendations. An example is presented in Table 12.3.

Table 12.2 Definitions of document terminologies related to practice recommendation (Aleksovska et al., 2021; D'Arcy, 2007; De Boeck et al., 2014; Joshi et al., 2019)

Terminology	*Definition*
Clinical practice guideline	Documents that are systematically developed using robust methodologies encompassing the identification of a relevant clinical question, methods of searching, selecting, and grading the evidence. CPGs are recommendations grounded on a synthesized body of evidence.
Practice standard	Established by an authority (i.e., professional organization) reaching a consensus on the minimum standards that, when met, results in the best outcomes, establishes the practice, and provides the greatest value. Typically used for organization accreditations and authoritative in nature.
Consensus statement	A document representing the collective opinions or recommendations of a professional organization or society's expert panel.
Position statement/paper	A policy report drafted by members of a professional organization or society that elucidates, explains, justifies, advocates, or recommends a certain course of action to approach a clinical issue.
Practice alert	A short statement quickly developed in response to a time-sensitive practice issue requiring immediate action or response.
Evidence summary	A concise report analyzing the best available evidence on a specific and focused practice-related issue. This document is typically developed using plain language to translate complex scientific findings in order for a broader audience to better understand.

Table 12.3 Definition and example of the Adopt, Contextualize, Adapt approach (adapted from Dizon et al., 2016)

Approach	*Definition*	*Example*
Adopt	This refers to accepting practice recommendations as they are, without any changes.	In the case discussed in this chapter, if the AHA recommends initiating rehabilitation within 24 hours of stroke onset, this recommendation will be followed as is. However, its universality assumes similar health systems and practices across countries. This may not be ideal for OT in the Philippines, given the differences in practice patterns worldwide.

Approach	Definition	Example
Contextualize	Contextualizing recommendations entails using the existing CPG recommendations while fitting them to the specific context where they will be implemented.	In the same case, while rehabilitation should be initiated within 24 hours, the term "rehabilitation" must be contextualized. In the Philippines, where not all hospitals have occupational therapists, rehabilitation may involve the most readily available therapy at the time of referral. Additional provisions should be outlined for advanced settings to ensure consistent health care delivery across the country.
Adapt	Adapting a CPG involves modifying existing recommendations to suit differences in values, context, or resources between the CPG's origin and the target country of implementation.	Considering the costs and availability of rehabilitation, particularly OT service, the recommendation from our sample case can be adapted to reflect these factors. Thus, referral or provision of rehabilitation service (e.g., OT, PT, or most readily available therapy) should be initiated within 48 hours of medical stability after stroke onset.

Evaluate

This phase involves evaluating one's EBP, identifying challenges and supports for applying evidence, and auditing the impact of evidence-based changes. Audits help identify strategies for sustaining and enhancing these changes. This subsection considers evaluation as an integral step in EBP and reflects on its impact on OT research in the Philippines.

With support from senior colleagues, Tanya proposed a change in the stroke unit's referral process. The hospital approved a six-month trial. The team informed staff about the recommendations through training, lunch meetings, and posters. After the trial, they evaluated the program through interviews, focus groups, and chart reviews. The results showed a 60% compliance rate and improvements in function and quality of life prior to discharge. Encouraged by these results, Tanya is preparing for a larger-scale implementation.

Process and outcomes evaluation

Integrating quality measures into OT service delivery requires a systematic and systemic approach, but this remains a challenge in the Philippines. Currently, aside from routine evaluations by OT professionals, there is no structured process for auditing practice at the clinical or national level.

Developing audit measures is imperative. While evidence suggests various methods such as surveys, interviews, focus group discussions, observations, and charting are common and feasible locally, issues like record availability, feedback response, behavior change, and practicality must be addressed. The audit process must consider the Philippines' social, cultural, economic, and political contexts, including who conducts, when, and how audits of OT practice are performed.

Choosing appropriate outcome measures is essential for evaluating changes in decision-making. For occupational therapists focused on participation in occupations, health, and well-being, context-specific tools are important. Although local outcome measures have been reported, their ecological validity in addressing practice gaps is not fully established (Sy et al., 2021). The utility and usability of these measures in clinical settings remain largely unknown.

Facilitation of change in practice

Managing change in practice can be challenging, as even minor changes, like changing scrub suit colors, can cause staff dissent. Introducing changes to processes, policies, and perceptions requires a leadership framework. Effective facilitation involves enabling acceptance of the change, and identifying and recruiting change champions is a promising strategy locally. A top-down approach can secure buy-in, while a participative approach helps develop strategies and ease in the change. Providing space for individual self-reflection within an organization promotes mutual investment in and support for the change. These strategies can facilitate cultural change in OT practice.

Sustainability in using research evidence to inform OT practice should be integrated into the initial planning. Identifying barriers and strengths to practice change is integral. As described earlier, Philippine OT practice and research patterns parallel each other. Leveraging this relationship through resource sharing between clinical and academic practice can ensure the sustainability of supporting research in OT.

Sustainability of knowledge generation and utilization

In a small community like OT in the Philippines, communities of practice can enhance research generation and utilization. Understanding the EBP needs of Filipino occupational therapists can inform curricula and lead to additional professional training for clinicians. Experiences and questions at the point of care can shape OT programs' research agendas and foster collaboration. Local funding from the DOST, DOH, and CHED supports these initiatives, while international funding is available from organizations like the WFOT, the RCOT, and the Swedish Association of Occupational

Therapists. However, these opportunities are not yet fully utilized. Filipino occupational therapists should leverage their collective potential to advance OT research in the Philippines.

Philippine OT research agenda setting

Our mapping of OT research provides an audit of Filipino OT research topics against international and local agendas. Comparing local results to WFOT's international research priorities (see https://wfot.org/resour ces/wfot-research-priorities), research in the Philippines often focuses on participation in everyday life, effectiveness of OT interventions, and EBP. However, research on OT in chronic conditions and professional issues is limited. Aligning with the United Nations' Sustainable Development Goals (SDGs), most research addresses SDG 3 Good health and well-being, SDG 4 Quality education, and SDG 8 Decent work and economic growth.

Locally, the 2015 PAOT research agenda (PAOT, 2015) provides a benchmark for current research trends, highlighting studies on culture, pediatric OT practice, and faculty development. However, interest in OT school practitioner profiles, career advocacy, and practice patterns is limited. Nationally, comparisons with the 2017–2022 National Unified Health Research Agenda (see https://www.healthresearch.ph/index.php/ nuhra) reveal that over half of the indexed undergraduate OT research focuses on holistic approaches to health, while global health innovations are least addressed.

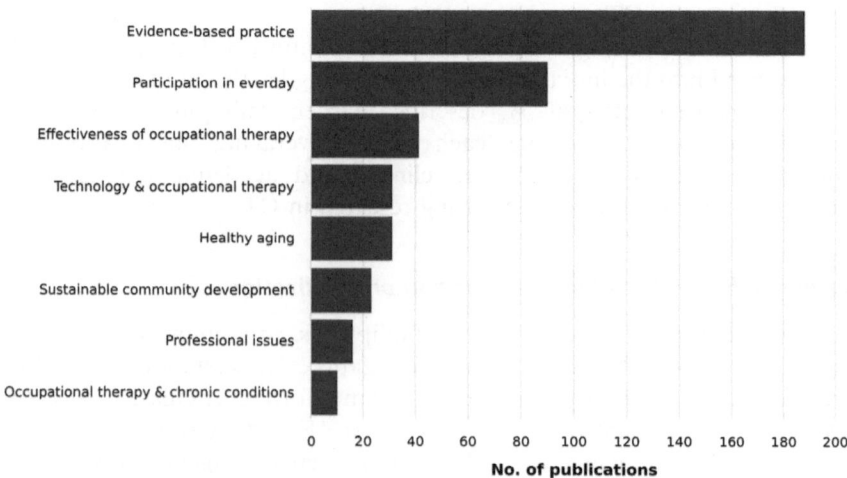

Figure 12.2 Filipino occupational therapy research addressing WFOT's international research priorities (n=430)

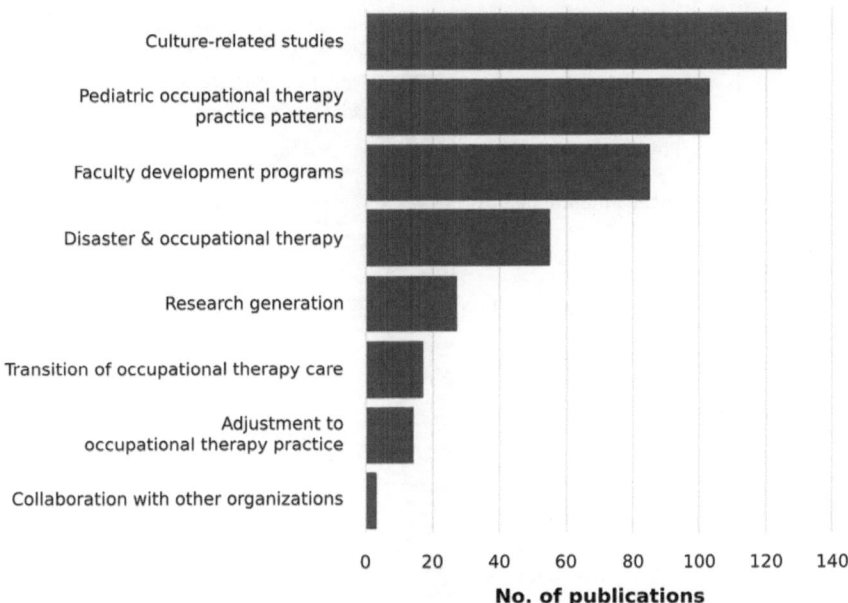

Figure 12.3 Filipino occupational therapy research addressing PAOT's research agenda (n=430)
Note: Agenda not reflected in the graph signifies no identified research addressing such.

These results highlight the need to redefine the OT research agenda in the Philippines. Future trends should address contemporary issues like global health, emerging technologies, occupational science, and artificial intelligence. The World Health Organization's Rehabilitation 2030 initiative (see https://www.who.int/initiatives/rehabilitation-2030) should also be considered. We must advocate for underexplored areas and ensure that future research aligns with both international and local health research agendas.

Reflecting on the ontology and epistemology of OT research in the Philippines vis-à-vis international and local research agendas, the PAOT research agenda needs an update with a contemporary, relevant, and critical perspective. Contextualizing Western evidence is positive but should be strengthened using methods beyond traditional paradigms. Research areas not traditionally explored like OT practice in provinces should be prioritized. Additionally, research on OT schools (i.e., practitioner profile, career advocacy) may need refocusing to align with the WFOT's research priorities. Future research should expand into chronic conditions, aging, sustainability, and technology. Leveraging innovations should address diverse health needs across the developmental lifespan and contexts.

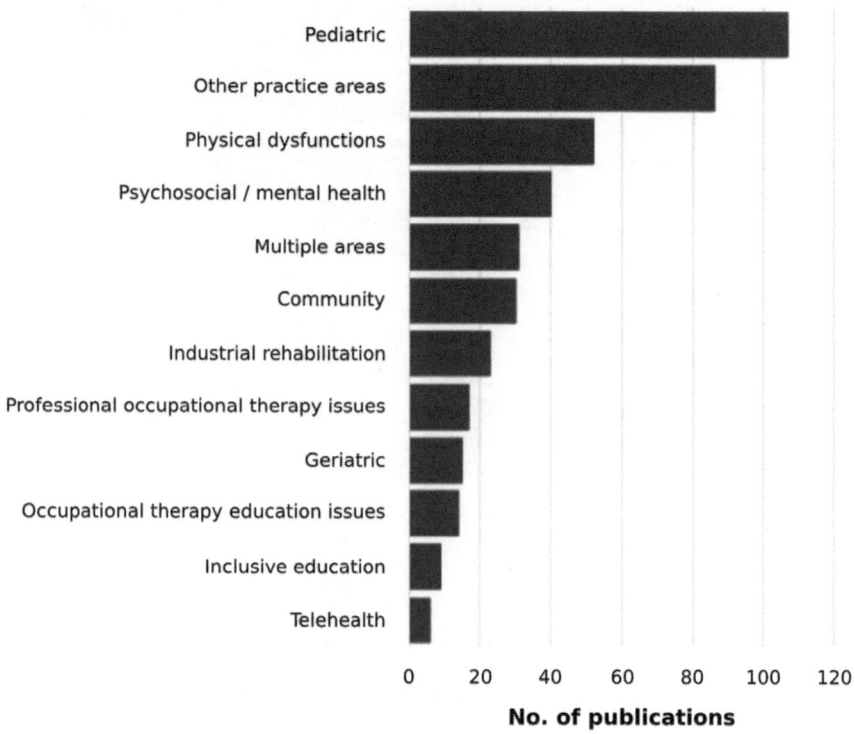

Figure 12.4 Researched occupational therapy practice areas (n=430)

Setting the OT research agenda in the Philippines should be a collaborative effort involving the PAOT, OT educational programs, and other stakeholders. A participatory approach and collective self-reflection will help shape future research directions. Adapting methods from the WFOT's research priorities (WFOT et al., 2017) can guide this process. Our collective commitment as research generators and consumers will be vital to advancing OT research in the Philippines.

Chapter summary

This chapter examined OT research in the Philippines, identifying key topics and gaps. It highlighted the need for enhanced evidence-based practice (EBP) training, considering ontology (nature of OT practice), epistemology (sources of knowledge), and axiology (values). Essential EBP steps—question formulation, evidence acquisition, critical appraisal, application, and evaluation—were discussed. The chapter explains adopting, contextualizing, and adapting international clinical practice guidelines (CPGs) to the local context using the SAGE Framework. It emphasizes the importance of collaboration among the Philippine Association of Occupational Therapists (PAOT), educational programs, and other stakeholders to develop a relevant research agenda that aligns with both international and local health priorities.

References

Aleksovska, K., Bassetti, C. L. A., Berger, T., Carvalho, V., Costa, J., Deuschl, G., Frederiksen, K. S., Jaarsma, J., Kobulashvili, T., Leone, M. A., Pavlakova, L., Romoli, M., & Vignatelli, L. (2021). Guidelines should be guidelines: Time to leave the terms "consensus" and "position" for other purposes. *European Journal of Neurology*, 28(8), 2461–2466. doi:10.1111/ene.14933.

Barker, T. H., Stone, J. C., Sears, K., Klugar, M., Leonardi-Bee, J., Tufanaru, C., Aromataris, E., & Munn, Z. (2023). Revising the JBI quantitative critical appraisal tools to improve their applicability: An overview of methods and the development process. *JBI Evidence Synthesis*, 21(3), 478–493. doi:10.11124/JBIES-22-00125.

Bukamal, H. (2022). Deconstructing insider–outsider researcher positionality. *British Journal of Special Education*, 49(3), 327–349. doi:10.1111/1467-8578.12426.

Cabatan, M. C., Gorgon, E. J., Guevarra, J. C., Santos, J. L., & Diongco, J. M. (2010). Helping Filipino occupational therapists become evidence-based practitioners—Discovering their learning needs. *Philippine Journal of Occupational Therapy*, 4(1), 12–22.

Carandang, K. A. & Delos Reyes, R. C. (2018). *Workforce survey 2017: Working conditions and salary structure of occupational therapists working in the Philippines survey.* PAOT.

CHED. (2017). *CMO 52: Policies, standards and guidelines for the BSOT education program.* CHED.

D'Arcy, Y. (2007, October 11). Practice guidelines, standards, consensus statements, position papers: What they are, how they differ. *American Nurse.* https://www.myamericannurse.com/practice-guidelines-standards-consensus-statements-position-papers-what-they-are-how-they-differ/.

De Boeck, K., Castellani, C., & Elborn, J. S. (2014). Medical consensus, guidelines, and position papers: A policy for the ECFS. *Journal of Cystic Fibrosis*, 13(5), 495–498. doi:10.1016/j.jcf.2014.06.012.

Dizon, J. M., Dizon, R. J., Regino, J., & Gabriel, A. (2014a). Evidence-based practice training for health professionals in the Philippines. *Advances in Medical Education and Practice*, 5, 89–94. doi:10.2147/AMEP.S54459.

Dizon, J. M. R., Grimmer-Somers, K., & Kumar, S. (2012). A pilot study of the evidence based practice training program for Filipino physiotherapists: Emerging evidence on outcomes and acceptability. *Internet Journal of Allied Health Sciences and Practice*, 10(2), 11.

Dizon, J. M. R., Grimmer-Somers, K., & Kumar, S. (2014b). Effectiveness of the tailored Evidence Based Practice training program for Filipino physical therapists: A randomized controlled trial. *BMC Medical Education*, 14(1), 147–147. doi:10.1186/1472-6920-14-147.

Dizon, J. M., Machingaidze, S., & Grimmer, K. (2016). To adopt, to adapt, or to contextualise? The big question in clinical practice guideline development. *BMC Research Notes*, 9(1), 442–442. doi:10.1186/s13104-016-2244-7.

Enriquez, A.L. (2019). Challenges of research ethics committees. *Philippine Journal of Allied Health Sciences*, 3(1). https://pjahs.ust.edu.ph/wp-content/uploads/2021/10/A4-Enriquez2019.pdf.

Gomez, I. N. B. (2019). The state of the journal. *Philippine Journal of Allied Health Sciences*, 3(1). https://pjahs.ust.edu.ph/wp-content/uploads/2021/10/A2-Gomez2019a.pdf.

Joshi, G. P., Benzon, H. T., Gan, T. J., & Vetter, T. R. (2019). Consistent definitions of clinical practice guidelines, consensus statements, position statements, and practice alerts. *Anesthesia and Analgesia*, 129(6), 1767–1770. 10.1213/ANE.0000000000004236.

PAOT. (2015). *The Philippine occupational therapy research agenda 2015*. https://paot.org.ph/pdf/research/Philippine%20Occupational%20Therapy%20Research%20Agenda%20(2015).pdf.

Rotor, E. R., & Gorgon, E. J. R. (2011). Teaching evidence-based practice: Preliminary outcomes of students' EBP-related attitudes and skills. *Philippine Journal of Occupational Therapy*, 4, 15–24.

Sackett, D. L., Rosenberg, W. M., Gray, J. M., Haynes, R. B., & Richardson, W. S. (1996). Evidence-based medicine: What it is and what it isn't. *BMJ*, 312(7023), 71–72.

Straus, S. E., Glasziou, P., Richardson, W. S., & Haynes, R. B. (2018). *Evidence-based medicine: How to practice and teach EBM*. Elsevier.

Sy, M. P., Yao, D. P., Panotes, A., Kaw, J., & Mendoza, T. (2021). Contemporary history: Progress and resilience of occupational therapy in the Philippines (2004–2020). *World Federation of Occupational Therapists Bulletin*, 79(1), 80–93.

Taylor, R. R. (2017). *Kielhofner's research in occupational therapy: Methods of inquiry for enhancing practice*. FA Davis.

Varpio, L., & MacLeod, A. (2020). Philosophy of science series: Harnessing the multidisciplinary edge effect by exploring paradigms, ontologies, epistemologies, axiologies, and methodologies. *Academic Medicine*, 95(5), 686–689. doi:10.1097/acm.0000000000003142.

WFOT. (2016). *Minimum Standards for the Education of Occupational Therapists 2016*. https://wfot.org/resources/new-minimum-standards-for-the-education-of-occupational-therapists-2016-e-copy.

WFOT, Mackenzie, L., Coppola, S., Alvarez, L., Cibule, L., Maltsev, S., Loh, S. Y., Mlambo, T., Ikiugu, M. N., Pihlar, Z., Sriphetcharawut, S., Baptiste, S., & Ledgerd, R. (2017). International occupational therapy research priorities: A Delphi study. *Occupational Therapy Journal of Research*, 37(2), 72–81. doi:10.1177/1539449216687528.

Chapter 13

Legislation affecting occupational therapy services and practice

Diana Jane Luib, Pauline Gail V. Martinez and Daryl Patrick Yao

Chapter objectives

1   Present international and national legislation and policies that shape occupational therapy services in the Philippines
2   Illuminate, through stories, advocacy in improving health and disability laws in the Philippines
3   Reflect on the influence of legislation and implementation on the practice of occupational therapy

Introduction

The practice of occupational therapy in the Philippines is guided by various legislative frameworks at international, national, and local levels. Understanding these laws and policies is essential for occupational therapists to facilitate optimal health, advocate for clients, and navigate the health sector. Additionally, comprehending laws that regulate the profession provides occupational therapists with a clearer professional identity. This chapter explores these legislations, shedding light on global perspectives that impact local practice and chronicling the national policies that govern occupational therapy in the Philippines. Moreover, it examines policies concerning key stakeholders and describes local initiatives promoting citizens' participation. Discussing these policies helps practitioners understand professional responsibilities and resources to effectively advocate for clients.

Global policies impacting occupational therapy services

To protect and promote human rights and improve the lives of people, the Philippines ratified[1] certain conventions, treaties, and frameworks. In this section, we examine international disability and health policies and standards.

DOI: 10.4324/9781003321217-13

The Convention on the Rights of Persons with Disabilities

The Philippines ratified the United Nations (UN) Convention on the Rights of Persons with Disabilities (CRPD) in April 2008 and is one of 186 countries that are parties to the treaty (UN, n.d.). Adopted in December 2006, the CRPD recognizes disabled persons as "subjects" with all human rights who can make decisions for their lives. This is a significant shift from viewing people with disabilities as "objects" of charity, medical intervention, and social protection (UN Department of Economic and Social Affairs [UN DESA], 2022). This Convention highlights the situation of individuals with disabilities, who have long been marginalized. While other human rights treaties, such as the Universal Declaration of Human Rights, arguably protect the rights of people with disabilities, they have not been entirely successful (Harpur, 2012). The provisions of the Universal Declaration of Human Rights are prone to interpretations that can exclude or undermine the rights of people with disabilities. The CRPD significantly reduces the potential for such exclusions and human rights violations (Harpur, 2012).

The CRPD aims to "promote, protect, and ensure the full and equal enjoyment of all human rights and fundamental freedoms by all persons with disabilities, and to promote respect for their inherent dignity" (UN General Assembly, 2006, Art. 1). It reaffirms the universal rights[2] of people with all types of disabilities in Articles 3–9 and introduces substantive rights[3] in Articles 10–30, ensuring that universal rights can be realized as intended (Harpur, 2012). The Convention protects people with disabilities from discrimination, guaranteeing access to health services, education, employment, and participation in other facets of culture and society.

The principles stated in the CRPD include "respect for the evolving capacities of children with disabilities and respect for the right of children with disabilities to preserve their identities" (GA, 2006, Art. 3). This is particularly important in the Philippines, where the practice of Occupational Therapy is primarily in the pediatric setting. Another is the obligation to promote the training of professionals and staff working with persons with disabilities to better provide the assistance and services guaranteed by those rights (UN General Assembly, 2006, Art. 4). Occupational therapy is part of the workforce that provides assistance to persons with disabilities, and the same convention strengthens the role of states in protecting the workforce.

The CRPD has a far-reaching influence on national and international policies. Most notably, it has informed the 17 Sustainable Development Goals (SDGs) of the UN's 2030 Agenda. The SDGs are a global call to end poverty, protect the environment and climate, and ensure peace and prosperity (UN Philippines, 2022). The 2030 Agenda also serves as a framework for achieving disability-inclusive development at local, national, or international levels (UN DESA, 2018). The SDGs explicitly reference people with disabilities in several indicators, including access to education, employment, transportation, public and green spaces, and data disaggregation by disability (UN DESA, 2018). While the 2030 Agenda relies on the international community to work collaboratively on the SDGs, accountability and review are mainly voluntary and country-led (UN General Assembly, 2015). Nevertheless, the SDGs demonstrate the global community's commitment to supporting developing countries in achieving these goals. The Philippines is obligated to align its policies with the rights stipulated by the CRPD.

Rehabilitation 2030 Initiative

The Rehabilitation 2030 Initiative of the World Health Organization (WHO, 2023) serves as a global call to action to improve access to rehabilitation services worldwide. Launched during the World Health Assembly in 2017, the initiative provides a non-legally-binding framework for strengthening rehabilitation services, including occupational therapy services, within the health system (Gimigliano & Negrini, 2017). Given global demographic trends, the increasing prevalence of non-communicable diseases, and the emergence of new infectious diseases, the Rehabilitation 2030 Initiative acknowledges the urgent need for rehabilitation to meet the broader goals of the SDGs (Seijas et al., 2023). As the Philippines is bound by the CRPD, endeavors toward this initiative also promote the health-related rights of people with disabilities. Awareness of the Rehabilitation 2030 Initiative can equip occupational therapy practitioners with a global perspective on rehabilitation, enabling advocacy for more streamlined services to improve outcomes for clients.

In many countries, rehabilitation is often under-prioritized and under-resourced (WHO, 2023). In the Philippines, rehabilitation services are frequently paid out of pocket due to insufficient financial coverage within the national health insurance system (Collantes et al., 2021). Moreover, access to and availability of rehabilitation services are inadequate, with facilities primarily located in major cities. Recognizing that this issue exists globally, the initiative identifies priority areas that member states should address. To address these areas, we need to strengthen advocacy efforts as well as invest and engage in research and innovation (Seijas et al., 2023).

National legislation: Policies, issues, impact, and developments

Exploring national legislation guides us in framing occupational therapy in the Philippines. National laws shape the identity and practice of occupational therapy professionals by fostering inclusivity and ensuring high standards of care. This section covers national disability and health policies affecting occupational therapy.

Disability policies

The key legislation protecting people with disabilities from discrimination is the Magna Carta for Persons with Disabilities (Republic Act [RA] 7277, 1992). Originally signed into law in 1992, RA 7277 acknowledges people with disabilities as beingpart of society, sharing the same rights as others. It aims to "give full support to the improvement of the total well-being of disabled persons and their integration into the mainstream of society" (RA 7277, Section 2a). This legislation covers rights and privileges related to employment, education, health, auxiliary social services, telecommunications, accessibility, and political and civil rights. It describes prohibition on discrimination in employment, transportation, and use of public accommodations and services.

The Magna Carta for Persons with Disabilities utilizes a hybrid view of disability. On one hand, it uses a medical view,[4] where it aims to "develop skills and potentials to enable them to compete for available opportunities" (RA 7277, Section 2a) and focuses on the rehabilitation of the disabled person (RA 7277, Section 2c). On the other hand, it reflects the social model of disability[5] and advocates for removing "all social, cultural, economic, environmental, and attitudinal barriers that are prejudicial to disabled persons" (RA 7277, Section 2e).

Equally crucial is the Accessibility Law (Batas Pambansa Bilang [BP] 344, 1983), which supplements RA 7277 by enhancing the mobility of persons with disabilities through required facilities in certain buildings, institutions, establishments, and public utilities. The Accessibility Law and Its Implementing Rules and Regulations set minimum requirements for accessibility and offer anthropometric measurements to guide design. An overview of infrastructure within its scope is provided in Table 13.1. Amendments to the accessibility law are currently being pushed in the House (House Bill 3448, 2022) and the Senate (Senate Bill 1700, 2023). Senate Bill 1700 proposes making information and communication technologies and services accessible to all persons with disabilities and creating *Access Audit Teams* [6] to monitor implementation.

The Magna Carta for Persons with Disabilities has been amended to clarify and expand the law in response to evolving needs. Key amendments are RA 9442, 10070, 10524, 10754, and 11228. RA 9442, signed into law in 2007, introduced Chapter 8 to Title 2, providing incentives and privileges to disabled Filipinos, including discounts on health, transportation, accommodations, and public services, as well as priority lanes and special discounts for basic commodities for those with a disability identification card. It also provides tax incentives to carers of disabled Filipinos and prohibits verbal and non-verbal discrimination and vilification against people with disabilities.

Table 13.1 Infrastructure within the scope of the Accessibility Law and Its Implementing Rules and Regulations

Infrastructure	Specific types
Residential buildings (government-owned only)	Duplex and single-detached houses School or company staff housing unit
Commercial and industrial buildings (government and private-owned)	Hotel, Inn, motel, pension houses Private or off-campus dormitories General wholesale and retail stores Shopping centers, supermarkets, public markets Restaurants, and dining and drinking establishments Office buildings Financial institutions Theaters, auditoriums, convention hall
Educational and industrial buildings	Schools, colleges, universities, vocational schools, seminaries Libraries, museums, exhibition halls, art galleries Hospitals, mental asylums, rehabilitation centers Jail, prison, reformatories, correctional institutions Homes for the aged, nursing homes, orphanages Police and fire stations Churches, temples, chapels, and similar places of worship
Public transportation	
Land transportation	City, provincial, and tourist buses; jeepneys Bus depots and terminals
Rail transportation	Railway systems in the country Train stations and terminals
Water transportation	Domestic passenger ships, ferry boats Ports and harbor facilities
Air transportation	Domestic passenger airplanes Airport terminal buildings, heliports

Box 13.1 Lack of Accessibility for Carlos

Carlos, a 25-year-old wheelchair user, aspires to pursue higher education. He has recently enrolled in a local university for a master's degree. Unfortunately, the campus lacks facilities for students with disabilities. The classrooms are inaccessible, with no ramps or elevators, making navigation difficult for Carlos.

RA 7277 emphasizes equal opportunities for persons with disabilities, including access to education. However, the university's failure to provide accessible infrastructure contradicts this legislation. Carlos faces exclusion as he struggles to attend classes and participate in academic activities.

Carlos also encounters difficulties commuting to the university. Public buses, jeepneys, and train stations lack ramps or lifts for boarding individuals with mobility disabilities. The lack of accessible transportation infringes on Carlos' right to move freely and independently.

Carlos' experience highlights the impact of the failure to implement key provisions from RA 7277 and BP 344. His educational aspirations are hindered by the systemic failure to create inclusive environments, impacting his ability to fully participate in society and realize his potential. This case underscores the need for proactive measures to ensure accessibility and equal opportunities as mandated by legislation.

RA 11228 mandates the automatic coverage of persons with disabilities in the National Health Insurance Program (NHIP)[7] of the Philippine Health Insurance Corporation (PhilHealth).

Subsequent amendments, enacted after the CRPD ratification, facilitated the establishment of a Persons with Disabilities Affairs Office (PDAO) in every city, municipality, and province or the appointment of a focal person for smaller municipalities (RA 10070, 2010). They also expanded employment opportunities within the government (RA 10524, 2013), increased privileges and incentives for disabled persons and their carers (RA 10754, 2016), and mandated health insurance coverage (RA 11228, 2019). Despite these laws, implementation remains problematic. Over 50% of local government units have no PDAO or focal person (Rocamora, 2021), limiting representation and monitoring of disability-related issues. Government employment opportunities are limited to those who pass the civil service examination, which only provides accommodations for visual, hearing, and mobility impairments (Civil Service Commission, 2019). Finally, the national health insurance has yet to cover rehabilitation services for many Filipinos with disabilities.

While several disability laws are presented in this subsection, this is not exhaustive. There are laws and policies specific to certain disability groups, such as intellectual and developmental disabilities, visual impairment, and hearing impairment.

Health policies

The Universal Health Care (UHC) Act (RA 11223, 2019) represents a monumental health policy reform in the Philippines. The UHC Act aims to grant every Filipino immediate eligibility and access to preventive, promotive, curative, rehabilitative, and palliative care for medical, dental, mental, and emergency health services, regardless of economic status.

The UHC Act mandates PhilHealth coverage for all Filipinos, protecting them against high medical costs. PhilHealth, the primary government health insurance agency, ensures equitable healthcare. The UHC Act commits to expanding PhilHealth benefit packages, encompassing a broad array of services from preventive and promotive care to diagnostics, curative, and rehabilitative services. This expansion seeks to address holistic health needs and reinforce primary care services, particularly at the community level. The Act emphasizes developing and deploying a competent health workforce, recognizing the integral role of healthcare professionals, as well as enhancing health facilities, thereby improving infrastructure to support health services. Section 37 of the UHC Act includes penal provisions,[8] applicable to occupational therapy practitioners, stating that healthcare providers engaging in unethical[9] or fraudulent[10] acts are punishable by a fine and/or suspension of contract for up to three (3) months.

The Mental Health Act of 2017 (RA 11036, 2018) is also relevant to the practice of occupational therapy. Occupational therapy practitioners working in mental health are regarded as *mental health service providers* in the Philippines. This Act enumerates the rights of mental health service providers, such as working in a safe and supportive work environment, continuing professional development, and managing and controlling all aspects of their practice, including the choice to accept or decline a service user for treatment, except in emergencies. Additionally, mental health service providers have the right to participate in the planning, development, and management of mental health services, contribute to the development and review of standards for evaluating mental health services, participate in the development of mental health policy and service delivery guidelines, and advocate for the rights of a service user when their wishes are at odds with those of their family or legal representatives. Occupational therapy practitioners possess the right to control all aspects of their practice and decline a service user for treatment. The Act also emphasizes informed consent. Service users must provide informed consent in writing prior to the implementation of any plan or program of therapy or treatment, including physical or chemical restraint.

In addition to these laws, the occupational therapy profession is subject to numerous rules and services from national and local agencies. The Department of Health (DOH) and other agencies such as PhilHealth, the Department of Social Welfare and Development (DSWD), the Department of Labor and Employment (DOLE), and local government ordinances mandate the inclusion of occupational therapy services in national and local health policies, integrating occupational therapy in health service delivery. The DOH, as the main authority on health, plays three major roles: 1) leadership in health; 2) enabler and capacity builder; and 3) administrator of specified services (DOH, n.d.). It published the National Objectives of Health 2017–2022, which declared its target to realize SDG 3, ensuring good health and well-being for all. A highlight of the expanded benefits is the extension of coverage through PhilHealth's Z benefit packages, which provides additional support for persons with disabilities requiring prolonged care and interventions (PhilHealth, 2012). These Z benefits cover occupational therapy and other rehabilitation services for persons who need Mobility, Orthosis, Rehabilitation, Prosthesis Help (Z MORPH), children with mobility impairment, and children with developmental disability (PhilHealth, 2013, 2017a, 2017b).

DSWD is the main government authority that develops and advocates for social welfare policies, standards, and programs, collaborating with partners and stakeholders to improve the quality of life of Filipinos (DSWD, n.d.). In its Administrative Order No. 9 series of 2010, DSWD mandated the inclusion of occupational therapy practitioners in DSWD centers and residential care facilities (DSWD, 2010). DSWD, in partnership with non-government organizations (NGOs), created avenues to deliver occupational therapy services for older people and children's care in Tagum City, Davao Del Norte (DSWD, 2010) as well as catering to children with disabilities in Alaminos, Pangasinan (Alaminos City Government, n.d.) and Cebu City (DSWD Region VII, 2016).

DOLE is the government authority that supports occupational therapy services for workers with work-related illnesses, injuries, or disabilities. The Employees' Compensation Program under DOLE provides financial assistance for rehabilitation services a worker may need (Employees' Compensation Commission, n.d.). Any claims must go through the Social Security System (SSS) or Government Service Insurance System (GSIS). Occupational therapy practitioners should direct clients to this benefit whenever applicable.

Local ordinances have also paved the way to access free occupational therapy services through community-based rehabilitation programs. For instance, the Mandaluyong City Government approved Ordinance No. 405 series of 2018, formalizing support for the project Therapy, Education and Assimilation of Children with Handicap (TEACH). This project focuses on delivering services to children with disabilities in collaboration with the PDAO and the DSWD (Mandaluyong City Government, 2008). Similarly, in Quezon City, City Ordinance No. SP-2617 series of 2017, amended by City Ordinance No. SP-2718 series of 2018, led to the establishment of the QC Kabahagi Center, which offers subsidized assessments, telecoaching, an inclusive arts program, a livelihood program for families of children with disabilities, and free group training/seminars for other concerned stakeholders (Quezon City Government, n.d.).

Occupational therapy–relevant laws

The rights and obligations of occupational therapy professionals and the law governing the relationships between occupational therapists and clients are written in the Philippine Occupational Therapy Law of 2018, RA 11241. This law regulates the registration, licensure examination, and practice of occupational therapy. It has been instrumental in shaping the profession's identity by separating it from physical therapy.

Prior to the Philippine Occupational Therapy Law, occupational therapy was regulated by RA 5680, known as the Philippine Physical and Occupational Therapy Law, since June 21, 1969. This old law created a Board of Physical and Occupational Therapy under the Professional Regulation Commission (PRC), regulating the registration of practitioners in both professions. While mainly a regulatory act, Section 27 in RA 5680 imposed criminal liability for the illegal practice of occupational or physical therapy. RA 11241 repealed RA 5680.

The Philippine Occupational Therapy Law includes provisions on the creation of the Professional Regulatory Board (PRB) of Occupational Therapy, licensure, examination, and registration, as well as the practice of occupational therapy. Article IV, which focuses on practice, prescribes the prohibition on illegal practice of Occupational Therapy, prohibited acts, Code of Ethics and Standards of Practice, Continuing Professional Development (CPD) Program, the integration of occupational therapists in one national organization, and Foreign Reciprocity. This law further defines prohibited acts as engaging in practice or representing oneself as an occupational therapist without a valid registration, professional license, or permit, allowing another to use one's certificate, using another's credentials, and violating the Code of Ethics (RA 11241, Article IV, Section 27). Violators face fines, imprisonment of two to five years, or both.

Decades in the making, the passing of the Philippine Occupational Therapy Law helped inform the public and distinguish occupational therapy from physical therapy. This distinction was crucial as occupational therapy had long been confused with physical therapy. In 2012, a significant incident occurred on national television, when a host erroneously defined occupational therapy as "one for the body and not for the brain," a statement the station later retracted and apologized for. Achieving recognition as an autonomous health profession was no easy feat. In the following case, you will learn about how the Occupational Therapy law came to be and the advocacy efforts that shaped its passage.

Box 13.2 Advocating for the Philippine Occupational Therapy Law: A brief history

On June 21, 1969, the bill drafted by Congressman Jose Aldeguer of Iloilo was passed into law, Republic Act No. 5680 or the Philippine Physical and Occupational Therapy Law. To gain better recognition of occupational therapy as a health profession and provide greater autonomy in the practice of occupational therapy, practitioners and the national organization of occupational therapy, the Philippine Academy of Occupational Therapists (formerly the Occupational Therapy Association of the Philippines), actively pushed for a revision to the legislation as early as 2004.

The amendment primarily entails a separation of the regulatory law for Occupational Therapy from Physical Therapy. The bill was first submitted on first reading in the House of Representatives in the 14th Congress and reached only the committee level and remained pending. It was refiled in the 15th Congress and still it did not reach plenary reading of the bill. In the 17th congress, the bill was co-authored by 26 congressmen and passed three readings, which meant the bill had been approved by the majority of the law makers after being read in three different sessions. The passing of the present law was lobbied by more than 30 occupational therapists and around 50 occupational therapy students for the year 2018–2019. The advocates planned the lobbying of the Occupational Therapy Bill for seven months through campaigns, actively attending congressional hearings and informing the public about Occupational Therapy. In 2018, occupational therapists and students went to each office of the 230 members of the House of Representatives to introduce the bill to the law makers and gain support. Similarly in the Senate, occupational therapists attended hearings, invited other stakeholders in the committee meeting and communicated in person with each of the 23 senators at that time. The bill was passed originally in the Senate and authored by Senator Antonio Trillianes through Senate Bill 454 on January 29, 2018. The bill was signed into law on March 11, 2019.

Under the Philippine Occupational Therapy Law, all practitioners must abide by CPD requirements, rules, and regulations set by the PRB of Occupational Therapy, in coordination with the professional organization and accredited educational institutions. CPD programs aim to improve professionals' competence and contribute to the general welfare, economic growth, and development of the nation. Occupational therapists must submit proof of CPD before renewing their professional identification card. CPD is described in more detail in Chapter 5.

The Philippine Occupational Therapy Law also outlines grounds for reprimand, suspension, or revocation of license to practice occupational therapy. Although specific penalties for violations were not detailed, individuals can be fined, imprisoned, or both. The law grants the PRB of Occupational Therapy the power to prevent anyone found guilty of immoral or dishonorable conduct or declared to be of "unsound mind" from obtaining a professional license. These provisions serve as bases for administrative cases filed in the PRC and do not preclude criminal complaints. While cases of medical negligence in occupational therapy practice are rare, the possibility of injuring a client underscores the importance of avoiding gross negligence in practice.

Gross or inexcusable negligence, defined under Article 365 of the Revised Penal Code, forms the basis for medical negligence against physicians. Though there are no documented cases of death or serious injury in occupational therapy, caregiver concerns about handling of children as clients, as exemplified in a 2012 television program, highlight the need to assess occupational therapists' potential liability under the said law, which may be classified as simple imprudence[11] rather than recklessness.[12]

Another critical consideration is the Child Abuse Law (RA 7610, 1992), which defines any act by deeds or words that debases, degrades, or demeans a child's intrinsic worth and dignity as child abuse. Given occupational therapy's prominent role in pediatric settings in the Philippines, this law is often used as the basis in cases where behavior management strategies are questioned. Presently, there is no jurisprudence[13] involving occupational therapists under RA 7610 in the Supreme Court of the Philippines.

Box 13.3 Behavioral intervention complaint

On March 27, 2012, a Philippine television (TV) show hosted by a public official aired a complaint about an occupational therapist's intervention for a client with attention deficit hyperactivity disorder (ADHD). The host called out occupational therapists and publicly criticized the intervention.

The technique involved a sensory integration strategy, involving wrapping the client in a heavy blanket. The Occupational Therapy Association of the Philippines submitted a formal complaint to the TV network for criticizing occupational therapy without seeking appropriate information on the intervention and the clinical reasoning behind it. On April 4, 2012, the network released a public apology, stating they did not intend to criticize "Physical and Occupational Therapy" and admitting the host's lack of information on managing clients with ADHD. The network committed to proper recourse for the program (Philippine Academy of Occupational Therapists, 2012).

The Data Privacy Act of 2012 (RA 10173, 2012) may subject occupational therapists to criminal liability concerning the storing and processing of personal health information. The Act significantly impacts occupational therapists since health information is routinely collected and used in practice settings. The law allows processing of sensitive personal information necessary for treatment, provided that adequate protection of personal information is ensured. Any other use of health information requires clients' consent. Practitioners must collect, use, and store clients' health information in a confidential manner and implement safeguards to protect it. Violating the Act are criminal acts, with corresponding penalties.

Chapter summary

This chapter provides an overview of the legal and regulatory landscape governing occupational therapy practice in the Philippines, emphasizing the role of legislation in safeguarding the rights and well-being of persons with disabilities and shaping the profession. It highlights the importance of policies as catalysts for change and the invaluable role of occupational therapists in advocacy. Besides equipping readers with knowledge of key policies, it underscores advocacy practices and the efforts of practitioners and students in claiming their professional identity. We hope the efforts illustrated serve as a model for future advocacy, promoting the profession and supporting persons with disabilities in the Philippines. We invite readers to examine the key legislation presented and reflect on these policies, their professional responsibilities, resources, and the transformative potential of policy engagement.

Reflective questions

1   What are the current implications or shortcomings of the Magna Carta for Persons with Disabilities and the Accessibility Law?
2   What amendments to the Accessibility Law would you propose to make the environment more inclusive for people with diverse disabilities?
3   How can occupational therapists advocate for the creation of inclusive environments in educational institutions and workplaces?
4   Data privacy regulations may prevent occupational therapists from sharing clients' personal information. However, what should occupational therapists do if they suspect that their clients are victims of abuse?
5   What strategies can occupational therapists employ to ensure compliance with data privacy regulations while effectively communicating with clients' caregivers or family members?
6   Should occupational therapists feature their clients on social media? If so, how should they go about this while protecting themselves from potential lawsuits?

7 Occupational therapists may need to physically manipulate their clients' bodies. How can they protect themselves from potential charges of sexual harassment?

Notes

1 To ratify means to make the law part of the national law by an act of the president, subject the same to the concurrence or consent of the Senate and House of Representatives, thereby incurring legal obligations at international law. A country that ratifies a treaty is a party to the treaty and is obliged to perform its obligations in good faith.
2 Universal rights are inherent rights to all humans.
3 Substantive rights are human rights possessed by people in a society.
4 The medical model of disability views disability as a physical or mental condition that deviates from standard body functioning.
5 The social model of disability views disability as a result of environmental and societal barriers that limit full participation and inclusion.
6 An Access Audit Team includes representatives from the Department of Transportation, Department of Information and Communications Technology, and persons with disabilities to participate in the assessment of accessibility of facilities.
7 The National Health Insurance Act of 2013 (RA 10606, 2013) mandates NHIP coverage for all citizens of the Philippines.
8 Penal provisions are punishment incurred by an individual for violating the law.
9 Unethical act refers to any actions, intentional or unintentional, that are against social and professional norms.
10 Fraudulent act refers to any act of misrepresentation or deception resulting in undue benefit or advantage on the part of the doer.
11 Simple imprudence is the lack of precaution displayed in cases in which the damage impending to be caused is not immediate or not clearly manifesting.
12 Reckless imprudence is a voluntary, but without malice, doing or failing to do an act from which damage results because of an inexcusable lack of precaution on the part of the person performing or failing to perform such act.
13 Jurisprudence are decisions made by the Supreme Court regarding the issues raised to the court and resolves questions of law or issues in its application

References

Accessible Environment for All Persons with Disabilities Act, Senate Bill No. 1700. (January 18, 2023). (Phil.).
Act to Enhance the Mobility of Disabled Persons by Requiring Certain Buildings, Institutions, Establishments and Public Utilities to install Facilities and Other Devices, B.P. Blg 344. (February 25, 1983). (Phil.).
Act to Enhance the Mobility of Disabled Persons by Requiring Certain Buildings, Institutions, Establishments and Public Utilities to Install Facilities and Other Devices – IRR of BP 344. (Phil.). https://www.dpwh.gov.ph/dpwh/references/laws_codes_orders/bpb344.
Act Expanding the Benefits and Privileges of Persons with Disability (PWD), Rep. Act No. 10754. (March 23, 2016). (Phil.).

Act Expanding the Positions Reserved for Persons with Disability, Amending for the Purpose Republic Act No. 7277, as Amended, Otherwise Known as the Magna Carta for Persons with Disability, Rep. Act No. 10524. (April 23, 2013). (Phil.).

Act Providing for the Mandatory PhilHealth Coverage for All Persons with Disability (PWDs), Amending for the Purpose Republic Act No. 7277, as Amended, Otherwise Known as the "Magna Carta for Persons with Disability," Rep. Act No. 11228. (February 22, 2019). (Phil.).

Act Providing for Stronger Deterrence and Special Protection against Child Abuse, Exploitation and Discrimination, and for Other Purposes. Rep. Act No. 7610. (June 17, 1992). (Phil.).

Alaminos City Government. (n.d.). Social services. http://www.alaminoscity.gov. ph/public-service/programs-and-projects/social-services/.

Civil Service Commission. (2019, July 24). CSC reminds gov't agencies: Provide PWD lane. Civil Service Commission. https://www.csc.gov.ph/csc-rem inds-gov-t-agencies-provide-pwd-lane.

Collantes, M. E. V., Zuniga, Y. H., Granada, C. N., Uezono, D. R., De Castillo, L. C., Enriquez, C. G., Ignacio, K. D., Ignacio, S. D., & Jamora, R. D. (2021). Current state of stroke care in the Philippines. *Frontiers in Neurology*, 12, 665086. doi:10.3389/fneur.2021.665086.

Continuing Professional Development Act of 2016, Rep. Act No. 10912. (July 21, 2016). (Phil.).

Data Privacy Act of 2012, Rep. Act No. 10173. (August 15, 2012). (Phil.).

DOH. (n.d.). DOH profile. https://www.doh.gov.ph/profile.

DOH. (2018). National objectives for health Philippines 2017–2022. https://doh.gov. ph/sites/default/files/health_magazine/NOH-2017-2022-030619-1%281%29_0.pdf.

DSWD. (n.d.). About us. https://www.dswd.gov.ph/about-us-main/.

DSWD. (2010). Administrative order no. 09 series of 2010. https://www.dswd.gov. ph/issuances/AOs/AO_2010-009.pdf.

DSWD Region VII. (2016, August 6). Physical & occupational therapy session to our special children in Reception and Study Center for Children (RSCC) [Tweet]. https://mobile.twitter.com/dswdfo7/status/765854989461786624.

Employees' Compensation Commission. (n.d.). Frequently Asked Questions. Department of Labor and Employment. https://ecc.gov.ph/frequently-asked-ques tions/.

Establishing Institutional Mechanism to Ensure the Implementation of Programs and Services for Persons with Disabilities in Every Province, City and Municipality, Amending Republic Act No. 7277, Otherwise Known as the Magna Carta for Disabled Persons, as Amended, and for Other Purposes, Rep. Act No. 10070. (April 6, 2010). (Phil.).

Gimigliano, F., & Negrini, S. (2017). The World Health Organization "Rehabilitation 2030—A call for action." *European Journal of Physical and Rehabilitation Medicine*, 53(2), 155–168. doi:10.23736/S1973-9087.17.04746-3.

Harpur, P. (2012). Embracing the new disability rights paradigm: The importance of the Convention on the Rights of Persons with Disabilities. *Disability & Society*, 27(1), 1–14. doi:10.1080/09687599.2012.631794.

Magna Carta for Disabled Persons, Rep. Act No. 7277. (March 24, 1992). (Phil.).

Mandaluyong City Government. (2008). An ordinance creating a "Mandaluyong City Children's Code". Ordinance No. 405, S-2008. https://www.mandaluyong.

gov.ph/updates/downloads/files/ORD%20NO.%20405,%20S-2008%20%20CHIL
DREN'S%20CODE.pdf.

Mental Health Act, Rep. Act No. 11036. (June 20, 2018). (Phil.).

National Health Insurance Act of 2013, Rep. Act No. 10606. (June 19, 2013).
(Phil.).

PhilHealth. (2012, July 3). Philhealth's Z benefits for catastrophic illnesses launched. https://www.philhealth.gov.ph/news/2012/z_benefits.html.

PhilHealth. (2013). PhilHealth Circular No. 0019 series of 2013. https://www.phil
health.gov.ph/circulars/2013/circ19_2013.pdf.

PhilHealth. (2017a). PhilHealth Circular No. 2017-0029. https://www.philhealth.
gov.ph/circulars/2017/circ2017-0029.pdf.

PhilHealth. (2017b). PhilHealth Circular No. 2017-0031. https://www.philhealth.
gov.ph/circulars/2017/circ2017-0031.pdf.

Philippine Academy of Occupational Therapists. (2012, April 4). Response from
TV5 (aired on Balitaang Tapat, April 4, 2012): "Nililinaw ng aming organisas-
yon na hindi intensyon ng news 4 ..." [Status Update]. *Facebook.* https://www.fa
cebook.com/PAOTInc/posts/response-from-tv5-aired-on-balitaang-tapat-ap
ril-4-2012-nililinaw-ng-aming-organ/335410549852108/.

Philippine Occupational Therapy Law of 2018, Rep. Act No. 11241. (March 11,
2019). (Phil).

Public Rail Transit System Safety and Accessibility Act of 2022, House Bill No.
3448. (August 10, 2022). (Phil.).

Quezon City Government. (n.d.). QC center for children with disabilities (Kabahagi).   https://quezoncity.gov.ph/departments/qc-center-for-children-with-disabili
ties-kabahagi/.

Rocamora, J. A. L. (2021, December 8). Over 50% of LGUs in PH have no PWD
office: NCDA. *Philippine News Agency.* https://www.pna.gov.ph/articles/1162167.

Rules and Regulations Implementing Republic Act No. 9442, an Act Amending
Republic Act No. 7277, Otherwise Known as the Magna Carta for Disabled
Persons, and for Other Purposes Granting Additional Privileges and Incentives
and Prohibitions on Verbal, Non-verbal Ridicule and Vilification Against Persons with Disability, Rep. Act No. 9442. (April 30, 2007). (Phil.).

Seijas, V., Kiekens, C., & Gimigliano, F. (2023). Advancing the World Health
Assembly's landmark resolution on strengthening rehabilitation in health sys-
tems: Unlocking the future of rehabilitation. *European Journal of Physical and
Rehabilitation Medicine,* 59(4), 447–451. doi:10.23736/S1973-9087.23.08160-1.

UN. (n.d.). Convention on the Rights of Persons with Disabilities. *Treaty Series,
2515, 3.*   https://treaties.un.org/Pages/ViewDetails.aspx?src=TREATY&mtdsg_
no=iv-15&chapter=4&clang=_en.

UN DESA. (2018). Disability and development report: Realizing the Sustainable
Development Goals by, for and with persons with disabilities. https://social.un.
org/publications/UN-Flagship-Report-Disability-Final.pdf.

UN DESA. (2022). Convention on the Rights of Persons with Disabilities (CRPD).
https://www.un.org/development/desa/disabilities/convention-on-the-rights-of-pers
ons-with-disabilities.html.

UN General Assembly. (2006). Convention on the Rights of Persons with Disabilities.
https://www.un.org/development/desa/disabilities/convention-on-the-rights-of-pers
ons-with-disabilities.html.

UN General Assembly. (2015). Transforming our world: The 2030 agenda for sustainable development. https://www.unfpa.org/sites/default/files/resource-pdf/Resolution_A_RES_70_1_EN.pdf.

Universal Health Care Act, Rep. Act No. 11223. (February 20, 2019). (Phil.).

UN Philippines. (2022). Our work on the Sustainable Development Goals in Philippines. https://philippines.un.org/en/sdgs.

WHO. (2023). Rehabilitation 2030 Initiative. https://www.who.int/initiatives/rehabilitation-2030.

Chapter 14

Ethical issues in occupational therapy practice

Kim Gerald G. Medallon and Caroline Fischl

Chapter objectives

1 Describe ethical principles and obligations relevant to occupational therapy practice in the Philippines
2 Reflect on ethical issues encountered in Philippine professional practice
3 Apply ethical principles in resolving dilemmas encountered in Philippine contexts

Introduction

Occupational therapy (OT) practice involves a thorough consideration of the transaction of the person, the environment, and occupation (Fisher & Marterella, 2019; Townsend & Polatajko, 2007). The dynamic interplay of these components creates unique contexts and situations where tensions may arise. These tensions place OT professionals in challenging positions due to conflicting allegiances to personal values, clients, colleagues, employers, and regulatory agencies (Durocher & Kinsella, 2021). Despite these challenges, OT professionals must promote equity and fairness while facilitating engagement in meaningful occupations for individuals, groups, and communities (Durocher et al., 2014; Nilsson & Townsend, 2010).

These tensions, known as ethical dilemmas, offer multiple courses of action, making it challenging to find a solution that benefits all parties (Kornblau & Burkhardt, 2012). OT professionals' backgrounds, core values, motivations, and accumulated experiences influence the way they perceive and act in a situation. A holistic resolution process is ensured when sociocultural and emotional considerations are guided by ethical and legal principles (Bailey & Schwartzberg, 1994). Table 14.1 presents these principles.

In addition, various theories can provide OT professionals a basis for decision-making (Kornblau & Burkhardt, 2012). These theories, which include *consequentialism, deontology, virtue ethics, rights-based ethics*, and *ethics of care*, are grounded in various moral beliefs and are interwoven

DOI: 10.4324/9781003321217-14

Table 14.1 Ethical and legal principles informing OT practice

Principle	*Definition*
Beneficence	To do good or provide benefit
Non-maleficence	To avoid inflicting harm and prevent situations that inflict harm or suffering on others
Respect for autonomy	To show regard for individuals' right to self-determination and the ability to decide for oneself
Integrity	To respect others' privacy (confidentiality), to keep promises and duties (fidelity), to tell the truth (veracity)
Justice	To treat all fairly
Utility	To maximize the good and attain the greatest benefit

with ethical and legal principles. *Consequentialism* focuses on the outcomes of an action, deeming a choice most ethical if it leads to the best outcome. The principle of utility, which seeks to maximize benefit for the most people, exemplifies consequentialism. *Deontology* places importance on the action performed and its adherence to established codes. In this theory, ethical actions highlight doing no harm (non-maleficence) and performing one's duty (fidelity). *Virtue ethics* stresses possessing acceptable traits like honesty and practical wisdom to follow through on one's intention. *Rights-based ethics* emphasizes that the most ethical actions involve upholding individual human rights. Lastly, *ethics of care* puts weight on interpersonal relationships and care in making decisions, promoting compassion and empathy (Scott & Reitz, 2015).

One's moral principles are shaped by comprehensive and collective views of the world. Acknowledging Filipino cultural nuances and traditions in decision-making can ensure a successful resolution of ethical dilemmas in Philippine contexts. Virtues such as *kagandahang loob, utang na loob, pakikiramdam, hiya*, and *lakas ng loob/bahala na* focus on preserving and strengthening human relationships (Reyes, 2015), in contrast to the individualistic perspective in Western traditions. Filipino OT professionals should recognize these cultural differences in decision-making (Lasquety-Reyes & Alvarez, 2015).

OT professionals must acknowledge that one ethical principle can counter another principle. For example, beneficence stresses providing good to others, but what is considered "good" can always be disputed (Williams, 1993). Doing "good" for one person (beneficence) may be harmful to another person (non-maleficence) or disadvantageous for a community or society at large (justice and utility). We may ask ourselves, *would it be ethical to use resources to manage a few when they could be used to provide OT interventions benefiting more people?* Such a dilemma prompts us to weigh our alternatives and probe our values system. Doing "good" could also threaten one's autonomy and integrity, such as providing OT intervention that a person has refused or disclosing details of OT intervention to a close family member without the client's consent. In these scenarios, OT professionals must carefully analyze behaviors, eventual outcomes, and intents of all involved parties.

After being introduced to various ethical underpinnings, it would be important to ponder on some critical questions emerging from these principles and theories, such as:

- How could a consequentialist perspective support decision-making when it is not always possible to foresee the outcome?
- In relation to deontology, can an act adhering to an established code be considered ethical if it results in a negative outcome?
- Are virtues culturally bound?
- Would focusing on the rights of an individual be beneficial for the care of people, and vice versa?
- In relation to the concept of *pakikisama* and *utang na loob*, would a collectivist approach to ethical dilemma resolution always take precedence among all alternatives in the Filipino context?

As OT professionals find themselves in unique contexts and situations, their responses can differ. Knowledge of these theories and principles supports professional reasoning and enhances reflective practice, contributing to a high standard of practice. With these issues and questions in mind, the OT professional should be guided by a Code of Ethics that embodies the philosophical base of the profession and reflects the current practice contexts.

Code of Ethics

Each OT professional organization should have its own Code of Ethics that incorporates societal needs, legal obligations, and cultural contexts to ensure high standards in the discharge of professional duties (Council of Occupational Therapists for the European Countries [COTEC], 2009). The Philippine Academy of Occupational Therapists (PAOT), the national association for OT professionals and students, adopted the American Occupational Therapy Association Code of Ethics with minor revisions (PAOT, 1998). This Code contains principles applicable to all components of the OT process and all the possible roles of OT professionals, which will be discussed in the succeeding paragraphs.

If a Code of Ethics should incorporate current societal needs, legal obligations, and culture, how often should it be updated?

OT professionals should ensure the well-being of service recipients, adhering to the principle of *beneficence* (PAOT, 1998). Services should be provided equitably, and compromising relationships or fraudulent activities should not be tolerated. Regardless of the setting or service delivery mode, OT professionals should anticipate potential risks to clients. Cultural factors can pose challenges to upholding beneficence. For instance, Filipino folk medicinal practices, perceived as effective in alleviating health concerns (Rondilla et al., 2021), may cause distrust in the healthcare system, including OT. OT professionals should strive to provide safe and evidence-based interventions while acknowledging the benefits of complementary and alternative services.

The client's *autonomy, privacy,* and *confidentiality* must be respected (PAOT, 1998). This is made possible by informing clients about the intervention process and treatment options and including them in the decision-making. In the Philippines, healthcare decisions are influenced by clients' family members who act as caregivers, patient advocates, and primary decision-makers (Genilo, 2021). OT professionals should navigate the Filipino family dynamics in communicating and making decisions with the client while respecting the individual's autonomy and privacy. The respect for autonomy, privacy, and confidentiality also applies to students in education and research participants.

Adhering to the principles of veracity and fidelity ensures the communication of accurate and appropriate information about one's own and others' services. The OT process with a client should be documented completely, correctly, and accurately. To treat others with fairness, discretion, and integrity, OT professionals should avoid engaging in any communication that is false or unjust. OT professionals should accurately represent their own and their colleagues' qualifications and contributions (PAOT, 1998).

OT professionals should commit to lifelong enhancement of competence to benefit the profession and its stakeholders. Principles related to *duty* include adhering to standards of practice, ensuring that services match one's qualifications, and channeling clients to appropriate professional services (PAOT, 1998). OT professionals must complete 15 units of continuing education every three years as a requirement to renew their professional license (Professional Regulation Commission [PRC], 2019). Beyond mere compliance with regulations, OT professionals should select continuing professional development (CPD) activities that maximize their strengths and benefit their clients.

OT professionals must comply with professional guidelines, institutional rules, and national laws, aligning with the principles of *justice*. This prompts prudent implementation of professional tasks within safe and secure contexts. In this way, clients can expect service delivery that meets professional standards.

According to the 2018 Revised Enforcement Procedures of the Occupational Therapy Code of Ethics (PAOT, 2018), the PAOT Committee on Standards and Ethics should investigate complaints of alleged violations of the OT Code of Ethics that may cause harm to the general public. Complainants should identify whether the violations were committed by a professional and/or by an institution and provide comprehensive details. Complaints may be dismissed if filed beyond the prescriptive period or if violations do not involve public risk. Disciplinary actions include probation, suspension, revocation, or denial of PAOT membership. The revised procedures focus on transforming erring members through educative letters and transformative plans, emphasizing continuous regulation and monitoring. Procedures may also involve reporting to the Professional Regulatory Board for Occupational Therapy under the PRC.

The next sections will describe the ethical obligations that OT professionals are to extend to clients, the profession, education, research, and society. Common ethical dilemmas perceived by OT professionals in these various contexts, as well as guides for reflection, are also presented.

Ethical obligations to clients

Intertwined with adherence to the Code of Ethics is the obligation to comply with professional standards. The OT Standards of Practice (PAOT, 1998) apply to all OT practice areas, settings, and services provided to an individual, group, or population. These standards ensure appropriate care for all recipients of OT services. OT practitioners must possess a current professional license and engage in CPD activities to maintain good professional standing.

Referral practices should include educating referral sources about the domain of concern of the profession, as well as collaborating with other professionals if their services are warranted. The OT process—encompassing *screening, assessment, intervention planning, intervention, transition services*, and *service discontinuation*—requires careful consideration of each client's unique context and thorough selection and implementation of procedures. Accurate and collaborative documentation of the OT process should be performed. OT practitioners should also evaluate the effectiveness of interventions and implement processes to promote continuous quality improvement. Additionally, OT professionals should engage in reflective practice while complying with these standards of practice. Reflective practice is described in Chapter 5.

At the start of the COVID-19 pandemic, service delivery options were explored to ensure that clients continuously received OT services in a safe and ethical manner. The PAOT released guidelines on the use of telehealth as an alternative form of service provision (See Chapter 9) and stressed maintaining the same standards of care for clients (PAOT, 2020a). The document also emphasized ethical considerations in identifying clients who may benefit from telehealth, checking the preparedness of stakeholders, and performing a thorough process for acquiring informed consent. Limitations in analyzing client conditions, ensuring security and privacy, and managing life-threatening situations when using telehealth must be considered (Cordero, 2023). Filipino OT professionals continue to offer telehealth services, adhering to these guidelines.

The return to in-person sessions necessitated strict adherence to safety measures for the welfare of all stakeholders. The PAOT released guidelines calling OT professionals to follow safety management protocols and reflect on the type of service delivery to be offered to clients depending on various factors such as outcomes, immediate necessity, and the presence of established institutional protocols (PAOT, 2020b). Table 14.2 contains a case study following the ethical decision-making process of clinic owners on the provision of OT services amidst the pandemic guided by the Prism Model of Ethical Decision-Making (VanderKaay et al., 2020).

Ethical obligations to the OT profession and other professionals

OT professionals should treat other professionals with fairness, discretion, and integrity, following the principles of fidelity and veracity. Despite inevitable differences in personal values and education leading to conflicting perspectives, the Code of Ethics (PAOT, 1998) calls its members to:

- Safeguard confidential information about colleagues and staff
- Accurately represent their qualifications, views, and contributions and that of their colleagues
- Refrain from using or participating in the use of any form of communication that contains false, fraudulent, deceptive, or unfair statements or claims

According to the PAOT Advisory on Continuing Education (PAOT, 2021), OT professionals are urged to engage in continuing education as part of their commitment to advance the profession and benefit stakeholders. It is advised that professionals should be prudent in examining the merits of these programs. The OT professional must also reflect one's motivations and overall capacity to implement the concepts gained from these programs to clients. Furthermore, OT professionals serving as resource persons should ensure that the publicly disseminated specifications of these programs are reflective and congruent to their qualifications and overall experience. OT professionals may further reflect on the following questions:

- Am I engaging in this endeavor out of mere compliance or for the greater benefit of my current and potential clients? (beneficence)
- In my current work setting, is there a prevalent need for this particular strategy or novel technique? (utility)
- As a resource person, do I have sufficient credentials to harness the skills and knowledge of others? Do I have the skill to clearly and accurately articulate to others the information I want to convey? (integrity and veracity)

Ethical obligations in education and to students

OT students should receive an education emphasizing professional behaviors and client-centered, values-based practice (Lecours et al., 2021; Silva et al., 2019; Hordichuk et al., 2015). OT educators should address pragmatic and ethical concerns affecting service delivery through teaching-learning activities and assessments aligned to professional practice using case studies, modeling, experiential techniques, and values clarification process. While direct instruction alone may not strongly influence professional behaviors, it complements core values, family upbringing, and religious beliefs (Medallon, 2023). To reinforce ethical behaviors, OT educators should present ethical dilemmas for discussion to clarify beliefs, values, and decision-making rationales.

OT educators should maximize clinical and community-based training during fieldwork. Practice with actual clients provides authentic learning opportunities for OT students to demonstrate competencies in professional reasoning, assessment, interventions, and case/project management while reconciling conflicting interests among stakeholders. This is achievable through partnerships between higher education institutions and affiliate institutions with OT practitioners. Risks to this partnership include the lack or high turnover of OT professionals and lack of interest, competence, or resources for student supervision. These risks can hinder the continuity and quality of OT educational programs. Therefore, both OT educators and practitioners must collaborate to equip students with the necessary knowledge and skills, emphasizing ethical principles and professional behaviors, to ensure the profession's sustainability in the Philippines.

Asymmetric power relations often characterize teacher-student relationships due to the expertise and degree of control possessed by the teacher. Such inequality of power can contribute to situations wherein abuses or injustices can occur. OT educators and clinical supervisors, therefore, have the ethical obligation to equalize this power imbalance by protecting students from harm and supporting students' autonomy and privacy. OT educators may further reflect on the following questions:

- Am I accommodating all learning types and preferences? (justice)
- Am I collaborating with my students to meet the program objectives and their personal learning goals? (beneficence and respect for autonomy)
- Am I taking all reasonable precautions to avoid harm to students? (non-maleficence)
- Am I communicating correct and accurate information (veracity)
- Am I demonstrating behaviors inside and outside the classroom where my integrity may be compromised? (integrity)
- Are my teaching and examinations aligned with relevant learning outcomes? (utility)

Ethical obligations in research

OT professionals are expected to engage in research and evidence-based practice. The ethical principles of *beneficence, non-maleficence, respect for autonomy, integrity, justice*, and *utility* are important in research, as reflected in the Declaration of Helsinki on the ethical principles for medical research involving humans (World Medical Association [WMA], 1964, amended 2013). Considering respect for research participants' autonomy and integrity, the PAOT Code of Ethics (1998) expects OT professionals to:

- *Obtain informed consent from subjects in research activities indicating they have been fully advised of the potential risks and outcomes*
- *Respect the individual's right to refuse involvement in research activities*
- *Respect the confidential nature of information gained from research and investigational activities*

In designing research, it is important to minimize risks (non-maleficence) to participants, the research team, and society in general. All conceivable risks, from participant selection to reporting of results, should be identified and addressed. Unavoidable risks must have plans for managing consequences. OT researchers should ensure that potential participants understand the risks and their consequences. Identifying societal risks involves analyzing the wider impact on other groups, the environment, and available resources (justice). The benefits of the research for the participants (beneficence), selected population, and society in general (utility) should outweigh the risks. A research project should not proceed if risks are neither identified nor addressed.

Participants should know their involvement is voluntary and they can withdraw at any time (respect for autonomy). To support decision-making, they should understand the research purpose and how it contributes to knowledge and society. For minors or those unable to consent, consultation with guardians or authorized decision-makers is required. Researchers

Table 14.2 Ethical decision-making process guided by the Prism Model (VanderKaay et al., 2020)

Process	Components	Key questions and actions to be performed
Process # 1: Considering the Fundamental Checklist	Client and Family Organization Professional Regulations Healthcare Team Theories/Evidence Law	*What are the current needs/concerns of clients?* • Some clients still prefer to receive services through telehealth; thus, it would still be provided. • Institutional protocols should be disseminated to the clients weeks before the resumption of in-person sessions for proper orientation. • Alternative forms of service provision should be provided to clients in case they will not pass the screening procedures upon entry. *What are the needed safety controls that the clinic must institute?* • In reference to the Department of Health and PAOT released guidelines, changes in the clinic's layout, along with overall process flow (e.g., documentation, payment, time allotment) should be made. • Personal protective equipment guidelines should likewise be oriented to both the therapist and clients. • The clinic should also coordinate with the Local Government Unit (LGU) if a special pass/permit would need to be sought prior to resuming in-person sessions.
Process # 2: Consulting Others	Colleagues Supervisors Legal Personnel Ethics Personnel Regulatory Bodies Others	*Have we consulted with other stakeholders on our proposed guidelines?* • It is important to seek the approval of all parties on the schedule containing the available day/s of therapists to adhere to safety guidelines and to balance it with income generation. • Legal consultation will be sought on the consent forms used, as well as guidelines to be followed when there is transmission of illness in the clinic. • The clinic should continuously communicate with the LGU and organizations if there are revisions in the set guidelines.

Process	Components	Key questions and actions to be performed
		What are we going to do now?
Process # 3: Doing What's Right	Meeting All Needs and Perspectives Accepting Limitations Assuming the Consequences	• Institutional guidelines, which stemmed from numerous consultations, will be disseminated and implemented. • The clinic acknowledges that the guidelines are a work in progress and accepts that there may be gaps that need modification along the way. It would also be accountable to possible consequences. • The clinic adheres to all national and professional regulations affecting the practice during the pandemic and beyond.

should support decision-making for persons with disabilities, ensuring their right to self-determination. Pre-existing relationships (e.g., clinician-patient, teacher-student, student-supervisor) can cause power imbalances and should be addressed before recruitment. Participatory approaches enhance participant autonomy.

To protect research participants' integrity, data collection and management plans should be clear. Identifiable information should be stored separately from de-identified data, and access to the different files should be assigned with various restrictions. Data storage and destruction plans should be established at the project's start. Personal data should be presented as aggregate data to prevent individual identification. While the Philippine Data Privacy Act of 2012 does not cover research data, researchers can seek ethical approval from institutional review boards.

Besides these principles, All European Academies (2017) include the principles of reliability (quality in the research) and accountability (responsibility for the process, outcomes, and wider impact). Research is described in Chapter 12.

Ethical obligations to society

Two principles, justice and utility, form the basis of OT professionals' ethical obligations to society. Justice involves the fair use of resources and the environment. Just OT professionals should protect the environment and contribute to sustainable development. Since healthcare is most sustainable when not required (Palstam et al., 2022), health promotion and disability prevention should be prioritized. OT professionals should empower people to manage their own health, streamline services to avoid redundancy, and use sustainable materials and methods (Palstam et al., 2022; Mortimer, 2010). The environmental impact of service provision (e.g., telehealth, home care, institution-based, community-based) should also be considered.

Equitable service provision is another key ethical obligation (PAOT, 1998). However, the shortage of OT professionals in the Philippines, exacerbated by migration, challenges fulfilling this obligation. Many Filipino healthcare workers, including occupational therapists, work overseas due to poor working conditions and better opportunities elsewhere (HRH2030 Program, 2020). Moreover, the 2017 PAOT Workforce Survey revealed that 91.71% of respondents work in private facilities, and only 3.62% of clinicians work in community practice settings (Carandang & Delos Reyes, 2018). This situation highlights the exclusivity of OT and the inaccessibility of OT for marginalized groups. Thus, equitable distribution of OT professionals across practice settings and the country would ensure all occupational issues are addressed, especially in community settings where problems may stem from poverty, homelessness, unemployment, drug use, and incarceration (Malfitano & Lopes, 2018).

What are the concrete solutions that must be in place to safeguard and improve the working conditions of OT professionals in the country?

What changes need to be made to occupational therapy in the Philippines in order for professionals to provide OT services that are fair and equitable and to reallocate resources that would result in the greatest benefit?

How to resolve ethical dilemmas?

Having knowledge of theoretical underpinnings and ethical principles, OT professionals should develop courses of action for ethical dilemmas. Various ethical dilemma decision-making frameworks are available, generally recommending the following steps:

1 Understand the context of a situation
2 Generate questions
3 Perform a thorough analysis
4 Identify various alternatives
5 Weigh the pros and cons
6 Choose a course of action
7 Monitor the effects of the chosen course of action

OT professionals should include all stakeholders in the analysis, whether they may be directly or indirectly affected by the decision. The nature of their participation, whether professional, personal, or economic in nature, provides additional nuances to the ethical dilemma being analyzed. Code of ethics, standards of practice, and existing laws and regulations should all be simultaneously considered in determining all types of violations that may have been committed. While multiple alternatives may be generated, the final course of action should be adherent to ethical principles and philosophies, and sensitive to moral, religious, and social beliefs.

OT professionals can use decision tables to ensure a comprehensive analysis of an ethical dilemma (Scott & Reitz, 2015). This involves listing all possible courses of action, along with their positive and negative consequences. The decision table can then be analyzed, alongside relevant codes, regulations, and institutional policies to facilitate making well-informed decisions.

Cases

To reinforce your understanding of the ethical principles, obligations, and issues discussed, reflect on the presented cases and work through your personal decision-making process. For each case, consider the following steps:

1. Articulate the ethical dilemma presented
2. Identify the relevant ethical principles, obligations, and issues
3. Recognize the involved parties
4. Generate and evaluate various courses of action, considering established laws and standards
5. Assess the implications of each action for the different parties involved
6. Choose the final course of action

Case 1

In the clinic where you are training, only one occupational therapist (your supervisor) is employed. To address the patient backlog, you are given a caseload and administrative work exceeding the requirements of your clinical training course. You feel unable to complain to your supervisor, but the workload leaves you no time to reflect on your learning needs and daily experiences. What would you do?

Case 2

As an occupational therapy student in clinical training, you often overhear your supervisor and other staff discussing patients' treatments and personal conditions during lunch breaks. Do you think this practice is appropriate? How would you handle such conversations if they occurred in your presence?

Case 3

You work in a private city clinic that serves clients from the provinces. Each appointment lasts about one hour unless arranged otherwise. One day, a client who has traveled far comes in with a doctor's referral. After reading the referral and conducting a screening, you realize you have no experience with the client's reported problem. Would you refuse service to this client? How would you manage the session?

Case 4

As an occupational therapist, you strive to choose and implement interventions that have been reported to be effective. However, your institution or community does not have enough funding to pay for subscriptions to scientific journals where you could gather current information about certain interventions. How would you deal with this dilemma?

Case 5

You are an OT researcher planning a study with school-aged children as primary informants. What ethical issues should you consider, and how would you go about acquiring consent?

Chapter summary

This chapter explored the theoretical underpinnings and various ethical principles essential to OT practice, providing a detailed description of the PAOT Code of Ethics in relation to these principles. It examined Filipino OTs' ethical obligations to clients, the profession, education and students, in research, and society in general. Reflection questions and cases were included to reinforce the understanding of ethical principles.

References

All European Academies (ALLEA). (2017). *The European code of conduct for research integrity*, revised edition. ALLEA.

Bailey, S., & Schwartzberg, D. (1994). *Ethical and legal dilemmas in occupational therapy*, 2nd edition. FA Davis Co.

Carandang, K. A., & Delos Reyes, R. C. (2018). *Workforce survey 2017: Working conditions and salary structure of occupational therapists working in the Philippines survey*. Philippine Academy of Occupational Therapists. https://paot.org.ph/pdf/other/Workforce%20Survey%202017%20Technical%20Report.pdf.

Cordero, D. A. (2023). Telehealth during the COVID-19 pandemic in the Philippines. *Family Practice*, 40(1), 207–208. doi:10.1093/fampra/cmac078.

COTEC. (2009). *Developing codes of ethics—COTEC policy and guidelines*. COTEC. https://coteceurope.eu/COTEC%20Docs/Code%20of%20Ethics.pdf.

Data Privacy Act of 2012, Republic Act No. 10173. (August 15, 2012). (Phil.).

Durocher, E., & Kinsella, E. A. (2021). Ethical tensions in occupational therapy practice: Conflicts and competing allegiances. *Canadian Journal of Occupational Therapy*, 88(3), 244–253. doi:10.1177/00084174211021707.

Durocher, E., Rappolt, S., & Gibson, B. E. (2014). Occupational justice: Future directions. *Journal of Occupational Science*, 21(4), 431–442. doi:10.1080/14427591.2013.775693.

Fisher, A. G., & Marterella, A. (2019). *Powerful practice: A model for authentic occupational therapy*. CIOTS, Center for Innovative OT Solutions.

Genilo, E. M. O. (2021). The Filipino family and health care decision-making at the end of life. *Concilium*, 5, 77–85.

Hordichuk, C. J., Robinson, A. J., & Sullivan, T. M. (2015). Conceptualising professionalism in occupational therapy through a Western lens. *Australian Occupational Therapy Journal*, 62(3), 150–159. doi:10.1111/1440-1630.12204.

HRH2030 Program. (2020). *Human resources for health migration*. Accessed May 5, 2022. https://hrh2030program.org/wp-content/uploads/2020/08/x12.8_HRH2030PH_Migration-policy-brief.pdf.

Kornblau, B., & Burkhardt, A. (2012). *Ethics in rehabilitation: A clinical perspective*, 2nd edition. SLACK.

Lasquety-Reyes, J., & Alvarez, A. (2015). Ethics and collective identity building: Scandinavian semicommunication and the possibilities of Philippine ethics. *Etikk i Praksis*, 9(2), 71–87. doi:10.5324/eip.v9i2.1866.

Lecours, A., Baril, N., & Drolet, M. (2021). What is professionalism in occupational therapy? A concept analysis. *Canadian Journal of Occupational Therapy*, 88(2), 117–130. doi:10.1177/0008417421994377.

Malfitano, A. & Lopes, R. (2018). Social occupational therapy: Committing to social change. *New Zealand Journal of Occupational Therapy*, 65(1), 20–26. doi:10.3316/informit.779763971754213.

Medallon, K. G. (2023). Attitude development from the perspectives of occupational therapy interns and clinical educators. *The Journal of Practice Teaching and Learning*, 19(3). doi:10.1921/jpts.v19i3.1745.

Mortimer, F. (2010). The sustainable physician. *Clinical Medicine*, 10(2), 110–111. doi:10.7861/clinmedicine.10-2-110.

Nilsson, I., & Townsend, E. (2010). Occupational justice—Bridging theory and practice. *Scandinavian Journal of Occupational Therapy*, 17(1), 57–63. doi:10.3109/11038120903287182.

Palstam, A., Sehdev, S., Barna, S., Andersson, M., & Liebenberg, N. (2022). Sustainability in physiotherapy and rehabilitation. *Orthopaedics and Trauma*, 36(5), 279–283. doi:10.1016/j.mporth.2022.07.005.

PAOT. (1998). *Occupational Therapy Code of Ethics*. Philippine Academy of Occupational Therapists. https://paot.org.ph/pdf/standardsandethics/Code%20of%20Ethics%20(1998).pdf.

PAOT. (2018). 2018 Revised enforcement procedures of the Occupational Therapy Code of Ethics. *Resolution No. 2018–2001*. https://paot.org.ph/pdf/standardsandethics/BR%202018-001%20Revised%20Enforcement%20Procedures.pdf.

PAOT. (2020a). Guidelines on the use of telehealth as an alternative form of occupational therapy service provision. *Resolution No. 2020–2001*. https://paot.org.ph/pdf/covid19/PAOT%20Guidelines%20on%20the%20Utilization%20of%20Telehealth.pdf.

PAOT. (2020b). Interim guidelines on the practice of occupational therapy amidst the coronavirus disease (COVID-19) situation in the Philippines. *Board Resolution No. 2020–2003*.

PAOT. (2021). *Continuing education on telehealth and OT professional competency advisory to members, fellow professionals, and stakeholders* (Advisory No. 2021–2001).

Philippine Occupational Therapy Law of 2018, Republic Act No. 11241. (March 11, 2019). (Phil).

PRC. (2019). Resolution No. 2019-1146. https://www.prc.gov.ph/sites/default/files/2019-1146%20CPD%20IRR.PDF.

Reyes, J. (2015). Loób and Kapwa: An introduction to a Filipino virtue ethics. *Asian Philosophy*, 25(2), 148–171. doi:10.1080/09552367.2015.1043173.

Rondilla, N. A., Rocha, I. C. N., Roque, S. J., Lu, R. M., Apolinar, N. L. B., Solaiman-Balt, A. A., Abion, T. J., Banatin, P. B., & Javier, C. V. (2021). Folk medicine in the Philippines: A phenomenological study of health-seeking individuals. *International Journal of Medical Students*, 9(1), 25–32. doi:10.5195/ijms.2021.849.

Scott, J., & Reitz, S. M. (2015). *Practical application for the occupational therapy code of ethics.* American Occupational Therapy.

Silva, L. C., de Almeida Troncon, L. E., & Panúncio-Pinto, M. P. (2019). Perceptions of occupational therapy students and clinical tutors on the attributes of a good role model. *Scandinavian Journal of Occupational Therapy*, 26(4), 283–293. doi:10.1080/11038128.2018.1508495.

Townsend, E., & Polatajko, H. (2007). *Enabling occupation II: Advancing an occupational therapy vision for health, well-being, & justice through occupation.* CAOT Publishers.

VanderKaay, S., Letts, L., Jung, B., & Moll, S. E. (2020). Doing what's right: A grounded theory of ethical decision-making in occupational therapy. *Scandinavian Journal of Occupational Therapy*, 27(2), 98–111. doi:10.1080/11038128.2018.1464060.

Williams, B. (1993). *Morality: An introduction to ethics*, Canto edition. Cambridge University Press.

World Medical Association. (1964, amended 2013). *WMA Declaration of Helsinki—Ethical principles for medical research involving human subjects.* https://www.wma.net/policies-post/wma-declaration-of-helsinki-ethical-principles-for-medical-research-involving-human-subjects/.

Chapter 15

Future directions of occupational therapy in the Philippines

Caroline Fischl, Michael Sy and Roi Charles Pineda

Chapter objectives

1   Articulate a vision and propose strategic directions for the future of occupational therapy in the Philippines
2   Inspire and motivate occupational therapy practitioners, educators, advocates, researchers, and leaders to collaborate with each other, stakeholders, and policymakers and contribute to the growth and development of the profession

The present

Through the stories in this book, Filipino occupational therapists illustrated the diverse spectrum of clients they encounter. Clients encompass individuals, often alongside their caregivers, as well as groups, communities, or populations, each with unique needs and circumstances. Here, the term "client" refers to recipients of occupational therapy services, provided in exchange for payment or pro bono. While a considerable portion of the clients in the Philippines are persons with disabilities, clients can also include individuals or communities vulnerable to disasters or dealing with the aftermath of disasters, as well as populations experiencing prolonged occupational deprivation, imbalance, or marginalization. Despite this diversity, the overarching goal of occupational therapy remains consistent: to enable clients to participate in meaningful occupations (*gawain*) in daily life while promoting health, well-being, independence, safety, and occupational balance. In the Philippines, occupational therapy encompasses the promotion of *ginhawa*—a sense of vitality (*sigla*), ease in dealing with life (*gaan*), life potency (*gana*), and joy (*ligaya*) (Chapter 7; Paz, 2008). Goal setting depends largely on clients' needs, abilities, capacities, preferences, and interests.

The *pamayanan*, with all its social networks and family structures, play a significant role in daily life, often influencing the goals and priorities of clients (Chapter 8). Within this context, the choice of *gawain* reflects an

DOI: 10.4324/9781003321217-15

intention to adhere (or not to adhere) to social or societal norms, leading to a sense of social connectedness (or disconnectedness). While independence in self-care is valued, familial support or paid caregivers may alleviate the need for full autonomy, allowing clients to focus on social participation and maintaining meaningful connections with others (Chapter 7).

Considering the spirit of *bayanihan*, which fosters interconnectedness of the community (Chapter 8), clients are motivated by their desire to not only engage in their own occupations but also ensure the family and community's ability to manage daily occupations. A holistic approach to occupational therapy intervention considers not only the individual client but also their familial and social contexts. This might involve supporting families in managing everyday life or preparing them to care for individuals upon discharge from therapeutic settings. For instance, in Chapter 7, the mother of a child newly diagnosed with autism resigned from work to provide more support for the child. Here, the occupational therapist prioritizes the family's needs to make caregiving more manageable. Conversely, an example of ineffective intervention is seen in Chapter 7, where an individual client in an acute mental health facility received occupational therapy focused on self-care and leisure activities without preparing family members to live with and care for the individual upon discharge. This shortcoming, brought upon by the limitation of short-term acute care, resulted in the client being unable to return to a home that is prepared to care for his needs. As a consequence, the client had to be admitted to a facility providing custodial care.

In contexts where familial support is missing or insufficient, individuals should have access to and be able to rely on institutional support as a fallback. It remains unclear whether stronger familial support develops due to inadequate institutional support in the Philippines or whether political systems fail to prioritize establishing or maintaining well-functioning institutions. However, in justice and correctional settings in the Philippines, efforts to assist CICL in acquiring skills crucial for reintegration into society post-release are insufficient (Chapter 11). Consequently, CICL endure prolonged occupational deprivation due to inadequate facilities or services for correction and both personal and vocational development. This inadequacy of institutional support leads to significant problems for both communities and populations.

The reality of poverty in the Philippines provides a strong illustration of the relationship between poverty and disability (Banks et al., 2017). People and communities in poverty are more vulnerable to health conditions and environmental hazards, which can lead to disablement. The vulnerabilities and lack of capacity elevate risk for disaster-related occupational disruption, which the case of relocated islanders to MARCH Village depicted (Chapter 10). Financial constraints also impact the access to and the continuity of occupational therapy services, potentially affecting clients' overall well-being and treatment outcomes. Even when telehealth provides a promising solution for reaching clients in more remote places (Chapter 9), these locations often also have high poverty and poor access to technology. Additionally, clients in the Philippines typically bear the responsibility for covering the costs of healthcare services themselves. When the family's primary income earner experiences injury or disability, it can disrupt established family roles and financial stability (Chapter 7). Unfortunately, even if the value of occupational therapy is understood and appreciated, competing subsistence needs of individuals, families, and communities may take priority.

These stories underscore the broader struggle within the profession in the Philippines, as some therapists prioritize enhancing physical and cognitive functions, akin to a medical model, while others work towards enabling participation in meaningful activities using a social model. Moreover, occupational therapists must navigate various institutional and demographic factors that influence client health and well-being. These include insurance coverage and government support systems, as well as socioeconomic aspects such as poverty, unemployment, and migration. Migration, for instance, can negatively affect the availability of occupational therapists in less urbanized regions or communities in the Philippines, thereby influencing the provision and accessibility of occupational therapy services (Chapter 3).

To address these challenges and ensure equitable service delivery, strong leadership and advocacy for policy development are crucial. Effective leadership within the occupational therapy profession can drive these advancements by inspiring and guiding practitioners, advocating for necessary policy changes, and ensuring that the profession identifies and adapts to meet new challenges. Additionally, occupational therapy education, practice, and research must undergo continuous advancement to meet evolving societal needs. This includes incorporating research tracks and specialized practice pathways in education programs, fostering critical thinking skills, and emphasizing occupation-based approaches over function-based ones. Practitioners also need to engage in CPD to stay updated on emerging demographic trends and technologies, including telehealth, as well as occupational therapy theories and evidence-based interventions.

A vision—Practice, Education, Advocacy, Research, and Leadership in synergism (PEARLs)

We propose the Practice, Education, Advocacy, Research, and Leadership in synergism (PEARLs) framework as a vision for occupational therapy in the Philippines. This framework aims to enhance the quality and reach of occupational therapy services across the nation. *Synergism* implies that the total effect of the interaction of these elements is greater than the sum of their individual effects (Merriam-Webster, n.d.). Thus, central to this vision is a commitment to collaboration. By fostering partnerships within the profession and with healthcare providers, educational institutions, community organizations, and policymakers, we can create a supportive network that enhances the impact of occupational therapy. Occupational therapists must work empathically with clients, their families, and other stakeholders to ensure that services are responsive to their needs and preferences. In the succeeding sections, each element of PEARLs—Practice, Education, Advocacy, Research, and Leadership—includes strategic directions necessary for the profession's growth and impact.

Inspired by the formation of a pearl, the PEARLs framework envisions the development of occupational therapy in the Philippines through continuous growth and refinement. Just as a pearl develops within a mollusk, layer by layer, until it achieves its unique pearlescent luster, each element of PEARLs represents layers of contributions to the profession's distinctiveness and value.

The Philippines, known as the Pearl of the Orient Seas, provides a fitting backdrop for the PEARLs framework. Just as the country is treasured for its beauty, diversity, and rich cultural heritage, the PEARLs framework aspires to cultivate a profession that is equally diverse and culturally rich. The synergy between the nation's identity and the vision for occupational therapy underscores a shared commitment to growth and excellence toward the well-being of all Filipinos.

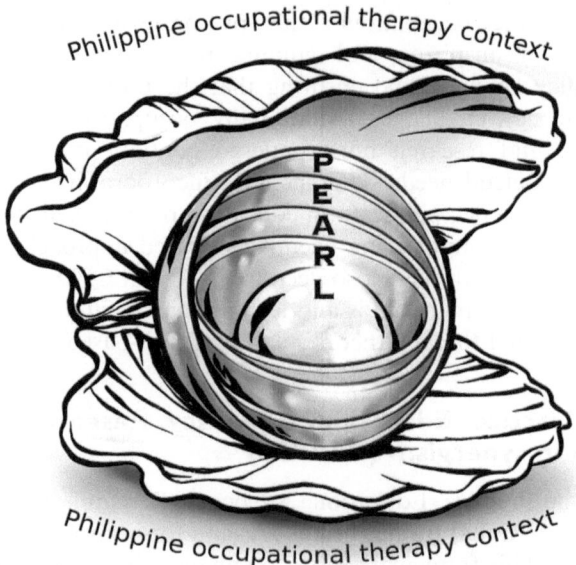

Figure 15.1 Practice, Education, Advocacy, Research, and Leadership in synergism (PEARLs) framework. The elements of the framework are in synergism (visualized by the alignment of P-E-A-R-L to create an organic gem) and formed and framed by the Philippine occupational therapy context (symbolized by a mollusk's shell).

Practice

Occupational therapy practice in the Philippines faces several key challenges, including a lack of consensus on the central focus of the practice. While many agree that occupation should be the primary focus, some practitioners prioritize improving function over the clients' meaningful occupations. To clarify the role of occupational therapy to clients, stakeholders, and policymakers, it is important to employ occupation-based methods (Fisher, 2013). In assessment, this entails using engagement in occupations to assess the quality of an individual's occupational performance (performance analysis) or to identify underlying person factors, body functions, or environmental factors that may contribute to diminished occupational performance (task analysis). In interventions, this involves utilizing occupations as therapeutic agents. However, the ability to apply occupation-based practice is influenced by staff culture and available resources within treatment settings.

Another key challenge is adopting an evidence-based approach. Access to research evidence is often constrained, particularly for consultants, private and community practitioners, and clinicians in small facilities, who lack subscriptions to research databases. Although hospitals may have libraries with access to literature, practitioners frequently seek assistance from educators and researchers or enroll in programs at advanced level to utilize library resources of higher education institutions (HEIs). It is important to recognize that evidence-based practice integrates best available research evidence with clinical experience, client preferences, and resources (Chapter 12). Thus, practitioners should meticulously document their clinical experience by recording outcomes of specific interventions for clients. Conditions surrounding a particular intervention should be well documented and comparable. Furthermore, occupational therapists should actively engage clients throughout the process in order to understand their preferences. Occupational therapists are often viewed as the experts in the Philippines, but it is vital to acknowledge that clients are the experts of their own occupations. When planning interventions, it is important to engage the client to make informed decisions about their own treatment, taking into account their preferences and available resources. This client-centered approach ensures that interventions are tailored to meet the needs and circumstances of each client, enhancing the effectiveness and relevance of occupational therapy services.

Access to occupational therapy services is often limited by geographical and economic factors, particularly in remote areas lacking sufficient resources and infrastructure. To address this challenge, occupational therapists should explore community-based programs as a means to expand access to occupational therapy in these underserved areas. Implementing community-based programs involves advocacy efforts and collaboration with local government units to garner support and resources for the initiative. By partnering with local authorities, occupational therapists can work towards establishing and sustaining programs that bring therapy services directly to communities in need. Another potential solution to address access barriers is telehealth. Utilizing telehealth platforms can facilitate remote delivery of occupational therapy services, overcoming geographical limitations. Similarly, implementing telehealth programs requires cooperation with local government units to ensure access to telehealth facilities and equipment. Collaboration with local authorities is essential to address the logistical, financial, and regulatory challenges associated with expanding occupational therapy services to remote locations.

Box 15.1 Giving choices to clients

When possible, I give my clients several choices: the optimal, the acceptable, and the affordable. The optimal involves renovations and adaptations to make the place accessible and safe. The changes support the client's performance long-term ... usually expensive but aesthetic. The acceptable involves adaptations that enable the client to do what they prioritized to do in a safe way. It is also costly but less expensive compared to the optimal. The affordable is a solution for the immediate needs, allowing the person to perform their identified occupations, but the adaptations may not be aesthetic.

— Occupational therapist who worked with home and workplace modifications

Learning new models of practice can pose challenges for some practitioners. However, it is important to recognize that the intervention process generally follows a structured framework, including assessment, goal setting and planning, intervention, and monitoring and evaluation. Throughout the intervention process, practitioners must engage in both professional reasoning and critical thinking to analyze and synthesize information, make decisions, and solve problems in client care. Practitioners can systematically gather and analyze data during the assessment phase, identify and prioritize client goals, develop intervention plans based on the identified goals, implement evidence-based interventions during the intervention phase, and monitor implementation and evaluate outcomes as well as adjust plans during monitoring and evaluation. Figure 15.2 illustrates the occupational therapist's roles across different stages of the intervention process, with examples drawn from previous chapters.

Another key challenge is the development of cultural competence and collaboration skills. In a diverse country like the Philippines, cultural competence is essential to ensure that occupational therapy interventions align with the unique cultural contexts and values of clients, leading to

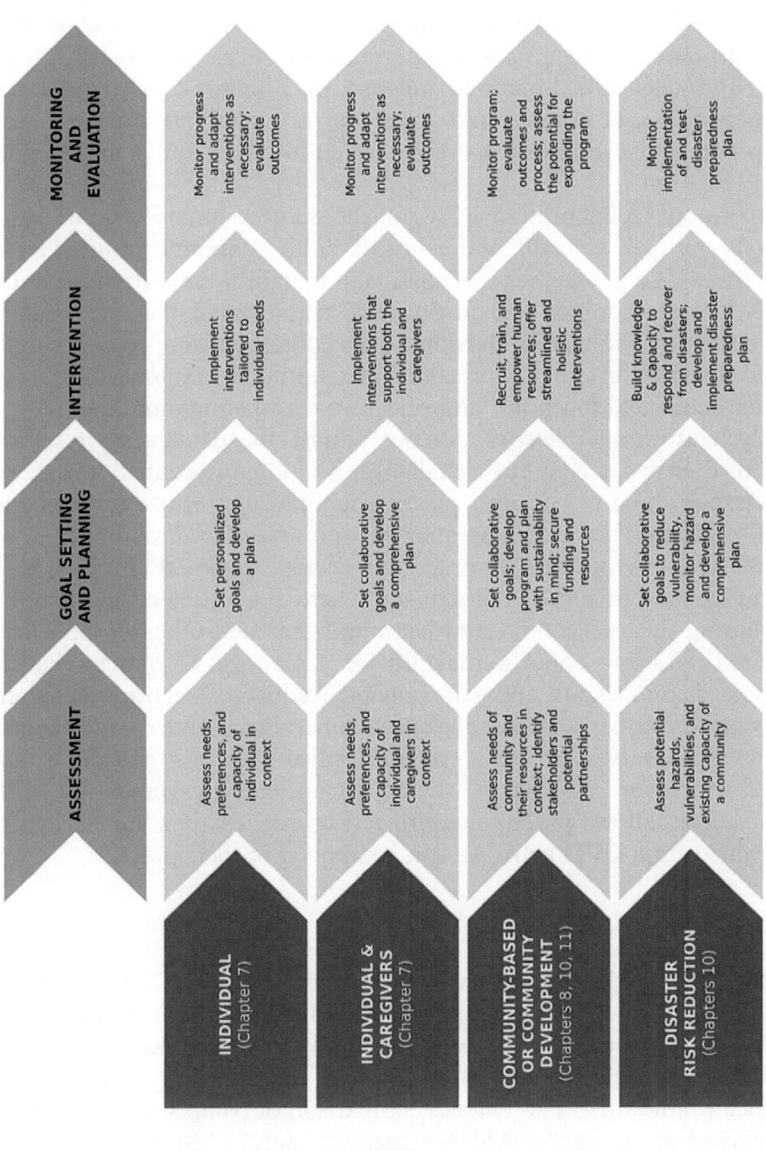

Figure 15.2 Occupational therapist's roles within the intervention process

meaningful and relevant outcomes. Moreover, Filipino occupational therapists must actively engage in interprofessional collaboration, leveraging diverse perspectives to effectively address the complex needs of clients.

These collaborations should extend beyond traditional partnerships with medical, rehabilitation, and teaching professions. Partnerships with engineering professions, for instance, are crucial for developing assistive technology and telehealth solutions tailored to Filipino communities. By incorporating local insights and expertise, occupational therapists can develop innovative solutions that are both culturally sensitive and technologically relevant.

Furthermore, collaboration with stakeholders, communities, and institutions is indispensable for addressing broader community and societal needs. By working together, occupational therapists can strengthen the capacity of communities and institutions, empowering them to become more resilient in the face of disasters. This collaborative approach should also incorporate sustainable practices that optimize resource utilization, minimize ecological footprint, and prioritize social equity and inclusion.

Lastly, cultivating reflective practice amidst the demanding responsibilities of their work is another challenge for Filipino occupational therapists. Despite these constraints, practitioners must prioritize finding time for self-reflection, as it is essential for professional development and learning. To support reflective practice, workplaces should create supportive and non-judgmental environments where practitioners feel comfortable sharing their reflections and learning from each other's experiences. Structured reflection opportunities provide a platform to discuss challenging cases, share insights, and gain valuable feedback. Practitioners should actively seek feedback from colleagues, supervisors, and clients to gain different perspectives on their practice, thus fostering reflection and growth. Moreover, workplaces should encourage engagement in CPD activities. This allows practitioners to reflect on how new knowledge or skills gained from CPD activities can be applied in their practice.

Education

To meet the mandatory approval requirements of the Commission on Higher Education (CHED, 2019), an education program should use an outcomes-based approach following the Philippine Qualifications Framework (PQF), which in turn is aligned to the ASEAN Qualifications Reference Framework. This enables comparison of competences within the Philippines and across the ASEAN member states (ASEAN Secretariat, 2024). The outcomes correspond to competences described in the PQF, which currently includes level descriptors in the subject area of occupational therapy at level 6 (bachelor's level) that outline competences of entry-level occupational therapists in the Philippines. These level descriptors are further detailed into performance indicators, aiding in formulation of learning outcomes. However, there are no level 7 (master's) and level 8 (doctorate) descriptors in the subject area of occupational therapy in the PQF.

To get voluntary international accreditation, most bachelor programs in occupational therapy align their learning outcomes with the competences outlined in the World Federation of Occupational Therapists (WFOT, 2016) document Minimum Standards for the Education of Occupational Therapists. This WFOT document defines minimum competences of entry-level occupational therapists around the world.

Given the current global landscape marked by rapid digitalization, the integration of artificial intelligence, climate change impacts, and ongoing armed conflicts, alongside persistent demographic-related challenges within the Philippines such as poverty, social injustice, crime, and unemployment, updating the competences for occupational therapists at bachelor's level is imperative. Furthermore, there is a need to define competences for occupational therapy at the master's and doctorate levels to advance the profession and enhance the quality of education.

To address these needs, the Philippines can draw inspiration from the European Qualification Reference Frameworks and Assessment Reference Frameworks developed by TUNING-CALOHEX (Kapanadze et al., 2024). The former provides a comprehensive description of occupational therapist competences at level 6 (bachelor's), 7 (master's), and 8 (doctorate). Meanwhile, the latter provides a breakdown of these competences into learning outcomes for level 6 and 7, and offers examples of relevant teaching, learning, and assessment activities. Spearheaded by the European Network of Occupational Therapy in Higher Education, this initiative involved a TUNING taskforce, composed of occupational therapy educators and students from European HEIs, and has undergone a rigorous consultation process with stakeholders and experts.

Collaborating with counterparts in the ASEAN member states and the Asia-Pacific region can further enrich occupational therapy education in the Philippines by identifying additional or more relevant competences. By building upon the WFOT standards, this collaborative effort ensures that occupational therapy practice remains adaptable to the evolving needs of individuals and communities in the ASEAN and Asia-Pacific regions.

The PQF and the WFOT minimum standards establish general competences for occupational therapists, both nationally and internationally. Consequently, it is the responsibility of Philippine HEIs to ensure that their education programs are attuned to the specific needs of the Philippine regions. In addition to the mandated objectives, programs should incorporate region-specific objectives tailored to local needs and cultural contexts in their curricula. By doing so, programs can effectively prepare occupational therapists to serve diverse communities across the country.

For instance, significant disparities in healthcare exist across regions, stemming from limited access to healthcare services in remote areas, extreme poverty, armed conflicts (Banaag et al., 2019), and lower health insurance coverage, leading to higher out-of-pocket payments (Ceballos, 2023). To address these challenges, each educational program must set program-specific objectives that directly target the unique needs of communities they serve and the regions in which they operate. Programs must also teach adapted service delivery models to improve access to occupational therapy in their respective regions.

In addition to region-specific objectives, programs must cultivate students' intercultural competence, defined as the ability to function effectively across cultures (Leung et al., 2014). This is relevant not only for the differing cultural norms between cultural groups across the country but also for the increasing number of foreign nationals residing in the Philippines. Intercultural competence not only facilitates effective client interaction but also contributes to national and international development efforts, particularly in addressing issues related to global disasters and climate change impacts, which necessitates collaborative approaches. Here, internationalizing the curriculum and facilitating internationalization activities for students and educators are imperative. Participation in international collaborations and exchange programs provides exposure to diverse perspectives, practices, and experiences, enriching the educational experience (Chapter 5).

A vision for occupational therapy education in the Philippines entails establishing programs at levels 7 (master's) and 8 (doctorate), necessitating the employment of occupational therapy educators with PhDs in Philippine HEIs. However, many PhDs currently work outside of the Philippines, favoring countries with greater political stability and better working conditions. These professionals are attracted to places offering adequate research opportunities, collaborations, learning, and professional growth, along with better living conditions and occupational balance.

To attract and retain these educators, Philippine HEIs must offer competitive salaries and benefits packages that reflect the value of PhD-level expertise. Additionally, institutions should prioritize research by investing in research infrastructure, funding research projects, and fostering a culture of innovation and collaboration among faculty. HEIs should foster interdisciplinary collaboration and a culture of inclusivity and diversity, while providing opportunities for professional development through mentorship programs, conference participation support, and continuing education resources. Recognizing contributions and creating a culture of appreciation is essential for retaining talent. HEIs should also promote flexible work arrangements and offer support services and wellness programs to promote occupational balance. Furthermore, Philippine HEIs could develop hybrid employment opportunities, leveraging experiences of visiting professorship programs and online education, supported by advanced digital communication technologies. By implementing these strategies while avoiding reliance on appeals to patriotism, Philippine HEIs can attract and retain talented educators, thus elevating the quality of occupational therapy education in the country.

Advocacy

The most important advocacy efforts needed to advance occupational therapy in the Philippines include policy development and implementation, public awareness and education, and the improvement of professional working conditions. These efforts should be led by the Philippine Academy of Occupational Therapists (PAOT) and its regional chapters. However, advocacy should also be seen as the responsibility of every occupational therapist. By working together and in collaboration with stakeholders on these key areas, the occupational therapy community can ensure the profession's growth and the delivery of high-quality services across the nation.

Collaboration with policymakers is crucial for developing and passing legislation that strengthens occupational therapy services in national healthcare policies and insurance coverage, and upholding the rights of clients in occupational therapy. To ensure consistency and quality of care across the country, advocating for national standards and guidelines for occupational therapy practice, including clinical practice guidelines (Chapter 12), is essential and can be achieved through collaboration with researchers and practitioners. Engaging and empowering stakeholders, including communities and organizations with clients and their families, ensures that their voices are heard in policy development. Additionally, advocating for the inclusion of occupational therapists in various policy-making bodies and committees would help to gain influence (Chapters 12 and 13). Efforts should focus on removing barriers to occupational therapy services, making them accessible to all individuals regardless of socioeconomic status, geographic location, or disability. Promoting equitable healthcare policies that address disparities is also critical to ensuring that all populations receive the occupational therapy services they need.

Launching national campaigns to educate the public about the benefits and importance of occupational therapy must be prioritized. Utilizing various media platforms, including social media, television, and print media, can help spread awareness. Organizing workshops and seminars for the general public, healthcare providers and policymakers can increase understanding and support for occupational therapy. Collaborating with educators to create courses where students can develop advocacy and communication skills as well as involving students in policy development are also important steps. Educators should design assignments in the form of newspaper opinion articles, commentaries, and responsible social media posts to further improve students' advocacy skills and sense of responsibility while simultaneously enhancing public awareness.

Lastly, occupational therapists should advocate for safe and fair working conditions that allow them to engage in evidence-based practice (Chapter 12), as well as continuing professional development (CPD) programs and reflective practice (Chapter 5). PAOT should advocate for fair wages and recommend appropriate professional fees to strengthen the position and elevate the value of the profession. It should support its members by offering training, networking, and mentorship opportunities, as well as resources like salary statistics that facilitate professional and career development.

Research

Occupational therapy research in the Philippines has made significant progress over the past decade, evidenced by a notable increase in the number of scientific articles published (Chapter 12). However, this progress remains constrained by several factors. Many of these researchers also hold roles as educators or practitioners, balancing heavy teaching or clinical responsibilities alongside their research activities. Moreover, a shortage of research funding further impedes the growth of research initiatives in occupational therapy.

PAOT's (2015) research agenda has been in place for nearly a decade. In light of the rapidly evolving landscape of healthcare and societal needs, it is imperative to revisit and update this agenda, especially in relation to the findings of their most recent workforce survey (Carandang & Delos Reyes, 2018). By doing so, research priorities can remain aligned with current, and responsive to emerging, needs and challenges faced by practitioners and the communities they serve. Updating the research agenda entails a comprehensive review of existing priorities and the identification of emerging areas of concern. This process should engage stakeholders from across the occupational therapy community, including practitioners, educators, researchers, clients, partners, and policymakers, to ensure diverse perspectives are considered. The updated research agenda should prioritize themes and topics that address pressing issues faced by occupational therapy practitioners and their clients. These may include innovations in treatment approaches, interventions for underserved populations, strategies for promoting health and well-being, and the integration of occupational therapy into broader healthcare and social systems. Additionally, promoting interdisciplinary collaboration and partnerships is important to maximize the impact of research efforts and leverage expertise from related fields.

In addition to updating the research agenda, there are specific areas where occupational therapy research in the Philippines can be further developed. First, there is a need to generate context-specific evidence for interventions to enhance evidence-based practice. This involves developing outcome measures tailored to Philippine cultures and contexts to assess intervention effectiveness. Qualitative research methods can be employed to explore clients' experiences, perspectives, and perceptions of occupational therapy interventions, shedding light on factors influencing treatment outcomes and client satisfaction. Additionally, conducting randomized controlled trials or quasi-experimental studies is essential to rigorously evaluate the effectiveness of specific occupational therapy interventions against standard care or alternative approaches.

Second, occupational therapy in the Philippines stands to benefit from research focused on defining unique concepts and terminology relevant to Philippine cultures and contexts and developing service provision models that address unique challenges, such as the need for remote access to occupational therapy (Chapter 9). This endeavor goes beyond simply adapting existing theories and practices. It requires theory construction that is aimed at generating new knowledge that reflects Filipino lived experiences and aspirations and is tailored specifically to the Philippine context. One example can be elucidating concepts that resonate deeply with Filipino culture and values but may not have direct equivalents in Western frameworks. For example, concepts such as *kapwa* [shared humanity], *hiya* [sense of shame or dignity], and *pakikisama* [social harmony] are integral to Filipino identity and interpersonal relationships. Given the importance of social interactions and environments to clients and in occupational therapy interventions, exploring how these concepts influence service provision can lead to the development of culturally sensitive interventions that better meet the needs of Filipino clients. Another example can be developing terminology and/or translations that accurately reflect the experiences and realities of Filipino clients for effective communication and understanding within the profession (Chapter 1). Moreover, research in occupational therapy can help tailor service provision models to address the unique challenges and opportunities in the Philippines. This involves considering factors like geographical diversity, socioeconomic disparities, cultural beliefs, and healthcare infrastructure.

Establishing a research ethics committee within PAOT would contribute to upholding ethical standards, protecting research participants, ensuring research quality, and promoting professional accountability among occupational therapists conducting research in the Philippines.

However, focusing solely on research within the discipline of occupational therapy is insufficient. Collaborations with other disciplines are indispensable for enhancing research capacity in occupational therapy. Multidisciplinary research is particularly crucial to comprehensively address societal needs. Such collaborative efforts not only highlight the valuable contribution of occupational therapy but also underscore its integral role within the broader context of healthcare and social services.

Ultimately, there is a pressing need to identify research gaps to guide future directions and ensure that evidence-based practice in occupational therapy continues to evolve and meet the diverse needs of clients and communities.

Leadership

According to the Philippine Occupational Therapy Law of 2018 (RA 11241), the Professional Regulatory Board (PRB) of Occupational Therapy holds significant powers and functions, including enforcing the law, supervising and regulating registration, licensure, and practice, maintaining a roster of occupational therapists, and issuing, suspending, and revoking registrations and licenses. The PRB is responsible for monitoring practice conditions and adopting measures to enhance the profession. Additionally, the PRB collaborates with CHED to ensure that HEIs comply with prescribed policies and standards for occupational therapy education (CHED, 2017). It also prescribes the Code of Ethics and Standards of Practice for occupational therapy endorsed by PAOT, sets guidelines for CPD, determines the subjects for licensure examinations, and investigates violations (Section 5). This array of powers and responsibilities places the PRB of Occupational Therapy, comprised of a chairperson and two board members, in a significant leadership role.

To further enhance the profession, the PRB should focus on developing more comprehensive and accessible CPD programs that incorporate emerging technologies and innovative practices, such as telehealth and virtual reality. To ensure these programs are effective and relevant, the PRB should promote evidence-based practice by integrating the latest research findings into CPD content. Establishing the Career Progression and Specialization Program and Credit Accumulation and Transfer System could support these efforts by recognizing specialized practice pathways and offering certifications in areas such as pediatrics and mental health, which are among the most commonly researched practice areas in the Philippines (Chapter 12).

The PRB should also regularly review and update the Code of Ethics and Standards of Practice for occupational therapy, and ensure their strict enforcement to uphold the profession's integrity. The current versions were both adopted with minimal revisions from the American Occupational Therapy Association in 1998 (PAOT, 1998a, 1998b). The Code of Ethics should reflect current societal needs, legal obligations, and cultural contexts (Council of Occupational Therapists for the European Countries, 2009), while the Standards of Practice should reflect current best practices and societal needs (Chapter 14).

Furthermore, the PRB should conduct regular workforce surveys to understand and address practice conditions, trends, and shortages. The latest survey (Carandang & Delos Reyes, 2018) highlights a need for more occupational therapists in specific geographical areas and practice settings. Consequently, the PRB should collaborate with the PAOT and government agencies to implement incentive programs and work with local government units to support therapists in rural and underserved communities, ensuring they have the necessary resources to deliver high-quality care.

In collaboration with the PRB of Occupational Therapy, PAOT plays a critical leadership role in setting professional standards and code of ethics, and advocating for the profession at a national level. According to RA 11241, all currently registered occupational therapists should automatically become members of the accredited national professional organization—PAOT—receive its benefits and privileges upon payment of the membership fees and dues (Section 30).

To advance occupational therapy, the PAOT should provide high-quality continuing education that can be credited as CPD units. This includes organizing regular congresses with good scientific programs, in collaboration with occupational therapy researchers. PAOT should offer CPD programs on a range of topics. Besides practice and education-related topics, PAOT should provide CPD programs related to advocacy, leadership, and management in occupational therapy to develop leaders and sustain leadership capacity. Topics related to career planning, budgeting, and financial planning are needed to promote professional development and entrepreneurial activities. Additionally, it should promote specializations through special interest groups (PAOT, 2020, n.d.) and develop specialized practice guidelines.

Enhancing public awareness of the benefits of occupational therapy is another key role of PAOT. This involves conducting outreach and advocacy campaigns, as well as educational campaigns for the general public through various media. The PAOT should lead educators, practitioners, researchers, and stakeholders in discussions to define occupational therapy concepts and terminology in native languages to improve communication and public understanding.

Furthermore, PAOT should continue to support collaborations with other healthcare and client organizations to improve service delivery and access. It should assist in policy development and implementation to ensure that occupational therapy services are well integrated into the broader healthcare and social services systems. Generating statistics on occupational therapist salaries and incomes is also important, as the information helps in making compensation competitive and fair and in recommending appropriate fees for private practitioners and consultants. Additionally, salary statistics can help in informed career decisions, conducting salary negotiations, and guiding students in making economic investments on their studies.

Given that the PAOT board of directors perform their roles on a voluntary basis, PAOT should collaborate with HEIs and employers to provide these volunteer board members with time in the form of outreach, networking, or competence development hours within their employment.

Conclusion

The stories shared in the book depict the dynamism of occupational therapy in the Philippines. On the one hand, the unappealing realities that the profession must navigate were laid bare. It can be easy to get disillusioned by all these threats to the profession in the Philippines—intellectual brain drain, health inequity, climate change and disasters, and political unrest, to name a few. On the other hand, the stories also show triumphs of occupational therapists amid these challenges; triumphs gained through the ingenuity, resourcefulness, *kabayanihan* [heroism], and sheer hard work and perseverance of occupational therapists.

However, ensuring the continued growth and relevance of occupational therapy despite the challenges of the modern age requires more than a single solution enacted by the actions of a few. There is a need for the collective action of the members of the profession and its stakeholders in *synergism* to implement a comprehensive strategy for the profession's future, as embodied by our proposed PEARLs framework.

Just like how pearls are formed, forming one layer at a time, this book has been a product of almost four years of conceptualization, ideation, discussion, and chronicling. With more than 30 Filipino occupational therapists and colleagues from other professions and disciplines who served as our contributors, it is our ambition to make this book a testament of our commitment to advance the profession to the future that lies ahead. While we acknowledge that our occupational therapy community is composed of sub-communities with different interests and priorities, we aim to encourage a fostering of a shared goal: to advance the profession for clients, populations, and sectors that we serve. We encourage our fellow occupational therapists to study the PEARLs framework and see how it can be applied in their own professional praxis. We also invite contributions, suggestions, criticisms, and discourses surrounding this proposed framework so we can achieve our shared goal together.

References

ASEAN Secretariat. (2024). ASEAN Qualifications Reference Frameworks. https://asean.org/our-communities/economic-community/services/aqrf/.

Banaag, M. S., Dayrit, M. M., & Mendoza, R. U. (2019). Health inequity in the Philippines. In A. Batabyal, Y. Higano, & P. Nijkamp (Eds.), *Disease, human health, and regional growth and development in Asia* (New Frontiers in Regional Science: Asian Perspectives, Vol. 38). Springer. doi:10.1007/978-981-13-6268-2_8.

Banks, L. M., Kuper, H., & Polack, S. (2017). Poverty and disability in low- and middle-income countries: A systematic review. *PLoS One*, 12(12), e0189996.

Carandang, K. A., & Delos Reyes, R. C. (2018). *Workforce survey 2017: Working conditions and salary structure of occupational therapists working in the Philippines survey.* PAOT.

Ceballos, X. D. (2023, November 11). Healthcare disparity seen in Mindanao— PIDS. *Manila Bulletin.* https://mb.com.ph/2023/11/11/healthcare-disparity-seen-in-mindanao-pids.

CHED. (2017, May 31). Policies, standards and guidelines for the Bachelor of Science in Occupational Therapy education (BSOT) program, *Memorandum Order No. 52, s. 2017* (Phil.). https://ched.gov.ph/wp-content/uploads/2018/04/CMO-No.-52-Series-of-2017-Policies-Standards-and-Guidelines-for-the-Bachelor-of-Science-in-Occupational-Therapy-Education-BSOT-Program.pdf.

CHED. (2019). *AQRF referencing report of the Philippines.* https://asean.org/wp-content/uploads/2017/03/AQRF-Referencing-Report-of-the-Philippines-22-May-2019_FINAL2.pdf.

Council of Occupational Therapists for the European Countries. (2009). *Developing codes of ethics—COTEC policy and guidelines.* https://coteceurope.eu/COTEC%20Docs/Code%20of%20Ethics.pdf.

Fisher, A. G. (2013). Occupation-centred, occupation-based, occupation-focused: Same, same or different? *Scandinavian Journal of Occupational Therapy*, 20(3), 162–173. https://doi-org/doi:10.3109/11038128.2012.754492.

Kapanadze, M., Fischl, C., Kraus, E., Viana-Moldes, I., Haworth, J., Hanßmann, K., Todorova, L., Costa, U. M., Rozalina, V., Charret, L., De Wachter, E., Gomes, M. D., Jackson, J., Lynch, H., González-Román, L., Poerbodipoero, S., & Vikström, S. (2024). *Occupational therapy.* https://www.tuning-calohex.eu/occupational-therapy.

Leung, K., Ang, S., & Tan, M. L. (2014). Intercultural competence. *Annual Review of Organizational Psychology and Organizational Behaviour*, 1, 489–519. doi:10.1146/annurev-orgpsych-031413-091229.

Merriam-Webster. (n.d.). Synergism. *Merriam-Webster.* Retrieved July 4, 2024, from https://www.merriam-webster.com/dictionary/synergism.

PAOT. (n.d.). *Position statement on special interest groups.* https://paot.org.ph/pdf/statements/Position%20Statement%20on%20Special%20Interest%20Groups.pdf.

PAOT. (1998a). *Occupational Therapy Code of Ethics.* https://paot.org.ph/pdf/standardsandethics/Code%20of%20Ethics%20(1998).pdf.

PAOT. (1998b). *Occupational Therapy Standards of Practice.* https://paot.org.ph/pdf/standardsandethics/Standards%20of%20Practice%20(1998).pdf.

PAOT. (2015). *The Philippine occupational therapy research agenda 2015.* https://paot.org.ph/pdf/research/Philippine%20Occupational%20Therapy%20Research%20Agenda%20(2015).pdf.

PAOT. (2020). *Guidelines on the institutionalization and governance of special interest groups (Board Resolution No. 2020–2003).* https://paot.org.ph/pdf/boardresolutions/PAOT%20Guidelines%20on%20the%20Institutionalization%20and%20Governance%20of%20Special%20Interest%20Groups.pdf.

Paz, C. J. (2008). Ginhawa: Well-being as expressed in Philippine languages. In C. J. Paz (Ed.), *Ginhawa, kapalaran, dalamhati: Essays on well-being, Opportunity/Destiny, and Anguish* (pp. 3–12). University of the Philippines Press.

Philippine Occupational Therapy Law of 2018, RA No. 11241. (2019, March 11) (Phil). https://www.officialgazette.gov.ph/2019/03/11/republic-act-no-11241/.

Philippine Qualifications Register. (n.d.) *Register of qualifications: Occupational therapy level 6*. https://pqf.gov.ph/PhQuaR/Qualifications?SearchQualification=Occupational+therapy&LevelCode=VI.

Ramugondo, E. L., & Kronenberg, F. (2015). Explaining collective occupations from a human relations perspective: Bridging the individual-collective dichotomy. *Journal of Occupational Science*, 22(1), 3–16. doi:10.1080/14427591.2013.781920.

WFOT. (2016, March). *Minimum Standards for the Education of Occupational Therapists 2016*. https://wfot.org/resources/new-minimum-standards-for-the-education-of-occupational-therapists-2016-e-copy.

Index

Pages in *italics* refer to figures, pages in **bold** refer to tables, and pages followed by "b" refer to boxes

community-based inclusive
   development 126–127
community-based rehabilitation 52, 124,
   126–127; matrix *126*, 164, **165**; process of developing programs 130, **131**;
   program 28, 31, *129*, 212; virtual 31;
   worker *129*, 133, 134, 149b
Comprehensive Community Health
   Program 28, 125
confidentiality 147, **221**, 224
consequentialism *see* ethics, theories
contextualization 115, 142, 176, 181,
   190, 196, **198**, 201
Convention on the Rights of Persons
   with Disabilities 125, **131**, 206–207
continuing professional development
   66, 69–70, 214, 244, 250–251; *see
   also* Philippine Occupational
   Therapy Law of 2018
Continuing Professional Development
   Act (RA 10912) 67
COVID-19 pandemic: education/
   research during 70, 188; resilience
   during 31, service delivery model
   during 116, 135, 147, 180, 225; work
   set-up 10

Data Privacy Act (RA 10173)
   215–216, 231
dark side of occupations 40, **42**;
decolonization 56
deontology *see* ethics, theories
disability; in the Filipino language 1,
   22b; models of 128, 208, 239; in
   relation to poverty 110, 114–115, 238
disability-inclusive development 127
disability policies 208, 210; *see also*
   Convention on the Rights of Persons
   with Disabilities; Magna Carta for
   Persons with Disabilities
disaster 154, 156; resilience 157, 164;
   risk elements of *155*, 156–157
disaster and development occupational
   perspective framework 158, *159*, 164
disaster risk reduction 157; cycle *155*;
   frameworks and policies related to
   159, 160b, **161**; preparedness plan
   161, 166; occupational therapy
   framework for 162
discrimination 44, 106, 125; protection
   from **131**, 206, 208
double marginalization 173

drug use 38, **42**

eating, as occupation 39–40
emigration *see* migration
Employees' Compensation
   Commission 111
empowerment: of communities 28, 133;
   of persons with disabilities 110, 128,
   131; *see also* community-based
   rehabilitation, matrix; leadership
ethical approval in research 192;
   see also occupational therapy
   research
ethical dilemma 221–222, 232; *see also*
   Prism Model of Ethical
   Decision-Making
ethical principles **131**, 170, **222**, 228
ethics; in education 227–228; in research
   228, 231; in telehealth 147; theories
   221–222; *see also* Code of Ethics
ethics of care *see* ethics, theories
evidence-based practice 109, 124, 194,
   228, 249–250; five steps of 187; JBI
   model 195
exposure *see* disaster, risk elements of

fieldwork placement *see* internship
fidelity *see* ethical principles
Filipino language *see* Philippine
   languages
Filipino values/virtues 222, 249; *see
   also* hiya; kapwa
Gibb's Reflective Cycle *see* reflective
   practice, models and theories
ginhawa 99–100, 237
Good Clinical Practice *see* ethical
   approval
graduate education 68–69

hazard *see* disaster, risk elements of
health insurance, private 111; *see also*
   PhilHealth
Health Research and Development
   Information Network 190
hidden occupations 40, **42**; *see also*
   dark side of occupations
history *see* kasaysayan
hiya 40, 45, 222, 249
Hospicio de San Jose 17

inclusion of persons with disabilities
   131: into the community 28–29; in